The Complete Home Health Advisor

© Copyright 1995 by Rita Elkins

ISBN 0-913923-96-6
Woodland Health Books
P.O. Box 160
Pleasant Grove, Utah 84062

Introduction

I have read many books on the care and feeding of the sick person, but I have never found **such a complete book** on the standard or allopathic control of infections and disease conditions that was able to skillfully intertwine the alternative methods of sickness control and even cure. The author, Rita Elkins, has obviously had training and experience in the use of all methods of treatment for the walking sickies in our country.

She describes the various complaints from acne to wrinkles with the confidence of one who has seen them all, and knows whereof she writes. Most medical authors write about the one way they were taught in medical school, whether it was allopathic, chiropractic, or naturopathic. This book gives the various treatments for the usual diseases, and allows the reader to decide — a little bit — which modality would best suit him or her. For instance, for chickenpox, the author gives the usual drug that medical doctors would like to try, but also the side effects are listed and the consequences of no treatment are also delineated. But right along with these "standard" methods are listed the herbs, vitamins, and minerals that could be helpful in this disease, and indicating that the side effects would be nil.

I think the beauty of this book, is that the patient could bring it along when they see the doctor and, when the diagnosis is made, could go over the possible choices of treatments. A patient could show the doctor that vitamin C could be of benefit in speeding the course of the chickenpox and because the alternative treatment is IN PRINT, maybe, just maybe, the doctor would say, "Well, okay, but watch it, and don't take too much."

The author is aware of the overuse of antibiotics, and although, many times an antibiotic would be appropriate (as the infection is due to a treatable germ,) herbal and vitamin remedies are listed with the idea in mind of improving the patient's immune system. In no other specialty is the overuse of antibiotics seen more than in pediatric practices in the United States, where the doctor is pushed into the use of antibiotics by the frantic, tired parents who hate to see their child suffer one more night. Eighty percent of ear infections do not need to be treated with antibiotics in the first place. Usually the child can be calmed with soothing ear drops, hydrotherapy, pain killers, and improving the immune system with vitamin C and Echinacea. If the child "learns" how to control infections, he will be less sick. The author wisely points out that there are reasons for sickness and a poorly functioning immune system is the chief reason for repeated infections. (After an ear infection, most of us have the parents stop the cow's milk.)

Let us remember that chiropractic methods are alternatives, and homeopathy is largely forgotten today. It constituted a large part of medical practice just 100 years ago. Both these modalities of treatment have been time tested. I have seen colicky babies and hyperactive children mellow right out after a visit or two with the chiropractor. Bedwetting can be reduced with their methods.

All in all, a useful, practical book. It is thorough and comprehensive in its coverage.

Lendon H. Smith M.D.

Contents

Acne

DEFINITION:

Anyone who has experienced acne knows firsthand that it can be a true adolescent calamity. Teenagers are already so sensitive about their appearance that a case of acne can come as a devastating blow. The good news is that today, more than ever, acne can be effectively treated. The best thing to do if you have acne is to see a good dermatologist and decide on how to tackle the problem.

Acne is a common skin disorder that usually affects teenagers characterized by blackheads, whiteheads, red bumps, and sometimes scarring. Acne can be extremely distressing both physically and emotionally, and can often have serious effects on self-esteem and social confidence.

Acne usually appears around age fourteen for girls and sixteen for boys. It generally disappears prior to age twenty; however, it has been known to continue into the forties. The presence of blackheads and whiteheads is typical in most cases of acne. Technically speaking, a blackhead is an inactive hair follicle which is blocked with oil but is not infected. If raised red blotches and whiteheads occur during an outbreak of acne, they indicate that infection is present.

In severe cases, whiteheads can multiply under the skin and rupture, which serves to aggravate the inflammation. Cystic acne, which causes areas of swelling, can leave noticeable scarring. Acne can be active for a period of months or even years.

CAUSES:

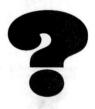

The exact cause of acne, regardless of age, is not completely understood. Hormonal changes have been linked to the occurrence of acne. Apparently these changes affect the oil glands and ducts of the skin and how they function in the production of sebum, a skin lubricant. Each hair of the body grows from a follicle which contains its own sebaceous gland. Occasionally, an overproduction of this oil results in a blockage within the follicle itself. Consequently, bacteria is allowed to grow, which causes an inflammation, resulting in a pimple.

Certain antiepilepsy drugs, phenothiazine, iodides, and steroids have also been known to cause occurrences of acne. Exposure to petroleum, certain chemicals, coal tar and oils can also result in acne. Acne can accompany diabetes. The role of diet, sleep and even hygiene in acne has recently been downplayed and is not considered to contribute significantly to the cause or onset of acne. It should be mentioned, however, that recently, the benefits of a low-fat diet have been stressed for overall good health. It stands to reason that lowering one's intake of dietary fat could contribute to the treatment of acne. There is some speculation that seafood that contains iodine may be linked to outbreaks of acne. Iodides are also contained in iodized salt, liver, tortilla chips, kelp, asparagus, broccoli and turkey.

In addition to the above factors, heredity plays a major role in the skin disorder, although how the condition is passed on is not completely understood. Some doctors have described acne as an inherited defect of the pores. There is also some speculation that acnelike conditions may be caused by stress, allergies or by taking birth-control pills.

SYMPTOMS:

Physical: Red bumps, pimples and whiteheads are usually found in the facial region in cases of acne; however, the neck, back, chest and buttocks can also be affected. This skin condition is characterized by the simultaneous healing of some blemishes and the appearance of new ones. A purplish scar is usually left as pimples heal, which will fade away in most instances. In more severe cases of acne, where healing is slow, some permanent scarring may occur; however, this is a rare occurrence, except in the case of cystic acne.

Psychological: The emotional factors that accompany acne should not be underestimated. During adolescence, the impact of acne can cause feelings of embarrassment, withdrawal and resentment. Talking about the subject with parents may be difficult, and even the most well-meant comment may cause feelings of anger or extreme sensitivity. Whatever you do, don't brush off the acne as being insignificant or try to minimize its impact on your child.

If you have a child who has experienced scarring from severe acne, treatment with dermabrasion or other cosmetic surgeries may be quite effective. Filling in scars with silicone or collagen is also an option, and should be discussed with a qualified plastic surgeon. Remember to be sensitive to a child who may be suffering from acne by educating yourself on medical and nutritional options.

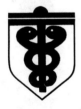

STANDARD MEDICAL TREATMENT:

In severe cases of acne, most doctors will prescribe an ointment which causes the skin to peel off and keeps new pimples from forming. If this therapy is not effective, small doses of antibiotics, such as tetracycline, may be administered for periods usually not longer than six months. Ultraviolet light from a sunlamp or from the sun itself is also considered beneficial. Vitamin A acids, and 13-cisretinoic acid, have also proved effective.

Your doctor will probably recommend using Acutane (isotretinoin), a prescription drug, that is effective in the treatment of severe cases, including cystic acne, and must be taken only under a doctor's supervision. It reduces the amount of oil in the skin, and shrinks the gland, therefore inhibiting oil blockage of the follicle.

SIDE-EFFECTS: Acutane: (isotretinoin): Anyone allergic or sensitive to vitamin A, any vitamin A derivative, or to paraben preservatives which are used in Acutane should not use the drug. Acutane has also been associated with severe headaches and visual disturbances caused by increased fluid pressure within the head. In addition, sensitivity to sunlight may occur during its use, and sunscreens and protective clothing should be worn. Do not use sunlamp therapy while taking Acutane.

Warning: Neither Acutane nor any form of isotretinoin should be used by pregnant women, and a pregnancy test should be administered before taking the drug. Nursing mothers should not use the drug.

Taking supplemental vitamin A increases the side-effects of acutane and should be avoided.

Alcohol and tetracycline should not be taken with the drug Retinoic acid (also known as Retin-A™), a synthetic derivative of the vitamin A, is considered an effective therapy if the acne is not severe. It comes in a gel, ointment or cream and works by causing the skin to peel.

SIDE-EFFECTS: Retin-A is an irritant and makes the skin more sensitive to sunlight; therefore, sunscreens of factor 15 should be used in conjunction with this drug therapy. If taking Retin-A, do not use sunlamp therapy. This drug may increase the ability of ultraviolet light to cause skin cancer.

Extreme weather, wind, and some cosmetics and soaps can cause severe irritation when using Retin-A. Do not use the preparation around the eyes, corners of the mouth or in the crevices to the sides of the nose.

NOTE: Medical research published in the *Journal of the American Medical Association* has suggested that regular application of Retin-A can have an anti-wrinkling effect on the skin. (See chapter on wrinkling.)

Warning: Retin-A (tretinoin) may cause birth defects and should not be used by pregnant women.

Success rating of standard medical treatment: very good. Current drugs available are quite effective in controlling acne. Caution must be exercised when taking any prescription drug, and side-effects should be discussed with your doctor and pharmacist.

HOME SELF CARE:

◆ Keeping the skin clean cannot be over emphasized. If possible, wash it with an unscented soap twice a day, but not more often.

◆ Mild exposure to sunshine is also beneficial; however if you are on an acne medication, you may experience an adverse reaction to sun exposure and should check with your physician before going out into the sun.

◆ Mild acne can be controlled with over-the-counter creams which contain benzoyl peroxide, such as Vanoxide, Oxy-5, Clearsil and Loroxide. It is interesting to note that the percentage of benzoyl peroxide does not necessarily determine the effectiveness of the product. When using these medications, a reddening of the skin is common.

◆ Use acne medications not only on the pimple, but also on the area of skin around it to prevent spreading.

◆ Using a warm washcloth to scrub the face helps to remove the oil plugs. For back pimples, use a back brush.

◆ Steam may also help to unclog pores, and hot compresses (not too hot) may have the same result.

◆ Avoid medications with bromides or iodides.

◆ Don't use different medications simultaneously. Using one medication at a time is recommended.

◆ Girls should avoid foundation makeup that is oil-based. Avoid cosmetic products with lanolins, isopropyl myristate, sodium lauryl sulfate, laureth-4 and D & C red dyes.

◆ Squeezing and picking the pimples will only aggravate the inflammation and is counterproductive. In the case of a pimple with a distinct whitehead, some doctors recommend removing the white core by gently squeezing and then using an antiseptic afterwards. They base this suggestion on the premise that the presence of the pus-filled core can slow down the healing process and should be removed if it is pronounced.

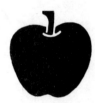

NUTRITIONAL APPROACHES:

One factor which is often ignored in the traditional treatment of acne is the importance of good intestinal functioning. Some health professionals insist that constipation or poor eating habits can contribute to toxicity, which can precede an outbreak of acne. To maintain a healthy and active colon, it is essential to eat food with a high fiber content that expedites waste products through the intestines.

Increase your intake of raw vegetables and decrease fats in the diet. (While the role of fats in acne is not considered a primary one, a diet which cuts fat has been proven to increase overall health, lower cholesterol levels, etc.) Eating plenty of whole grains and drinking a great deal of water, carrot, and citrus fruit juices is recommended for treating acne. Eat plenty of cherries, which naturally cleanse the blood of toxins.

◆ *Chromium:* Contributes to reducing skin inflammations and improves glucose tolerance. Some studies indicate that skin glucose tolerance was impaired in people suffering from acne.

◆ *Zinc gluconate:* Aids in the process of tissue healing.

◆ *Vitamin A:* Strengthens the epithelial layer of the skin, and can be taken in a beta carotene form in combination with fish oil formulas. Consult your physician for a safe dosage.

- *Vitamin B-complex (extra vitamin B2, B6, niacin, biotin)*: Contribute to maintaining good skin tone and fighting infection.
- *Vitamin C with bioflavonoids*: Boosts the functions of the immune system.
- *Niacin*: Promotes better blood circulation to skin.
- *Vitamin E*: Helps prevent scarring and works to regulate the balance of vitamin A in the body. Selenium in combination with vitamin E has been found to help improve skin conditions.
- *Zinc*: Important for inflammation control and tissue regeneration.
- *Acidophilus*: If taking an antibiotic for acne treatment, some form of acidophilus is recommended to replace "friendly" intestinal bacteria.

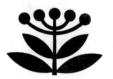

HERBAL REMEDIES:

- Wash the affected areas with a tea made from calendula or use a bar of calendula soap.
- Red clover and lavender can be used on the face as a steam poultice, or in a wet compress made from the tea.
- A steam sauna made with strawberry leaves is soothing and helps to promote tissue healing.
- A poultice of chaparral, dandelion and yellow dock root can also be applied to affected areas.
- *Lavender*: Aids in killing germs and promoting the growth of new cells.
- *Alfalfa*: Contributes to fighting infection and can be taken internally in capsule form.
- *Golden seal*: Has detoxifying and anti-bacterial properties to help control infections.
- *Burdock root*: Helps to purify the blood and can be taken in capsule form.
- Basil oil applied to the skin kills bacteria and is an old Indian remedy for acne. It can usually be purchased in health food shops.
- *Chaparral*: Known as a good herbal antibiotic which can be used topically and taken internally.
- *Echinacea*: Considered an immune system stimulant which inhibits inflammation.
- *Oregon grape*: An herb which has traditionally been used in the treatment of a variety of skin diseases.
- *Sassafras*: may help in adjusting hormone levels, which can affect the outbreak and severity of acne.
- *Stillingia*: A glandular stimulant which should be used with caution.
- Tea tree oil in rose water can be applied as a lotion to help dry out excess oil and promote skin healing.
- The following herbs taken in combination may be useful: red clover blossoms, sheep sorrel, peach bark, barberry bark, echinacea, licorice root, Oregon grape

root, stillingia root, prickly ash bark, burdock root, kelp and rosemary leaf.

NOTE: Traditional Chinese medicine treats acne with herbs and diet that increase body fluids. This approach is referred to as Ayurvedic medicine and may provide an alternative approach to conventional medical treatments for acne.

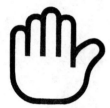

PREVENTION:

◆ While acne is often considered to be a hereditary disorder, good facial hygiene and a low-fat diet, with an emphasis on complex carbohydrates, fresh fruits and vegetables, can assist in prevention.

◆ Keep the bowels functioning properly by eating a high-fiber diet and by drinking plenty of pure water. Adding psyllium to the diet can help prevent constipation.

◆ If you are taking birth-control pills, discuss the possibility of acne with your doctor.

Age Spots

DEFINITION:

As if wrinkling isn't bad enough, the appearance of age spots also reminds us that time and exposure to sunshine are taking their toll on our skin. Age spots are unattractive but otherwise harmless spots that commonly appear after the age of 45. A true age spot is nothing more than a large freckle. Age spots are also commonly referred to as sun spots or liver spots although, oddly enough, they have nothing to do with liver function.

Age spots look like flesh colored or tannish, frecklelike flat spots. They are most noticeable on the backs of the hands and the face, although they can grow on the chest, arms, abdomen and especially the back. With time, age spots get larger, thicken and become darker, resembling small moles. They eventually turn brown and occasionally, black.

Age spots can grow into greasy, wartlike blemishes with distinctive edges. When they reach this level of maturity, they are referred to as seborrheic keratoses. The appearance of these dark blotches can cause alarm in that they can resemble early forms of skin cancer. Age spots can also become De Morgan spots, which are red, pinpoint like blemishes that appear on the trunk of the body. Age spots are usually of no medical significance.

CAUSES:

Age spots are the result of pigmentary changes in the skin brought about by a combination of exposure to the sun and aging. With age, some skin cells over-produce melanin, which causes darkened areas. A buildup of waste products from damaged skin cells is also thought to account for the appearance of an age spot.

SYMPTOMS:

Physical: Age spots look dark and blotchy, and can appear as smooth or raised molelike blemishes. They can appear suddenly on the backs of the hands, face, arms and forehead. The backs of the hands are particularly susceptible and can become covered with several of these blemishes with time.

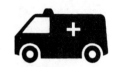

MEDICAL ALERT:

If an age spot appears to increase in size or has a bizarre color change, consult your doctor immediately. Such changes can signal skin cancer.

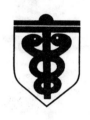

STANDARD MEDICAL TREATMENT:

Usually, medical treatment is only sought out when the spots have advanced to the point of keratosis. Freezing the blemishes with liquid nitrogen is the most common treatment. Surgical removal under a local anesthetic is another option, although less commonly done. Chemical peeling, burning, or electric needle removal are also used to remove age spots. Retinoic acid, used in the treatment of acne, has also been used on age spots.
SIDE-EFFECTS: Liquid nitrogen can burn healthy tissue and result in weltlike areas of inflammation. It should be administered only by a qualified physician.

Success rating for standard medical treatment: very good. The use of liquid nitrogen is very effective in removing age spots, and decreases the risk for development of skin cancer.

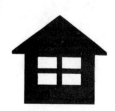

HOME SELF-CARE:

◆ Avoid excess exposure to sun or use a strong sunscreen, especially if you are fair-skinned.
◆ Age spots can be camouflaged with a cosmetic cover stick. A product called Covermark is effective.
◆ Bleaching age spots is an option. Straight lemon juice can be applied twice daily with a cotton ball, or an over-the-counter cosmetic preparation can be purchased, such as Porcelana or Esoterica.

- Hydroquinone applied with a cotton ball can also lighten the spots; however, the results are gradual.
- The use of Lac-hydrin lotion, a non-prescription preparation, can help to enhance the action of lightening agents through lactic acid, which promotes the shedding of the upper layers of skin.
- Castor oil may be applied to larger, rougher legions to help to soften the crust-like appearance of these more mature spots.

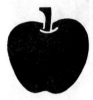

NUTRITIONAL APPROACHES:

- Vitamin C with bioflavonoids: Acts as an antioxidant and helps in tissue repair.
- Vitamin E and aloe vera gel can be applied to the spots to help shrink them and prevent irritation or scarring.
- Cosmetic creams with alpha-hydroxy compounds may help to gradually remove outer layers of the skin, which may lessen the appearance and pigmentation of age spots.

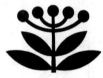

HERBAL REMEDIES:

- *Ginseng, gotu kola, licorice and sarsaparilla* are all considered anti-aging herbs which contribute to increased energy and the healthy function of the endocrine system. These herbs help to regulate hormonal changes, which usually initiate different processes of aging.
- Apply a paste of *chaparral* directly on the age spot and cover at night with a gauze bandage. Chaparral can help to heal and diminish several kinds of skin disorders.

PREVENTION:

- Use a sunscreen of at least factor 15 and apply at least 10 minutes before exposure to the sun. Routinely using sunscreens is the most effective way to avoid developing sun spots or age spots.

AIDS (Acquired Immune Deficiency Syndrome)

DEFINITION:

Aids is a 20th century worldwide epidemic, and everybody seems to be talking about it. It is a blood-born disease, caused by the HIV virus (human immunodeficiency virus). This virus specifically attacks the body's immune system and eventually disables its defense mechanisms. As a result, other disease organisms can overwhelm the immune system. Consequently, death usually occurs from a secondary infection, such as pneumonia or other opportunistic disease. The only good news about AIDS is that it is generally a disease caused by specific avoidable behaviors.

In Africa, AIDS is considered primarily a heterosexual disease; however, in the United States, male homosexuals, bisexuals, intravenous drug users, and hemophiliacs, who need frequent transfusions, make up the primary risk group for AIDS. AIDS can also be transmitted from an infected pregnant woman to her newborn. It is important to understand that AIDS is not present in all individuals who are infected with HIV; AIDS will usually develop in between 1 and 5 percent of those who test positive for HIV. Many infected individuals have no obvious signs of the disease and can remain without symptoms for an indefinite period of time.

AIDS is classified as a fatal disease. Eighty percent of those that have been diagnosed with AIDS since 1984 have already died. As of yet, there is no curative treatment or vaccine for AIDS, however, the symptoms and complications of AIDS respond in a variety of ways to antibiotics, antivirals, radiation and anticancer therapy.

CAUSES:

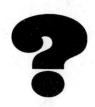

The HIV virus has been isolated from blood, tears, semen, saliva, breast milk, nervous system tissue, and female genital tract secretions. The major methods of transmitting the disease are through sexual contact including penis to anus, vagina, or mouth; through tainted transfusions or needle sharing; and from a pregnant woman to her fetus. In very rare instances, infection can occur through accidental needle injury, kidney or organ transplant, or artificial insemination.

Male homosexual activity has accounted for most cases of AIDS in the United States and comprises approximately 60 percent of the AIDS population. The percentage of AIDS cases contracted from heterosexual relationships is on the rise, and may also be connected to drug use. The disease is far less likely to pass from woman to man during conventional intercourse than from man to woman. The frequency of sexual contact also plays an important role in raising the risk of contracting AIDS. Prostitutes are much more likely to become infected, and also raise their risk because many of them are also intravenous drug users. There is some suggestion that venereal diseases, such as genital herpes, may predispose one to the HIV infection.

NOTE: The AIDS virus has not been shown to spread from sweat, tears, urine, or feces. It has not been proven that you can contract AIDS from casual contact such as a dry kiss, a handshake, a telephone receiver, a swimming pool, a toilet seat, or through bedbug or mosquito bites.

SYMPTOMS:

NOTE: It can take up to two to five years for the symptoms of AIDS to appear after contracting the infection.

Physical: When the HIV virus becomes activated, symptoms vary significantly from case to case. They included persistent fatigue, weight loss, swollen glands, unexplained fever, night sweats, chronic diarrhea, dry coughing, short-lived illnesses sometimes resembling mononucleosis, skin disorders such as dermatitis (especially in the facial area), thrush, and enlarged liver or spleen.

Other conditions that can affect those with the AIDS virus are shingles, tuberculosis, herpes simplex, and salmonellosis. Fifty percent of AIDS patients contract pneumonia. Thirty percent come down with cancer of the connective tissues (Kaposi's sarcoma) and 12 percent with other opportunist infections listed above. The virus may also affect the brain and cause dementia.

When AIDS is in a progressed stage, diseases such as cancers (especially Kaposi's sarcoma), and infections such as pneumonia, severe diarrhea or other life-threatening conditions can occur.

A person who has been infected with the HIV virus, but does not actually have AIDS, may experience weight loss, fever and enlarged lymph nodes. These symptoms are referred to as ARC, (AIDS-Related Complex).

Psychological: because this disease, more than any other modern infection has caused widespread fear and panic, the psychological effects to both the carrier and those with whom he or she interacts are profound. Dispelling myths dealing with the way the disease is spread can help create a more relaxed relationship with the AIDS victim. The victim himself not only has to cope with the disease itself, but also with its social stigma. Consequently, feelings of alienation, isolation and loneliness may result. Counseling is recommended through self-help groups and organizations offering support (see AIDS hotline below).

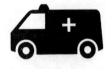

MEDICAL ALERT:

If you think you have been exposed to the virus, get tested. Do this not only for your own knowledge, but to also avoid spreading the virus.

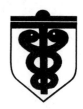

STANDARD MEDICAL TREATMENT:

Confirmation of the presence of the HIV virus involves the testing of a blood sample for the presence of antibodies to HIV.

Determining the presence of the virus itself is more difficult. A negative test result may occur in a person carrying the virus if it was contracted recently. A repeated test after six months is recommended for someone at risk.

There is no known cure for AIDS. A number of antiviral drugs such as AZT™ (zidovudine) and acyclovir are currently in use. AZT has serious side-effects; however, it does inhibit the progression of the disease. Supportive therapy for complications resulting from AIDS include using antibiotics such as pentamidine for pneumonia. If Kaposi's sarcoma is present, anticancer drugs and radiation are used, but are rarely curative.

SIDE-EFFECTS: AZT (zidovudine): Anemia, reduced white blood cell count, headache, nausea, sleeplessness, muscle aches, chills, and dizziness. AZT also attacks blood cells, which are produced in the bone marrow. The effects of AZT on a pregnant women or nursing mothers are not known.

Note: After prolonged treatment with AZT, the AIDS virus can become more resistant to the medication

Warning: Combining AZT with certain drugs can cause kidney damage and should be done only with your doctor's approval. Acetaminophen and aspirin can increase the toxicity of AZT.

SIDE-EFFECTS: Acyclovir (zovirax): Dizziness, nausea, vomiting, headache, diarrhea and aching joints, loss of appetite, fluid retention, swollen glands, and fever.

Warning: Do not take this drug if pregnant or nursing without your doctor's permission.

Success rating of standard medical treatment: poor. While extensive testing is being done on a variety of antiviral drugs and vaccines, to date, medical therapies are severely limited in their effectiveness. While AZT is the drug of choice for most doctors treating AIDS, it is not always effective and has severe side-effects.

MEDICAL UPDATE:

◆ More than 70 drugs are currently being tested which are designed to slow or stop the virus, or to help bolster the body's immune system. The National Cancer Institute has conducted studies with a new drug called dideoxyinosine or DDL. This anti-AIDS drug may be more effective in combating the AIDS virus with less side-effects than AZT. Another drug which shows promise for victims of AIDS is n-acetylcysteine or NAC, a drug routinely prescribed for bronchitis. This drug seems to inhibit weight loss along with the growth of the virus.

The AIDS virus is spreading rapidly throughout Africa, Asia and Latin America. In less than two decades, 25 percent or more of the people in some of these countries could become infected with HIV. Census bureau statistics are chilling, to say the least. Up to 90 percent of all prostitutes in Kenya are HIV-positive. Approximately 20 percent of all teenage boys entering the army in Thailand are HIV-infected. This alarming spread of the AIDS virus creates a potential danger for all countries and will take an enormous toll in the next few decades.

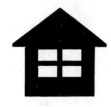

HOME SELF CARE:

◆ Keep your spirits up by getting plenty of rest, sunshine and good food.

◆ Obtain fresh air on a regular basis, and get moderate exercise that your doctor has approved.

◆ Educate yourself on the availability of support groups (see hotline number at the end of this section).

◆ Be aware of the difficulty that dealing with this disease can cause others, and educate yourself and them on the facts about AIDS, rather than the myths.

◆ Keep yourself updated on the latest treatments available.

◆ Use massage therapy or acupuncture to help relieve troublesome symptoms.

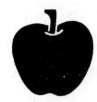

NUTRITIONAL APPROACHES:

◆ Because AIDS makes you so susceptible to getting other diseases, the primary focus of any nutritional therapy is to build up the immune system as much as possible. Protecting and strengthening the immune system is the best defense, in combination with drug treatment. Studies confirm that individuals who have AIDS have experienced repeated stress on their immune systems, such as having other sexually transmitted diseases (herpes), repeated exposure to hepatitis, intravenous drug use or frequent infections.

◆ Nutritional deficiencies, including lack of vitamin A, zinc, and pyridoxine may cause a decreased output of the thymus gland, which functions to provide resistance to disease. For the immune system to function properly, adequate levels of vitamin A, thiamine, riboflavin, pantothenic acid, pyridoxine, folic acid, vitamin E, vitamin C, magnesium, iron, zinc, and several amino acids must be maintained. Building up the immune system is the most important single factor in helping to combat the disease.

◆ A diet high in raw foods is recommended (fruits and vegetables); in addition, fish liver oils, onions, yellow vegetables, dark green vegetables, seeds, whole grains, and alfalfa are recommended. Drinking freshly juiced fruits and

vegetables with the addition of garlic and onion is recommended.
- ◆ *Avoid:* Processed foods, salt, bacon, hot dogs, pickled products, potato chips, soda pop, lunch meats and cheeses, alcohol, caffeine and sugar.
- ◆ *Chlorophyll:* Works to purify the blood of toxins produced by invading pathogenic organisms.
- ◆ *Egg lecithin:* Contributes to cellular strength and integrity.
- ◆ *Garlic:* Helps to boost the body's defenses through immuno-stimulation. Garlic is also considered a natural antiviral agent.
- ◆ *Selenium:* Works to take up free radicals, which are produced when disease is present.
- ◆ *Germanium:* Helps to oxygenate tissues and is believed to contribute to interferon production.
- ◆ *Polyporus umbellatus:* A Chinese tonic mushroom which increases resistance to infection.
- ◆ *Vitamin B complex, especially B12 and B6:* antistress vitamins which are important for normal brain functions.
- ◆ *Vitamin C with bioflavonoids:* There has been some experimentation with vitamin C administered intravenously for AIDS. Check with your physician about this option. Vitamin C can help protect the liver and also has antiviral and antibacterial properties.
- ◆ *Vitamin A (carotenes):* Check with your doctor for a proper dosage. Vitamin A promotes healing and helps to fight infection.
- ◆ *Vitamin E:* An antioxidant that improves tissue repair.
- ◆ *Zinc:* Some studies have shown AIDS patients to be low in zinc, which benefits the immune system. The picolinate form seems to be the most efficiently absorbed.
- ◆ *Manganese:* Essential for iron-deficient anemia and boosts the immune system.
- ◆ *Chromium:* Helps in maintaining energy
- ◆ *Catechin:* Has antitoxin properties and is considered useful in viral infections.
- ◆ *Acidophilus:* Replenishes friendly bacteria destroyed by antibiotic therapy.
- ◆ *Evening primrose oil:* Improves the functioning of white blood cells.

Herbal remedies:

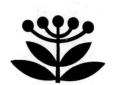

- ◆ *Black walnut:* Helps to balance mineral assimilation and also assists in oxygenating the blood.
- ◆ *Burdock:* Acts as a blood purifier to help remove toxins.
- ◆ *Echinacea:* Helps clear the lymphatic system and has immune-enhancing properties.
- ◆ *Pau d'arco:* Boosts liver function and is considered a good immune system builder.
- ◆ *Silymarin:* Expedites liver damage repair, which can occur as a complication of AIDS.
- ◆ *Mullein:* Helps to strengthen the immune system.
- ◆ *Ginkgo:* Good for stimulating circulation and brain function.
- ◆ *Golden seal:* Helps in assimilation of vitamins and minerals, and is considered an

herbal antibiotic.

◆ *St. Johnswort:* May help to inhibit retroviral infections.
◆ *Licorice:* Used extensively in the Orient for immune function enhancement.
◆ *Aloe vera juice:* Contains carrisyn, believed to stimulate T-cell production, which is directly attacked by the AIDS virus.
◆ *Siberian ginseng:* Helps with endocrine function and helps to promote stamina.
◆ *Native American* medicine uses leptotania and osha root to treat serious diseases; however, there is no literature available on their specific functions. These herbs have been traditionally utilized in fighting virus-associated diseases.
◆ *A combination of the following herbs taken together, may be useful:* burdock, turkey, rhubarb, sorrel, and slippery elm.

PREVENTION:

◆ Practice abstinence from sexual contact or remain in a monogamous relationship with a partner who is free from the virus.
◆ Avoid having sexual contact or intercourse with persons known or suspected of having the AIDS virus. Those who have had several sexual partners are at higher risk for carrying the virus.
◆ Casual sexual activity of any kind can be hazardous. Regular use of condoms can decrease the risk; however, the safety of a condom cannot be guaranteed.
◆ Do not use intravenous drugs. If IV drugs are used, never share needles or syringes.
◆ Do not have sexual contact with people who are IV drug users. People who test positive for the HIV virus should not donate blood, plasma, organs, any kind of tissue, or sperm.
◆ There should be no exchange of body fluids during any kind of sexual activity, including oral sex. Use a condom when having sexual intercourse. The effectiveness of condoms in preventing the HIV infection has never been conclusively proved; however, their consistent use may reduce the incidence of transmission, since contact with body fluids is known to increase the risk of contracting AIDS.
◆ Any implement that could become contaminated with blood should not be shared, such as razors, toothbrushes etc.
◆ If in doubt about blood supply for an upcoming surgery, donate blood for yourself ahead of time. The screening of blood supplies and the use of disposable needles has greatly decreased the incidence of AIDS contaminated blood.
◆ Keep your immune system strong. Avoid steroids, the indiscriminate use of antibiotics, and exposure to radiation or harmful chemicals. Eat a healthy diet that is low in fat and protein and high in complex carbohydrates, fresh fruits and vegetables.

Aids Hotline: 1-800-342-2437

Allergies

Definition:

Nothing can spoil the loveliness of spring like an allergy to pollen. For allergy victims, beautiful blossoms, green grasses and leafy trees can trigger miserable sneezing attacks, not to mention itchy, watery eyes and swollen sinuses. If you suffer from allergies, don't sit around wondering "why me?" There are plenty of good treatment options that can make life worth living again.

An allergy is a disorder that occurs when the body overreacts to the presence of a substance it thinks is a foreign invader. A variety of substances which are eaten, inhaled, or which come into contact with the surface of the skin can cause an allergic reaction. An allergy is actually a malfunction of the immune system, which attacks invaders such as dust or pollen with sticky proteins, known as antibodies. It is this inappropriate defense mechanism which causes the flair-up of allergic symptoms. When the immune system is triggered by an allergen, antibodies produce histamine and serotonin, which cause inflammation resulting in watery eyes, itching, sneezing etc.

The intensity of an allergic reaction can range from simple hay fever, hives, and asthma to life-threatening shock. The term "allergy" is often misused. Skin irritations resulting from contact with certain chemicals, burning eyes resulting from pollution, and coughing which is caused from exposure to cigarette smoke are not necessarily the result of a true allergic reaction.

Causes:

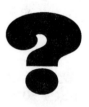

Allergies can be caused by certain foods, pollens, pets, dust mites, and insect venoms. In infants and small children, cow's milk can cause an allergic response. While the exact causes of why a particular individual becomes allergic to certain substance such as cow's milk remains unclear and somewhat controversial, heredity is a major determining factor. Other foods typically associated with allergies are wheat, eggs, citrus fruits, beef, veal, shellfish and nuts.

Pollens which come from ragweed and other plants can also cause seasonal allergies. Certain types of grasses are considered common allergens. In addition, contact with dog, cat and horse dander frequently causes allergic reactions. Mold and house dust are also culprits, and insect bites and stings can bring on severe, life-threatening allergic reactions. Drug sensitivities, such as allergies to penicillin, which is made from a mold, and reactions to bee stings can produce anaphylactic shock in an allergic individual, a condition which can be fatal.

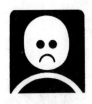

SYMPTOMS:

Physical: Allergies can include one or a combination of the following symptoms: hives, which can cause itchy, swollen palms; skin rashes, which almost always itch; sneezing; runny nose; itchy watery eyes; nasal congestion; asthma; swelling of the mouth or throat; and diarrhea, which typically affects allergic infants. Persistent sinusitis, irritable bowel syndrome, and arthritic-like pains may also be symptoms of a masked allergy.

Psychological: Some doctors have made a connection between emotional stress and the onset of an allergic reaction. This type of allergy must be treated for both its physical and mental causes. Allergies have a strong psychological component. Often just the suggestion of a certain weed, or even the sight of a silk plant can produce an allergic reaction.

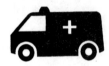

MEDICAL ALERT:

A violent reaction to a bee sting, insect venom, penicillin, aspirin, some vaccines, shellfish or nuts is probably anaphylaxis. It is a grossly exaggerated immune system reaction which causes the entire respiratory tract to swell, including the bronchial tubes and the larynx, which cuts off breathing. A drastic drop in blood pressure also occurs and the heart and kidneys can cease to function. Symptoms of anaphylactic reaction are flushed face, fear, dizziness, weakness, swelling of the eyes, face or tongue, nausea and vomiting, abdominal cramps or pain, difficulty breathing wheezing, tightness of the chest, difficulty swallowing, and unconsciousness.

Warning: If you have any of the above symptoms, seek out medical care immediately. In the future, wear a medical ID tag and carry an adrenalin kit if appropriate.

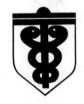

STANDARD MEDICAL TREATMENT:

Routine treatment involves a combination of avoiding the offending substance and of relieving symptoms. Antihistamines will usually be recommended by your doctor. Terfenadine (Seldane) is a commonly prescribed antihistamine which causes less drowsiness than other conventional antihistamines. Other standard treatments include steroid nasal sprays, eyedrops and inhalers.

In more severe cases of allergies or when asthma is involved, corticosteroid drugs such as prednisone may be used to treat asthmatic symptoms and severe nasal congestion. Cortisone can be prescribed under several brand names such as hydrocortisone, triamcinolone, methylprednisolone, meprednisone, paramethasone, fluprednisolone, dexamethasone, betamethasone, and fludrocortisone. Nebulizers or spray medicines can also be corticosteroids, such as beconase and vancenase.

Cromolyn sodium (nasalcrom, intal, gastrocrom, opticrom), a rather new allergy treatment, can come in inhaler, nasal spray or eyedrop form. Cromolyn does not treat symptoms that are present, but rather prevents the future onset of allergic reactions by stabilizing mast cells so histamine is not released. This drug is effective only on the areas to which it is applied. The drug must be taken on a daily basis before exposure to the allergen occurs.

Corticosteroid, cromolyn and antihistamine eyedrops are also available to control, itchy, red, watery eyes.

Allergy shots, available from your doctor or allergy specialist, may also prove helpful. This option should be explored with a physician, although its success rate varies, depending on the type of allergy being treated.

Over-the-counter antihistamines such as benedryl, chlortrimeton, dimetane, and PBZ are also frequently used. All of these may cause some drowsiness and should not be combined with sleeping pills or alcohol. Antihistamines interfere with the normal functions of the brain and can also cause mental dullness and a feeling of depression. Pregnant or nursing women should not use antihistamines without their doctor's approval.

Nasal sprays such as Afrin, Dristan, etc., should be used very sparingly, if at all. They can cause an intensified reverse effect, which only worsens the problem and creates an even greater reliance on these sprays. If the sinuses are severely blocked, this type of nasal spray is sometimes used to open the passageways so that other nasal medications can be used more effectively.

SIDE-EFFECTS: Seldane (terfenadine): Headache, nervousness, nosebleeds, dry nose and mouth are a few reported side-effects. Less common effects include rapid heartbeat, palpitations or other cardiac abnormalities, depression, and sleeplessness. Unlike other antihistamines, this drug does not interact with other drugs, or with alcohol.

Warning: Do not take this drug or any antihistamine when pregnant or nursing without the permission of your physician. Do not take this drug if you have had an allergic reaction to it in the past, if you have asthma, glaucoma, or stomach problems.

SIDE-EFFECTS: Prednisone or any steroid therapy should be discussed with your doctor in depth due to a number of possible side-effects. Dosage must be carefully monitored. Corticosteroid therapy can cause infections, gastric disturbances, water retention, heart failure, potassium and calcium loss, bruising, and irregular menstrual cycles.

Warning: Do not take any corticosteroid when pregnant or nursing without your doctor's permission. Do not become vaccinated against any infectious disease when on the drug due to its interference with physiological reaction to the vaccination. Do not increase, decrease or stop the dosage without specific instructions from your doctor. Steroids may cause a significant loss of potassium and they can interfere with laboratory test results.

SIDE-EFFECTS: Cromolyn sodium: Skin rashes, itching, dizziness, headache, nausea, urinary difficulty.

Warning: Cromolyn should never be used to treat an acute allergic attack. Its purpose is strictly preventative.

Dosages should be carefully monitored if kidney or liver disease is present. If taking the eyedrop form, soft contacts should not be worn. Pregnant or nursing women should check with their doctors before taking the drug.

Success rating of standard medical treatment: good. Most allergies can be helped with medication; however, treatment is usually to relieve symptoms and does come with specific side-effects, especially in the case of steroid therapies. Allergy shots have remained controversial and should be investigated thoroughly before initiating treatment. So far, there is no known cure for allergies.

MEDICAL UPDATE:

◆ Recently children in West Germany were found to be more allergy prone than those in East Germany. The higher rates of allergies among young people in West Germany have been seen as a possible result of the large number of automobiles that produce gas fumes which contain nitrogen dioxide, which is known to be associated with increased rates of hay fever in areas where the pollen count is high.

◆ Doctors in the Netherlands have recently found that using a goose-down comforter or pillow can cause severe allergic reactions. Goose down or goose feathers can contain significant numbers of dust mites, which are considered highly volatile allergens.

◆ A new drug called budesonide (rhinocort nasal inhaler) has recently received FDA approval for its use in helping to control allergy symptoms.

HOME SELF-CARE:

◆ A nasal wash with warm saline solution can help relieve soreness and encourage drainage.

◆ Eyedrops like Visine can help control redness, but are not recommended on a long-term basis. These preparations can have a rebound effect if used longer than three days, and actually cause more eye redness. (See chapter on conjunctivitis.)

◆ Installing an air-purification system of industrial quality may also be beneficial.

◆ Dehumidifiers can bring relief from pollens, molds and pet dander.

◆ Air conditioning your house or environment is very effective in controlling molds, pollens and dust mites. The cool temperature along with air-filtering devices cuts down on the presence of these allergens.

◆ Use a fungicide like Clorox to keep the growth of mold and mildew in check.

◆ Throw out rugs and carpets that carry pet dander and dust mites.

◆ Replace your furnace filters often. These can become heavily laden with dust and pollen.

◆ Use synthetic pillows, which can be washed, and keep sheets and pillow cases

changed often.
◆ Wear a mask when dusting or mowing the lawn.
◆ Stop smoking.
◆ Avoid using aspirin, which has been reported to allow food allergens to be more effectively absorbed by the body.

NUTRITIONAL APPROACH:

◆ Avoid foods such as wheat, eggs, dairy products, caffeine, chocolate, shellfish, strawberries, tomatoes, and citrus fruits.
◆ Avoid consuming FD&C yellow #5 dyes, along with BHT-BHA, monosodium glutamate and vanillin.
◆ If taking any corticosteroids, eat high potassium foods such as bananas or melons.
◆ Take a good multi-vitamin supplement with extra A, B complex (pantothenic acid, B6, B12) and vitamin C: All of these help to strengthen the immune system and control the production and release of histamine.
◆ *Vitamin C with bioflavonoids:* Essential for maintaining cell and tissue integrity which may be compromised when histamine is released.
◆ *Calcium and magnesium, manganese, potassium and zinc:* Help to reduce immune stress created by allergens.
◆ A natural antihistamine can be made by cutting orange peels into small strips and soaking them in apple cider vinegar for several hours. Drain the mixture and cook in honey until soft. Keep in the fridge and use as needed.
◆ *Quercetin (a bioflavonoid):* Helps to increase immune responses.
◆ *Tyrosine:* An amino acid which has been used to treat allergies from hay fever and grass pollens.
◆ *Brown rice and stone fruits:* Help with elimination, and are non-allergenic foods.
◆ *Raw honey:* Contains pollen dust and may help build resistance to certain allergens.
◆ *Brewer's yeast, grapefruit and wheat germ* blended together works to strengthen cell walls and provide natural immunity. If you have a sensitivity to yeast products, do not use brewer's yeast.

HERBAL REMEDIES:

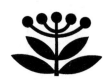

◆ *Bee Pollen:* May help to gradually modify allergic reactions to pollens and build immunity. Take a very small amount of bee pollen at first to determine your sensitivity to it, and then slowly increase the dosage according to instructions provided.
◆ *Blessed thistle:* Helps to loosen mucus and phlegm and strengthens lung tissue.
◆ *Pleurisy root:* Also helps to thin and loosen mucus and can facilitate the elimination of toxins through the pores.
◆ *Burdock:* Works as a blood purifier that clears toxins through the lymphatic system.
◆ *Garlic:* Contributes to fighting infection and is considered an antiviral compound.

- *Golden seal:* A natural antibiotic that can reduce nasal or congestion. (Do not use if allergic to pollens.)
- *Ground ivy:* Helps to reduce phlegm and dry out secretions.
- *Marshmallow:* Helps in the relaxation of bronchial tubes, which can constrict if allergens are present and cause an asthmatic reaction.
- *Lobelia:* Acts as an expectorant to move mucus out of the body, and can help relieve spasms in the bronchiole tubes.
- *Stinging nettle plant:* Can be used as a tea or in a freeze-dried extract to treat allergic reactions.
- *Ma huang:* Works as a natural antihistamine.
- An *eyewash* for allergy-irritated eyes can be made out of bayberry and red raspberry teas. Use an eye cup for application.
- *Angelica:* Helps the immune system in the formation and use of antibodies.
- A *combination* of the following herbs taken together may be useful: ephedra, white willow bark, valerian root, lobelia, golden seal, bee pollen, capsicum (take bee pollen in a very small dosage at first to check for sensitivity).
- *Alternative treatments:* Acupuncture is also accepted in some circles as being an effective treatment for certain types of allergies. If this option is explored, it should be done with a licensed and recommended acupuncturist.

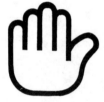

PREVENTION:

- Do not introduce cow's milk, citrus juices, eggs, meats, nuts or wheat too early into an infant's diet. Check with your doctor or allergist for a recommended time table for introducing new foods.
- Breast feed infants whenever possible for at least six months.
- Keep your immune system healthy by avoiding junk foods, caffeine, tobacco, alcohol, white sugar and white flour foods, and salt.
- Taking a good vitamin C supplement with bioflavonoids can help to boost the immune system.
- Eat lots of high-fiber foods and drink plenty of water. There is some evidence that allergies may be caused by an excessive accumulation of waste in the system, due to a poor diet, which can promote inappropriate immune responses.

Asthma and Allergy Foundation of America
1717 Massachusetts Avenue, Suite 305
Washington, D.C. 20036
202-265-0265

Alzheimer's Disease

DEFINITION:

Within the last decade, Alzheimer's disease has received a great deal of attention. Public awareness of this disorder has resulted in the formation of various support groups that can provide an invaluable service to anyone who must cope with this disorder. With Alzheimer's disease, becoming forgetful is only the tip of the iceberg.

Alzheimer's disease is a progressive, degenerative condition which involves the deterioration of nerve cells in the brain, resulting in memory loss and disorientation. If you have ever worked with a person suffering from Alzheimer's disease, then you are aware of how frustrating and tragic its effects can be.

The disease is considered the most common cause of senility in the older population, and is thought to be responsible for 75 percent of dementia in those 65 years and older. The disease progresses over several years. Unfortunately, the intellectual and personal decline that typically results from Alzheimer's cannot be arrested as of yet. The disease affects over 1.5 million Americans and is responsible for 20 percent of patients in nursing homes or chronic care facilities. The disease rarely appears before age 60; however, up to 30 percent of people over 85 suffer from Alzheimer's.

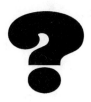

CAUSES:

The causes of Alzheimer's remain unknown, although several theories exist which range from exposure to aluminum to the existence of prolonged infection. Recently, speculation that Alzheimer's disease may be caused by a specific virus have been proposed.

Reduced levels of acetylcholine, a brain chemical, have been found in people suffering from Alzheimer's disease. In addition, nerve fibers in the brain become tangled and certain areas of brain tissue can shrink during the course of the disease. A genetic factor may also play a role in the disease and is currently being investigated. This hereditary link has been strengthened by the fact that the disease is more prevalent in Down's syndrome cases. In addition, approximately 15 percent of victims of Alzheimer's have a family incidence of the disease.

There has been significant speculation that an intake of aluminum from foods, antacids, cookware or antiperspirants may play a role in contracting Alzheimer's disease. The same speculation exists concerning silicon. There is no scientific evidence accepted in the medical community which confirms this connection; however, autopsies of Alzheimer's victims have shown excessive amounts of aluminum and silicon in the brain.

In addition, a deficiency of vitamin B12, zinc, potassium, selenium and boron was also found to exist. Consequently, there is evidence to suggest that increased contact with aluminum in combination with a lack of certain vitamins and minerals may predispose one to the disease (refer to aluminum sources below).

Regarding the possibility of a viral component, similarities between Alzheimer's disease and Creutzfeldt-Jakob disease have been noted by some, who see a slow-growing viral connection with both disorders. Another correlation that has recently been investigated is the finding that women with Alzheimer's had lower estrogen levels than healthy women of the same age.

SYMPTOMS:

Physical: There are three general stages to the disease. Initial symptoms include increasing forgetfulness, which may be typified by the almost obsessive writing of lists. As the disease progresses, forgetfulness becomes severe memory loss, particularly when dealing with short-term events, although long-term memory may not be affected. Disorientation may also occur, and it is not uncommon for a victim of the disease to lose his way home. Mathematical calculations may also become difficult, indicating a decrease in intellectual ability, in addition to becoming unable to find the right words (dysphasia).

Anxiety, mood swings and apprehension may become evident and personality changes can also become apparent. During the final stage of Alzheimer's, severe disorientation and confusion are the rule. Hallucinations and paranoid delusions may also occur. Symptoms of this disease typically intensify at night. Involuntary actions, incontinence of urine and feces, belligerence, and violent behavior are not uncommon, although some victims become more docile and withdrawn. Wandering, and neglecting appearance or hygiene require that the victim have full-time supervision. Once bedridden, the Alzheimer victims life expectancy is short.

Psychological: In their initial stages, victims of Alzheimer's usually try to compensate for their forgetfulness and will sometimes try to solicit others to help them. Depression and anxiety brought on by memory loss are common and should be addressed. As mentioned earlier, personality changes are common. Those caring for someone suffering from Alzheimer's should definitely take advantage of support groups available. The disease can be devastating to families. Often the caregiver in this situation will need as much psychological support as the patient. Emotional as well as financial stress can result as the disease demands more care, and self-help groups should be used. Counseling is recommended to prevent the possibility of abuse due to the stressful nature of this disease. Because the victim of Alzheimer's cannot be reasoned with, the caregiver needs external support and advice. (See information at end of this section).

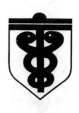

STANDARD MEDICAL TREATMENT:

The only way to absolutely diagnose Alzheimer's disease is with a brain biopsy or post-mortem examination of brain tissue. An EEG (which records brain wave patterns) will show slower waves; however, the rest of the diagnosis is purely clinical. There are no lab tests that can prove the existence of the disease. Alzheimer's disease is particularly difficult to diagnose; consequently, some symptoms of dementia can be misdiagnosed as Alzheimer's. Senile dementia, unlike Alzheimer's disease, can be caused by treatable conditions such as hypothyroidism, vitamin B12 deficiency, alcoholism, pernicious anemia, a series of strokes, or a brain tumor. In some cases, the elderly may experience severe depression, which can mimic Alzheimer's disease in several of its symptoms. Overmedication of the elderly is another factor which should be addressed as a possible cause of Alzheimer-like symptoms.

No medical treatments, including attempts at restoring acetylcholine nerve cell function have proven successful. The provision of good nursing care is vital, which includes a good diet, social interaction and using tranquilizers if behavior becomes difficult.

Success rating of standard medical treatment: very poor. Conventional medical approaches to Alzheimer's disease are very limited.

MEDICAL UPDATE:

◆ Recently a team at John Hunter Hospital in Newcastle reported that high levels of aluminum exist in some canned soft drinks. Their studies reveal that the aluminum content of non-cola drinks in cans was almost six times that found in bottles. For cola drinks, the amount was three times higher. Apparently, the acidity of soft drinks erodes the protective covering which lines the cans. As a result, aluminum dissolves into the beverage.

◆ Treatment with two drugs, sandostatin and tetrahydroaminoacridin, may prove helpful in treating the symptoms of Alzheimer's and should be discussed with your physician.

HOME SELF-CARE:

◆ Because one who suffers from this disease is usually very limited in his or her ability to be self-sufficient, a heavy burden falls to the caregiver. Because that care is so intensive, contact should be made with the Alzheimer's disease society for specific instruction and support (see address at end of this section).

◆ Make sure that symptoms assumed to be Alzheimer's disease are not simple cases of dementia. A high number of elderly people are nutritionally deficient or on a number of prescription drugs which may precipitate confused states of mind. Try to stay off any unnecessary drugs and eat a nutritionally sound diet.

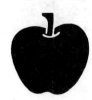

NUTRITIONAL APPROACHES:

◆ A good dietary regimen with an emphasis on a high-fiber diet, which stresses fresh fruits and vegetables, sprouts, seeds, nuts, pressed oils, millet, brown rice, oat bran, whole grains, fish, and other low fat foods is recommended.
◆ Do not stress the immune system by consuming alcohol, nicotine, caffeine, white sugar processed foods or red meat
◆ *Lecithin:* Contains choline, which stimulates the production of acetylcholine and may help with short-term memory.
◆ *Manganese, zinc, and iodine:* All play a vital role in proper brain function.
◆ *Selenium:* Also beneficial for proper brain function.
◆ *Sulphur and phosphorus:* Help to promote good nervous system health.
◆ *Coq10 and germanium:* Help carry oxygen to brain cells.
◆ *Vitamin B complex, B6 and B12 and B15:* Important for healthy brain cell activity and myelin sheath production in nerve cells. Some studies confirm that serum vitamin B12 levels are significantly lower in patients with Alzheimer's disease.
◆ *Vitamin E:* Helps transport oxygen to brain cells.
◆ *Vitamin C, calcium and magnesium* may help reduce aluminum accumulations.

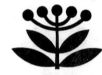

HERBAL REMEDIES:

◆ *Ginkgo:* Improves blood supply to the brain and combats the effects of atherosclerosis.
◆ *Alfalfa and burdock:* Improve cerebral circulation, which helps to oxygenate the cells and promote better brain function.
◆ *Capsicum:* Helps in supplying nutrients to the brain.
◆ *Chaparral:* Contributes to removing metals from the blood.
◆ *Ginseng, gingko, suma and gotu kola:* Increase the efficiency of the brain.
◆ *Lady's slipper:* Supplies nutrients to the nervous system.
◆ *The following herbs in combination may be useful:* Lily of the valley, periwinkle, mullein, juniper berries, pan pien lien.

PREVENTION:

◆ Avoid sources of aluminum which are commonly found in food additives (cake mixes, processed cheese, frozen dough, etc.). Check ingredient lists. Baking powder can have from 5 to 50 milligrams of sodium aluminum phosphate per teaspoonful.

Other sources of aluminum include:
　　pickling salts
　　some salad dressings

table salt
some white flours
some water sources
douches
some feminine hygiene products
some lipsticks
antacids (there are a
number available which are aluminum-free)
some brands of buffered aspirin
antidiarrheal medications
aluminum coated cookware (cooking tomato-based ingredients, which
are acidic, can cause some leeching into the food from the pot or pan)
some antidandruff shampoos
aluminum cans and other containers, especially soda pop cans

While the origins of the disease remain a mystery, keeping active and staying involved during post-retirement years has been known to prolong life and enhance its quality. Join senior citizen clubs, travel, exercise and keep yourself busy.

Eat a diet high in antioxidants such as carotenes, flavonoids, vitamin C, zinc and selenium.

Alzheimer's Disease Society
2 West 45th Street, Room 1703
New York, New York, 10036
212-719-4744

Association for Alzheimers and Related Diseases
70 East Lake Street
Suite 600
Chicago, Illinois 60601-5997
800-572-6037
800-621-0379

Anxiety or Panic Attacks

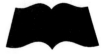

DEFINITION:

A panic attack can be an extremely terrifying and intense physical and emotional experience. Panic attacks can be so devastating that people who suffer from them will often radically change their life-styles to avoid triggering one.

An anxiety or panic attack results in an extremely negative emotional state, which is characterized by feelings of intense fear and apprehension. Anyone suffering from an anxiety attack feels a sense of impending doom, although in most cases, there is no actual physical threat present. While anxiety, if kept within limits, is a normal part of life, when it begins to disrupt one's ability to participate in day-to-day activities, it is considered a psychological illness. Anxiety attacks also cause a variety of physical symptoms that can easily be mistaken for serious disorders like heart attacks.

Normal activities such as driving, finding oneself far from home, stepping into a crowded room or going shopping may trigger a set of physical and emotional symptoms which reinforce the anxiety or panic. Frequently, the person who has suffered a panic attack relates that attack to what they were doing at the time. As a result, they may want to avoid shopping, driving, etc. for fear that another attack will occur.

It is not uncommon, however, to have one panic attack and then never experience another.

Anxiety disorders are rather common and affect roughly 4 percent of the American population. Younger adults are more susceptible, and the disorder affects men and women equally. A panic attack can last from 5 minutes to an hour and usually averages about 20 minutes in length. Anxiety attacks can lead to phobias such as agoraphobia, in which the person rarely leaves home for fear of losing control in public.

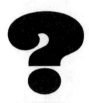

CAUSES:

Often, victims of anxiety attacks have a heightened level of arousal in the nervous system so that their reactions to certain stimuli are more intense. One area of the brain referred to as the locus ceruleus controls emotion, and when it is stimulated, it creates anxiety. Accordingly, panic attacks may be seen as a form of epilepsy in which the locus ceruleus becomes overstimulated and discharges impulses in excess.

People prone to depression seem to suffer more from panic attacks. This implies that a neurochemical imbalance may be the cause of both disorders. Typically, people who experience feelings of panic for no obvious reason find it more difficult to adapt to changing situations and environments.

Heredity is a factor in that these attacks seem to run in families. Some psychoanalysts believe that anxiety disorders stem from repressed or unresolved childhood conflicts. Feelings of insecurity and the lack of reassuring love and nurturing have also been cited as possible causes for panic or anxiety attacks which surface later in life. Perfectionists also seem more susceptible to these kinds of disorders.

There is some speculation that inner ear disorders can contribute to feelings of anxiety or phobias.

SYMPTOMS:

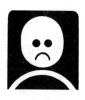

Physical: An anxiety or panic attack can produce the following symptoms: tightness in the chest; rapid, pounding heartbeat; throbbing or stabbing pains in the chest; breathlessness; heavy sighing or deep inhaling; headaches; neck and back spasms; inability to relax; restlessness; pallor; sweating; clammy skin; fatigue; nausea; diarrhea; difficulty swallowing; belching and vomiting. In addition, one may feel the urgent need to urinate or defecate and also experience dizziness, hyperventilation, yawning or a tingling sensation in the limbs.

Psychological: Someone who is experiencing a panic or anxiety attack feels that something terrible is about to happen to them immediately. Usually that fear has to do with the idea of losing control in public. Often, people who are having a panic attack say or do irrational things and may refer to unseen sources of danger. As a result of their impaired social function, many panic attack victims become irritable, increasingly dependent on others, easily fatigued, withdrawn, frustrated and may suffer from insomnia or bad dreams. In severe cases, the person feels cut off from themselves or from the real world.

MEDICAL ALERT:

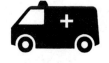

Whenever an anxiety attack or a phobia has progressed to the point where it interferes with everyday functioning, get professional help. If you feel incapacitated, contact local phobia centers, who will often send phobia aides to help you in your own home.

STANDARD MEDICAL TREATMENT:

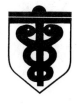

Counseling and psychotherapy are routinely prescribed, along with anti-anxiety drugs such as benzodiazepines. Beta-blockers (Inderal, tTenormin) can also help to control the adrenalin surges that accompany anxiety attacks. Clomipramine is considered one of the best treatments for panic attacks and is a relatively new antidepressant. Alprazolam (Xanax), which is derived from Valium, is also routinely used; however, it is highly addictive and when it is withdrawn, panic attacks can recur.

Success rating of standard medical treatment: fair to good. Much of this rating depends on the individual approach of your doctor or therapist. Often, physicians will rely on tranquilizing or antidepressant drugs to control these disorders and badly ignore counseling or self-help measures. Becoming dependent on drugs should be a last resort, and can in itself contribute to more anxiety and stress.

Drugs which block the action of adrenalin, such as beta-blockers, may help to control the physical symptoms of panic attacks but do nothing to remove the fear itself. Finding a good psychotherapist trained to deal with these kinds of disorders is preferable to becoming dependent on drugs. Using biofeedback, self-hypnosis and nutritional and herbal support are recommended.

Side-effects: Clomipramine (Anafranil): High or low blood pressure, abnormal heart rates, drowsiness, heart attack, confusion, hallucinations, disorientation, anxiety, delusions, restlessness, excitement, numbness, tingling in the limbs, lack of coordination, convulsions, tremors, loss of appetite, and blurred vision. These are only a few of the possible side-effects of this family of antidepressants.

Warning: Pregnant women or nursing mothers should not use clomipramine unless their doctor specifically recommends it.

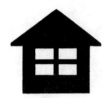

HOME SELF-CARE:

◆ Find support groups that have been organized to provide a forum for sharing feelings and contributing to overcoming phobias through a network of mutual sharing and counseling. Your local mental health organization will have a number of support groups that you can contact.

◆ Condition yourself in moments of oncoming panic to invoke positive reassurances about the situation. A therapist or support group can provide a long list of possible and helpful phrases to use.

◆ When you feel a panic attack coming on, immediately recognize it for what it is and kick in a conditioned response such as singing a particular song, popping in a favorite tape, or counting backwards. Learn to help yourself. If your mind is powerful enough to create feelings of overwhelming panic when there is no real danger, then it is powerful enough to quell those imaginary fears.

◆ Exercise daily. Exercise is a wonderful outlet for pent-up tension or anxiety. Choose something you enjoy and learn to express your emotional fears in a constructive physical way such as jogging, swimming, or racquetball. If you feel you cannot leave your home, get a treadmill or pop in an aerobics tape.

◆ Get a regular massage and if you feel an attack coming on, have your companion give you a deep shoulder and neck massage.

◆ Investigate therapies such as self-hypnosis, breathing exercises, music therapy, and biofeedback. Any of these may offer valuable advice on how to control the mind and subsequently the body in avoiding feelings of panic or anxiety.

◆ Aromatherapy may have some benefit for anxiety disorder victims. Sniffing certain aromas can have the immediate affect of calming and relaxing the nerves and creating a feeling of well-being. Some of the smells which typically produce a state of happiness are cookies or bread baking, cinnamon and ginger, baby powder, and a freshly cut lawn, etc. You may be able to find a bottled aroma that can be carried with you to help you feel calmer during times of stress.

◆ Become involved with community groups, church groups, etc., which give you something constructive to do. Teach adults how to read, visit the bedridden, get on a computer network, start a home business, learn to serve others, concentrate on spiritual enrichment, and learn to truly love by connecting with a higher power.

NUTRITIONAL APPROACH:

◆ Avoid caffeine in any form such as colas and other soft drinks, chocolate, coffee, tea and some medications. People who are prone to panic attacks and anxiety disorders will sometimes also be sensitive to caffeine.
◆ Do not eat white sugar or highly sweetened foods. Sporadic fluctuations in blood sugar can create feelings of anxiety and stress. Eat complex carbohydrates such as whole grains and avoid empty calorie junk foods and cold cereals.
◆ *Vitamin B complex and B6 injections:* All of the B vitamins are vital to the proper functioning of the nervous system and mental health. Strong supplementation of the B vitamins can improve brain function and help in reducing anxiety and stress.
◆ *Calcium/magnesium:* Has a calming effect and helps to decrease feelings of nervousness. Take the calcium citrate form for better absorption.
◆ *L-tyrosine:* An amino acid which can help alleviate symptoms of stress and also promotes sleep.
◆ *Vitamin C with bioflavonoids:* Important for healthy adrenal gland function. During periods of prolonged stress, the adrenal gland may become overworked.
◆ *Gaba with inositol:* Acts as a natural tranquilizer.
◆ *Lecithin:* Helps to protect nerve fibers in the brain and spinal cord.

HERBAL REMEDIES:

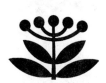

◆ *Gotu kola:* Helps to relax the nerves and supplies energy to the body to combat fatigue.
◆ *Black cohosh:* An antispasmodic and sedative that helps to relax and calm the central nervous system.
◆ *Neroli oil:* A natural sedative and antidepressant which has been used traditionally as a remedy for hysteria. It also helps to control heart palpitations.
◆ *Valerian:* A potent herbal tranquilizer.
◆ *Jamaican dogwood:* Combats, insomnia, tension and nervous anxiety.
◆ *Linden:* Helps to decrease nervous tension.
◆ *Skullcap:* Functions as a relaxant and restorative for the central nervous system.
◆ *Wood betony:* Has a sedative and calming effect and is excellent for feelings of fearfulness and exhaustion.
◆ *Vervain:* Considered a relaxing nerve tonic.

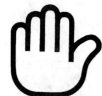

◆ *Damask rose:* Soothes the nerves and is a natural antidepressant. Can also help to prevent anxiety-induced vomiting.

PREVENTION:

◆ If anxiety attacks run in your family, recognize them for what they are. If you experience one, educate yourself on anxiety disorders, get counseling if you need it, and be determined not to let panic attacks compromise the quality of your life.
◆ Eat nutritionally, get exercise and learn to control your thoughts through biofeedback or other methods.
◆ Learn to relax by setting aside a certain portion of each day for relaxation techniques.

The Phobia Society of America
133 Rollins Avenue Suite 4B
Rockville, MD 20852-4004

Arthritis

DEFINITION:

Arthritis may be the oldest and most treated disease in the history of mankind. For generations, tonics and potions have been created and sold with the promise of curing this disease, and most people who suffer from it will try anything at least once. Arthritis is characterized by inflammation of joints with accompanying pain, swelling, stiffness and redness. The term does not refer to a single disease, but rather to a number of joint diseases which may result from a variety of causes. Osteoarthritis, which typically strikes older people, is the most common form. Rheumatoid arthritis, which can occur at any age, is one of the most destructive forms of the disease Gout is yet another form of the disease, and has been successfully treated.

Arthritis may be limited to only one joint or may affect many. It can range from mild aching to severe, debilitating pain, which can result in eventual joint deformities. It is the leading cause of physical disability in the United States. Approximately 50 million people suffer from the disorder. If you suffer from arthritis, there are several self-care options you can adopt that make the disease much more manageable.

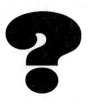

CAUSES:

While rainy weather does not cause arthritis, it definitely seems to aggravate the condition. Arthritis may be caused by a number of circumstances such as endocrine disorders, a defect in the immune system, genetic predisposition, a complication of other diseases, or as the result of an infection. In addition, injury or surgery, excessive mobility, age-related changes in the joints, and altered biochemistry may also cause arthritis. Osteoarthritis, which is a natural consequence of aging joints, attacks the knees, hips, and fingers. It occurs when the cartilage cushion which lines the joints becomes stiffer and rougher; consequently, bone can actually overgrow the joint area, causing swelling and decreased mobility. In its final stages, the pain may actually subside; however, the joint is no longer functional.

Rheumatoid arthritis is the most severe type of the disease and is classified as an autoimmune disorder. The body's immune system acts against the joints and surrounding tissue the same way it would attack an unwanted invader. Joints in the hands, feet and arms become extremely painful, stiff and eventually deformed. This type of arthritis can affect the entire body.

Gout is a disorder associated with a type of arthritis in which uric acid, a waste product, accumulates as crystals in the joints and causes inflammation.

SYMPTOMS:

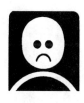

Physical: The following symptoms are typically experienced by arthritis sufferers: early morning stiffness, swelling, recurring tenderness in one or more joints, changes in the ability to move a joint, redness or a feeling of warmth in joints, unexplained weight loss, fever, or weakness associated with joint pain or discomfort. In cases of rheumatoid arthritis, symptoms may disappear during periods of remission. Emotional stress does not cause arthritis, but does seem to worsen its symptoms.

MEDICAL ALERT:

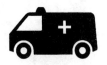

Lyme disease, which is caused by a tick bite, can be misdiagnosed as arthritis (refer to chapter on Lyme disease).

STANDARD MEDICAL TREATMENT:

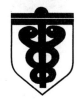

Drug therapy, exercise and rest comprise conventional medical treatment for arthritis. There is no known cure for this disease. Frequently, nonsteroidal anti-inflammatory drugs will be prescribed for pain control, such as naprosyn, feldene, clinoril, indocin, tolectin, or ibuprofen. Some studies have indicated that non-steroidal anti-inflammatory drugs successfully suppress the symptoms of arthritis, but may actually accelerate the progression of the disease.

SIDE-EFFECTS: *Ibuprofen (Motrin™, Advil™, Haltran™, Medipren™, Midol™, Nuprin™)*: stomach upsets, stomach ulcers, dizziness, ringing in the ears, lowered blood sugar, kidney dysfunction, abnormal heart rhythms.

Warning: Ibuprofen increases the action of sulfa drugs, phenytoin, antidiabetics, phenobarbital, and anticoagulants. Check with your doctor if you are using any of these.

◆ Do not use this if you have kidney trouble.

◆ Do not take this if you are pregnant or nursing without your doctor's approval.

◆ Do not take aspirin with this drug.

The side-effects of Naproxen (Naprosyn™, Anaprox™) are almost identical to those of ibuprofen.

Cortisone injections: Injecting cortisone directly into a painful joint can dramatically reduce pain and swelling for months. This procedure should be done only if your doctor recommends it, and is qualified to administer a joint injection.

The Side-effects of any corticosteroid are in the chapter on Allergies.

SIDE-EFFECTS: *Allopurinol (zyloprim)* is prescribed for gout (see Chapter on gout): rashes, nausea, vomiting, drowsiness, inability to concentrate, and stomach pain are some known side-effects.

Warning: Do not take this drug if you are pregnant or nursing.

Do not take with iron, or any vitamin containing iron, or liver damage may result.

Do not take megadoses of vitamin C with this drug as kidney stones may form.

Surgical options: Recently, hip and knee replacements used in advanced stages of arthritis have proven to be quite effective and should be discussed with a physician as a last-resort measure. Synovectomy involves the removal of diseased synovial membrane which surrounds the joint. Several orthopedic procedures can help to realign deformed fingers or toes.

Success rating of standard medical treatment: fair to good. Drugs that can alleviate painful symptoms can be effective; however, as in the case of any other incurable disease, options are limited.

MEDICAL UPDATE:

◆ Ask your doctor about using the drug carafate, which is commonly prescribed for ulcers. It can give the same relief as aspirin or an anti-inflammatory without stomach lining damage.

◆ A team of anesthesiologists at the general hospital in Denmark have recently discovered that acupuncture can significantly improve joint mobility and reduce pain in patients suffering from arthritis in the knee joint. Classic Chinese acupuncture points were used and the needle method was employed. Unquestionably, skilled acupuncture can reduce pain and improve joint movement and should be investigated as a treatment option that is preferable to taking pain killer drugs.

◆ A study conducted by the National Public Health Institute in Finland found that male smokers have about eight times the risk of developing rheumatoid arthritis as non-smokers. Exposure to tobacco smoke may trigger the production of rheumatoid factors which, when combined with male hormone, may contribute to the development of arthritis.

HOME SELF-CARE:

◆ Arthritis is one of those diseases which can respond to a number of inexpensive home self-care treatments.

◆ If you smoke, stop. Smoking is directly related to contracting and aggravating arthritis in males.

◆ A combination of rest and exercise is beneficial; however, long periods of bed rest may increase stiffness and muscle deterioration. At the same time, excessive exercise can promote increased joint inflammation. A regimen should be designed with your doctor to suit your needs. Stretching, strengthening and endurance exercises should be incorporated into the program.

◆ If your stomach can tolerate aspirin, it works as an inexpensive anti-inflammatory. Aspirin acts as a blood thinner and should be taken under a doctor's care.

◆ Ibuprofen is also an effective anti-inflammatory but should be used with caution to prevent stomach problems. Acetaminophen (Tylenol™) is less effective as an anti-inflammatory.

◆ Heat, administered as warm baths, hot tubs or wet compresses helps to relieve chronic pain.

◆ Hot wax treatments, in which paraffin wax is melted and placed over a painful joint, is an old remedy which has proven helpful for some.

◆ Raw lemon rubs and hot castor oil packs are traditional treatments for arthritis.

◆ An ice bag may be used after acute pain or injury to the joint has occurred. Apply for 15 to 20 minutes, remove for 10 minutes, and repeat as necessary.

◆ If you are overweight, stress on weight-bearing joints is increased and weight loss would be beneficial.

◆ Relaxation sessions through books and audio-tapes can help alleviate muscle tightening and cramping.

◆ Flotation tanks or relaxed swimming produces pain relief through stress reduction. Pool exercises are also excellent.

◆ Physical therapy through the use of exercise, heat, cold, diathermy, ultrasound etc. are all beneficial in improving the mobility of the joints, and will help to reduce pain to some extent.

◆ Use a good muscle ointment at night before going to bed to help with morning stiffness.

◆ Regular eucalyptus ointment massages can feel wonderful and help to alleviate stiffness and pain.

NUTRITIONAL APPROACHES:

◆ *Avoid foods* such as potatoes, tomatoes, peppers, eggplant, and milk products.
◆ *Avoid red meat*, which causes uric acid buildup and can cause joint inflammation.
◆ *Increase your intake of* carrots, celery, cabbage or tomato juice.
◆ *Cod liver oil or salmon oil:* Contains omega-3 fatty acids which provide substantial amounts of vitamin D, important for bone growth, and vitamin A, which may act as an anti-inflammatory. Fish oils also compete with certain fatty acids that are thought to trigger arthritis inflammation. Vitamin A and D can be toxic if taken in large amounts. Consult with your doctor on dosages.
◆ *Decrease vegetable oils high in omega-6 fatty acids.* Olive oil and canola oil may be used in moderation.
◆ *Vitamin A, B6, E, zinc and copper:* These compounds are needed for the maintenance of normal cartilage, which cushions the joints.
◆ *Vitamin C:* Studies have confirmed that people with rheumatoid arthritis are deficient in vitamin C. The toxicity of vitamin C is very low and it is believed to bring about some degree of regression in the disease. Vitamin C also helps to strengthen capillary walls in the joints and to counteract bleeding; consequently, it may be beneficial in conjunction with aspirin therapy.
◆ *Pantothenic acid:* A deficiency of this acid in rats appeared to cause a failure in the growth of cartilage and initiated arthritis-like symptoms.
◆ *Folic acid and zinc:* Research has shown that victims of rheumatoid arthritis had lower blood levels of zinc, folic acid and protein.
◆ *Calcium plus magnesium:* Helps to prevent bone loss.
◆ *Histadine:* Has anti-inflammatory properties which can reduce pain and swelling. This amino acid is also used to stimulate tissue growth and repair.
◆ *Methionine:* An essential amino acid that is important to the structure of cartilage and can act as a natural anti-inflammatory.
◆ A *low-sodium diet* helps counteract water retention in tissues, which can aggravate the swelling that accompanies arthritic inflammation.

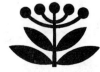

HERBAL REMEDIES:

◆ *Angelica compress:* Warms and stimulates muscles and can soothe painful joints. Soak flannel cloths with a strong angelica tea and use them as a warm compress on painful joints.
◆ *Devil's claw:* Natural analgesic and antiinflammatory which can be taken in capsule form. It has been compared to cortisone but has none of the side-effects of a steroid.
◆ *Garlic:* helps to prevent the formation of free-radicals, which are believed to damage the joints.
◆ *Willow bark:* Contains salicin, which is an antiinflammatory and works like aspirin to reduce pain.

◆ *Bromelain:* Helps to reduce inflammation and swelling.
◆ *Yucca:* Precursor to synthetic cortisone and wonderful for the control of swelling and irritation.
◆ *Comfrey:* Helps to purify the system of any toxins, which can make joint pain worse.
◆ *Alfalfa:* Can help with pain control and is a wonderful source of vitamins and minerals.
◆ *Chaparral:* Helps to dissolve uric acid accumulations where gout is present.
◆ *Celery:* Also helps to remove uric acid deposits from joints.
◆ *Burdock:* Helps to reduce joint swelling.
◆ *The following combination of herbs may be useful:* Yucca, willow, alfalfa, burdock, black cohosh, sarsaparilla, parsley, redmond clay, slippery elm, comfrey, pan pien lien and capsicum.

PREVENTION:

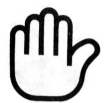

◆ Risk factors for arthritis include obesity, lack of exercise, or injury to a joint.
◆ Keeping fit with a regular exercise program, watching your weight and protecting joints from injury are all effective preventative measures.
◆ Eat a diet that is low in animal fats and proteins to avoid creating a build-up of uric acid, which can cause painful joint conditions.

The Arthritis Foundation
1314 Spring St. N.W.
Atlanta, Georgia 30309
404-872-7100

Asthma

DEFINITION:

The feeling that you just can't get enough air has got to be one of the worst sensations there is. Unfortunatley, asthma victims know all too well how this feels and will do just about anything to prevent an attack. The whys and wherefores of asthma are still not totally understood and, in many cases, the disease continues to baffle medical science.

A person experiences an asthma attack when the airways in the lungs decide to constrict, making the process of breathing much more difficult. Asthma is considered a respiratory disease characterized by recurring attacks of breathlessness, which are accompanied by wheezing, especially when exhaling. There are two main categories of asthma: extrinsic, in which an allergy causes the attack, and intrinsic, in which there is no apparent external cause. During an asthma attack, the bronchiole tubes, located within the lungs, constrict as a result of a kind of muscle spasm. In addition, mucus may clog the smaller tubes, trapping stale air. An asthma attack can vary in its severity, and is usually unpredictable. An attack can last from less than an hour to over a week, with occurrences usually sporadic in nature.

More than 10 million Americans suffer from asthma, 4 million of which are children. Asthma can occur as young as age three, or even younger, and in some cases diminishes with time. Over half of the children suffering from asthma will outgrow the disease. The rate of asthma is higher for boys. The disease is rarely fatal, but can be quite unsettling. Asthmatic episodes are responsible for over 8 million lost school days each year. This particular disorder appears to be becoming more prevalent in the U.S. and other developed countries. Asthma is considered an incurable disease; however, attacks can be avoided or relieved with treatment.

CAUSES:

In the case of most children and in some adults, asthma may occur after a cold, respiratory infection, or case of the flu. The majority of asthma attacks are triggered by an allergen, such as pollen, cat dander, feathers, cigarette smoke, certain foods, molds, etc. These allergens cause an intensified response of the bronchiole tubes and constriction results. Asthma attacks can also be brought on by certain drugs, especially aspirin, and by vigorous exercise, typically in cold air. Just running up stairs too fast, or becoming anxious and apprehensive can initiate an asthma attack.

There is a strong disposition for asthma is certain families. Often, no specific reason for a particular asthma attack can be found, and many asthmatics breathe normally in-between attacks. In cases of chronic asthma, emphysema can occur. Even today, the mechanics of asthma are not fully understood. Bronchiole tube constriction is controlled by nerves, and why these nerves make the tubes constrict is somewhat of mystery.

SYMPTOMS:

Physical: An asthma attack usually comes on suddenly. The most obvious symptoms of asthma are difficult breathing, a feeling of tightness in the chest without actual pain, and wheezing, which can be easily heard, or only detectable with a stethoscope. Exhaling is even more difficult than inhaling, and as a result, increased anxiety can worsen the bronchiole tube spasms. Frequently, coughing accompanies an asthma attack due to the presence of mucus; therefore, expelling that mucus can be beneficial.

In an extremely severe attack, breathing can become so labored that it may cause sweating, rapid pulse rate, and blueness in the face and lips, which is a condition called cyanosis, resulting from low oxygen levels. An attack this severe, can be fatal. It is common during an attack for an asthmatic to hunch over in order to facilitate breathing. In addition, the asthma victim will not be able to lie down, and may be unable to speak. Most attacks will last about an hour, although shortness of breath and wheeziness can persist for up to a week. It is common for asthmatics to have continual runny noses and other respiratory ailments.

Psychological: An asthma attack may be brought on by a period of emotional stress or upset. Emotions, both positive and negative, such as excitement, laughing too hard, crying, anger or sadness can be involved. While not altogether understood, periods of psychological anxiety or exertion can produce the same effect as the presence of an allergen for certain asthmatics. It is also true that asthmatics may be overly anxious about exposure to smoke, exercise, cold air, etc., triggering an attack. It is not uncommon for changes in temperature, the presence of cold, humid air, hair spray, paint thinners, bleach, perfumes, etc. to cause an asthma attack. As a result, serious consideration of life-style and how it affects the asthmatic must be taken to remove substances and habits that may cause an attack.

MEDICAL ALERT:

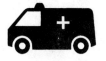

For an acute attack, find any inhalers or drugs the asthmatic usually takes if not already in use, and help administer medication. Help the asthmatic find a comfortable position, which is commonly sitting up, leaning slightly forward. Stay calm and be reassuring. Call the appropriate physician if necessary, and in severe cases, drive the person to the hospital or call for an ambulance if transportation is not available.

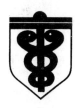

STANDARD MEDICAL TREATMENT:

Your doctor will want to take blood samples, X-ray the chest, examine sputum, and in some cases, perform hypersensitivity tests to determine allergic reactions in diagnosing asthma.

Immunotherapy in the form of allergy shots may be recommended; however, this particular treatment remains controversial and often is not successful. The most effective use of allergy shots seems to be for asthmatics who are allergic to pet danders and grasses.

Asthma medications commonly prescribed include:

Cortisone: An effective anti-inflammatory which can be used in liquid, tablet, or aerosol spray. Intravenous cortisone is used only in severe cases. Cortisone drugs commonly prescribed are beclomethasone (vanceril, beclovent,), triamcinolone, medrol and decadron.

Cromolyn sodium: This substance is not a steroid medication. Used in an inhaler, this preparation is useful for mild allergy-induced asthma. It is not a bronchodilator and must be taken regularly on a preventative basis.

Cromolyn (Intal) can help to stabilize sensitive airways.

Bronchodilator inhalers: These drugs are used in aerosol form or in metered dose inhalers. They work like adrenalin and include isoetharine, albuterol, metaporternol, and isoproterenol. These are effective, particularly for exercise-triggered attacks. Common inhalers are ventolin, proventil, alupent, and metaprel.

Theophylline bronchodilators: Help to relax and open airways and are fast-acting. Most individuals with chronic asthma use this type of sustained-release drug therapy. Common forms of the drug are accurbron, aerolate, asmalix, bronkodyl, theoclear, theolair and theostat.

Epinephrine or adrenaline: Given through injection or inhalation, the effect is almost immediate. Because of its side-effects, this treatment is usually used only in severe cases and must be overseen by a physician.

Psychotherapy to help asthmatics deal with emotional stress is sometimes recommended in cases where anxiety is directly related to the incidence of asthma attacks.

If the asthma attack is severe enough to require hospitalization, an intravenous injection of aminophylline may be administered. A fine-mist breathing apparatus may also be used to administer drugs. The use of a mechanical respirator in conjunction with muscle relaxants is another option.

SIDE-EFFECTS: *Cortisone:* All cortisone derivatives are steroid drug therapies and must be carefully monitored.

Note: Inhaled or nasal spray steroids are preferable to oral steroid preparations which are very toxic.

SIDE-EFFECTS: *Cromolyn:* Restlessness, weakness, anxiety, fear, tension, tremors, dizziness, urinary difficulties, headaches, abnormal heart rhythms and high blood pressure.

Warning: Bronchodilators should be used with caution by people with cardiac abnormalities, high blood pressure, stroke, diabetes, glaucoma, thyroid disease or prostate disorders. They should also be avoided by pregnant or nursing women.

SIDE-EFFECTS: *Theophyline:* Nausea, vomiting, diarrhea, restlessness, irritability, excitability, muscle spasms, heart palpitations, irregular heart beats, and headache.

Warning: Do not take theophylline without your doctor's permission if you suffer from stomach ulcers or heart disease.
Do not use if you are pregnant or nursing.

Note: Most bronchodilating inhalers can become somewhat addictive and the cycle of constricting and dilation can be aggravated, as in the case of some nasal sprays designed to shrink swollen sinus passages.

Success rating of standard medical treatment: fair to good. Bronchodilators can be a life saver for asthmatics, however they can become addictive and less effective with prolonged use. Steroid preparations are also effective but have toxic side-effects.

The actual causes of asthma still remain a relative mystery, and until that factor is discovered, total understanding of the disease is limited.

MEDICAL UPDATE:

◆ A new type of metered dose inhaler called Maxair autohaler is now available and is considered to be superior to other types of inhalers. Ask your doctor about this new pharmaceutical product.
◆ A new drug called salmeterol xinafoate (Serevent) has recently received FDA clearance and is designed to control asthma by using twice. It is particularly good for asthma that is exercise-induced.

HOME SELF-CARE:

Asthma is considered a reversible disease to some extent, and through the following suggestions it can be controlled and minimized.
◆ Do not smoke and stay out of smoke-filled rooms.
◆ Avoid exposure to any offending substances such as dust, molds, pollens, pet dander, chemicals, etc.
◆ Stay away from products stuffed with animal hair or pillows stuffed with feathers.
◆ Be careful when starting a fire. Wood stoves and fireplaces can trigger an asthmatic attack due to smoke particulates which can be released into the room.
◆ Protect yourself against sudden blasts of cold air by covering your nose and mouth with a scarf.
◆ If you have exercise-induced asthma, build up slowly to the pace you wish to maintain, breathe through your nose so as not to dry out your throat, and use asthma medication 15 minutes prior to exercising. Swimming is an excellent exercise for asthmatics.
◆ Install an air purifier and central air-conditioning in your home.
◆ When in the car, use the air-conditioner on the recirculation setting, so as to not bring in pollens etc., from the outside.
◆ Watch the kinds of foods you eat (refer to nutritional approach section).
◆ Use pain relievers that are non-aspirin, preferably acetaminophen.
◆ If you find yourself without medication and an attack is coming on, ingest caffeine in the form of strong coffee, etc., which may help to diminish the intensity of the attack.
◆ Certain yoga techniques have been found to be beneficial in promoting relaxed inhaling and exhaling.
◆ Sleep in a propped-up position, which facilitates breathing.
◆ Drink plenty of water to keep the respiratory tract secretions fluid. The less medication taken, the better.
◆ Traditional Chinese medicine and Ayurvedic medicine (healing methods of India) have specific dietary regimens designed for asthma.

◆ Avoid antihistamines, as they tend to dry out secretions, which may perpetrate the production of mucus.
◆ A number of studies usually not cited by traditional medicine indicate that low stomach acid may be linked to asthma in children. In addition, food additives including the dyes tartrazine(ornabe) yellow, amaranth, both reds and pate blue, preservatives such as sodium benzoate, 4-hydroxybenzoate, esters and sulphur dioxide have also been linked to asthma attacks.

NUTRITIONAL APPROACHES:

◆ Eliminate milk and milk products from your diet. Milk proteins can increase the production of mucus secretions in the bronchiole passageways. Check ingredient labels for non-fat dry milk, etc.
◆ Watch culprit foods such as eggs, wheat, nuts, and seafood.
◆ Watch your intake of salt, which can promote fluid retention.
◆ Avoid ice-cold beverages and ice cream. Extreme cold can sometimes trigger an asthma attack.
◆ Beware of food additives such as MSG and metacisulfite, which in some cases can bring on an attack. Sulfites are commonly found in beer, wine, shrimp, dried fruits, potato chips and sausages. Also avoid BHA and BHT, food additives FD&C yellow #5 dyes, and tryptophan.
◆ Test strips to detect the presence of sulfites in foods are now available. For information, write to: Sulfitest, Center Laboratories, 35 Channel Drive, Port Washington, NY 11050 or call 1-800-645-6335.
◆ Diet should be strong on fresh fruits, vegetables, oatmeal, sprouts, onions, garlic, honey, and complex carbohydrates.
◆ *Magnesium:* Some research has implied that low magnesium levels may play a role in some types of asthma, and may be linked to mucus production.
◆ *Calcium:* Helps in proper transmission of nerve impulses.
◆ *Selenium:* Helps to keep the heart strong.
◆ *Beta carotene:* Enhances immunity, which is often compromised in cases of allergic disorders.
◆ *Vitamin A:* Aids in tissue repair and immunity; can be taken in the form of salmon oil capsules.
◆ *Pantothenic acid (B5):* Considered an anti-stress vitamin
◆ *Vitamin B6:* This supplement has been found to reduce the severity of asthma attacks. (Check with doctor so doses will not be toxic.) Injections are the most effective form.
◆ *Vitamin B12 tablets or lozenges:* Can be used to boost immunity
◆ *Vitamin E:* A strong antioxidant that helps in tissue repair.
◆ *Vitamin C with bioflavonoids:* Contributes to maintaining connective tissue strength and is a natural anti-inflammatory.

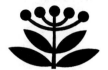

Herbal remedies:

◆ *Roman chamomile:* Anti-inflammatory and antispasmodic. Helps control allergic reactions in the respiratory tract.
◆ *Comfrey:* Acts on the respiratory system to move mucous and reduce congestion.
◆ *Licorice:* Functions to some extent like a natural corticosteroid.
◆ *Fenugreek:* Helps to expectorate mucous and contributes to fighting infection.
◆ *Garlic:* Used for centuries by Chinese herbalists to inhibit and prevent the formation of allergic antibodies in the immune system. Helps clear congestion from the lungs
◆ *Gumplant:* Antispasmodic and an expectorant.
◆ *Slippery elm:* Helps to alleviate inflammation of the mucous membranes.
◆ *Lobelia:* Helps to relax and clear airways of mucus. Using lobelia extract in drops can help control attacks.
◆ *Marshmallow:* Helps to soothe and relax irritated bronchiole tubes.
◆ *Ground ivy:* Helps to reduce and dry mucus.
◆ *Capsicum:* Helps in dissolving thick mucus and protects airways from irritation.
◆ *Elecampane root:* Sweeten with honey and take as a hot tea.
◆ *Chinese ephedra:* Traditional Chinese medicine has valued ephedra for centuries in treating asthma. It is a natural source of ephedrine, a bronchodilator, and can be used in capsule form, as a tincture or as a tea. American ephedra is not as effective.
◆ *Chinese scullcap:* Compares to a nonsteroid anti-inflammatory and can function in an anti-asthmatic capacity.
◆ *Echinacea:* Stimulates the immune system.
◆ *Ginkgo:* Considered an adaptogen herb, which helps in dealing with stress.
◆ *The following herbs taken in combination may be useful:* mullein, comfrey, cayenne, horehound, marshmallow, and lobelia.
◆ *Onions:* Act as an anti-inflammatory for irritated bronchiole tubes.

Prevention:

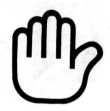

◆ Because asthma, like allergies, runs in families, prevention is often difficult. Avoiding substances that trigger attacks can greatly decrease the incidence of asthmatic episodes.
◆ Avoiding potential allergens found in food dyes, preservatives, junk foods, dairy products, dusts and pollens can also help prevent asthma-inducing sensitivities.
◆ Not letting an initial asthmatic reaction get out of control through the use of inhalers, herbs etc. can also help in avoiding prolonged irritation of the bronchiole tubes which makes subsequent attacks more likely.

Asthma and Allergy Foundation of America
1717 Massachusetts Avenue, N.W.
Washington, DC 20036
202-265-0265

Athlete's Foot

DEFINITION:

Athelete's foot can be both bothersome and persistent. It certainly isn't limited to just atheletes and, like most fungi, it can hang around far too long. It is a common skin disorder that affects the feet especially in the area between the toes and at times, the toenails. Athelete's foot is the most common of fungal infections and is also called ringworm of the feet. The fungus thrives in a warm, moist environment. As a result, closed, sweaty shoes provide the perfect location for it to thrive. The disease is common during and after adolescence. Unless it is particularly troublesome, it does not usually require professional attention.

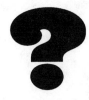

CAUSES:

Athelete's foot is caused by a form of ringworm fungus called a dermatophyte. People who spend long periods of time in sweaty socks and shoes are susceptible; hence, the name athelete's foot. The fungus can also develop and spread in locker rooms and showers. Using snug, poorly ventilated shoes can provide the ideal environment for the fungus to proliferate. Athelete's foot is slightly contagious and can be contracted from others through the shedding of fragments of infected skin. It is also believed that the use of antibiotics, radiation or certain drugs which kill beneficial bacteria can facilitate the spread of the fungus. Immunity plays a significant role in susceptibility, in that frequently people who are constantly exposed to the fungus never contract the disease.

PHYSICAL SYMPTOMS:

The fungus usually attacks the fourth and fifth toes, although the sides or soles of the feet, can become infected as well. The skin can become red, flaky, cracked, blistery, and itchy, and a burning sensation is also common. In some cases, an unpleasant smell can accompany the disorder. Exposure to sweat or water will make the top layer of skin appear white and soggy during the infection. If the condition is severe enough, at least a month's worth of treatment is needed to overcome the fungus. A condition called dyshydrosis may mimic athlete's foot. Eczema may also resemble athlete's foot; however, it will not usually attack the toe web between the fourth and fifth toe. If the nails are affected, a cure is more difficult and oral therapy may be required. Athelete's foot rarely strikes anyone under 10. If a child has similar symptoms, consult a physician.

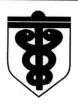

STANDARD MEDICAL TREATMENT:

Over-the-counter antifungal preparations are usually effective in controlling athlete's foot and will initially be recommended by your doctor. There are three general types containing either miconazole nitrate (Micatin™ products), tolnaftate (Aftate or Tinactine), or fatty acids,(Desenex™). Tolnaftate is generally considered better in preventing than curing athlete's foot.

The application of a 30 percent aluminum chloride solution is also beneficial for its drying properties, and can be made up by your pharmacist. This should be used for two weeks after the infection is gone. Don't use this if the skin is raw or cracked, or intense stinging will occur.

If the condition is persistent, your physician may prescribe haloprogin (halotex), ciclopirox (Loprox™), or ciclopirox (Lotrimin™) in a cream or ointment form.

Note: Creams can trap moisture. Another form of the medication may be preferable.

SIDE-EFFECTS: *Ciclopirox* (Lotrimin™): Side-effects are rare and usually mild. If taken externally, redness, stinging, blistering and itching can occur. Taking the drug orally may cause diarrhea, vomiting and cramps.

If the nails become infected, ketoconazole, an oral drug, may be recommended. If this therapy is not successful, permanent removal of the nail may be required.

SIDE-EFFECTS: *Ketoconazole: (nizoral):* nausea, vomiting, abdominal pain, headache, dizziness diarrhea, male impotence and reduced sperm count.

Note: Taking an antacid will decrease the potency of this drug, by decreasing its absorption. Check with your doctor before taking any antacid.

Warning: This drug has been associated with liver inflammation and damage. Pregnant or nursing mothers should not take this drug.

Success rating of standard medical treatment: good. Most over-the-counter preparations usually control athlete's foot; however, when the fungus attacks the nail, medical treatment is often ineffective.

HOME SELF-CARE:

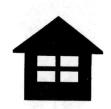

◆ Wash the affected area with soap and water at least twice a day and dry thoroughly, especially between the toes. Put on clean socks, preferably cotton ones.

◆ Avoid wearing vinyl or plastic shoes which do not allow for moisture evaporation. Leather and cotton are preferable to rubber or wool, which may induce sweating. Sandals or canvas shoes are recommended while fighting the infection.

◆ Use extra hot water to wash socks so as to control the fungal infection

◆ Use a powder preparation to help keep feet dry. A powder can be placed in your shoes also. To avoid the mess of applying powder directly, place it in a plastic bag, then put your foot in the bag and shake it around.

◆ A baking soda paste can also be beneficial. Make sure to rinse thoroughly and dry completely after an application

◆ Air your feet as much as possible. A hair blower can be used to dry both your feet and your shoes. Exposure to sunlight is also good.

◆ Change your shoes every other day and make sure they air out.

◆ A disinfectant such as Lysol™ can be used directly in the shoes as long as they dry our completely before wearing

◆ Foot compresses can be used to soothe the infected areas. Domeboro powder or burrow's solution can be used, and are available without a prescription. Soak the area with a cotton cloth for at least 15 minutes.

◆ A salt-water foot soak may also prove beneficial. Use 2 teaspoons of salt per one pint of warm water. Soak for 5 to 10 minutes, and dry thoroughly.

◆ Keep your toenails clean by using a wood orange stick rather than a metal nail file.

NUTRITIONAL APPROACHES:

◆ *Acidophilus:* Replenishes friendly bacteria that can help to inhibit the growth of pathogenic organisms. Can be found in live active culture yogurt or may be purchased in liquid or tablet form

◆ Avoid a diet high in sugar and fat.

◆ *Lemon juice or apple cider vinegar* applied to the infected area has been helpful in some cases, but stings if skin is raw.

◆ *Vitamin B complex, high potency* (use a yeast free source): Contributes to tissue repair and boosts immune defenses.

◆ *Vitamin C with bioflavonoids:* Helps to strengthen the immune system and is important in connective tissue regeneration and capillary wall strength.

◆ *Zinc:* Can inhibit the growth of fungus.

◆ *Selenium:* Helps to strengthen the immune system.

◆ *Liquid chlorophyll:* Acts as a blood purifier and is an excellent supplement for facilitating the removal of toxins caused by bacteria and fungi.

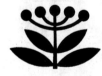

HERBAL REMEDIES:

◆ *Figwort:* Works as a skin medication when used as a poultice or wet compress that can be made from soaking a gauze pad in figwort tea.

◆ *Garlic:* Aids in killing fungus and can be taken internally in the form of capsules and applied as an oil on the rash. Some burning is usual if used externally.

◆ *Black walnut:* Use extract externally to help in killing skin fungus. May also be taken internally according to instruction.

- *Chaparral:* Works as a natural antiseptic when used externally. May also be taken internally.
- *Horsetail:* Contains silicon and calcium to help in healing skin problems.
- *Tea tree oil* used externally can help promote healing and fight the infection.
- *Myrrh:* An antifungal herb that can be used as a foot wash by mixing it with warm water.
- *Pot marigold:* Antifungal and anti-inflammatory. Can be used as a cream, ointment or in a footwash.
- *Powdered whey and slippery elm* mixed to a paste with water and applied as a poultice directly on the infected area can promote drying and soothe irritated tissue.
- *Thyme oil:* Six drops to a cup of water rubbed on the feet at least three times daily.
- *Aloe vera gel:* Helps to soothe and heal irritated skin.

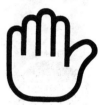

PREVENTION:

- Prevention is by far the most effective way to control athlete's foot.
- Keep your feet clean and dry.
- Using disinfectants on shower floors and locker rooms may help to prevent the condition.
- If you must walk in public shower areas, wear slippers or shower shoes to avoid coming in contact with the fungus.
- Nutritionists wholeheartedly agree that keeping the immune system strong through a healthy diet and lifestyle can provide protection against exposure to infection of any kind.

Backache

DEFINITION:

Having your back "go out" can put a damper on your day and totally ruin any plans you might have had. A bad backache cannot be ignored and in some cases, will literally sweep you off your feet. Back pain is suffered by the majority of people at one time or another, who understand the cliche, "oh my achin' back" all too well.

Lower back pain is the most common kind of backache and can result from a variety of causes. The most common kind of back pain involves a persistent dull pain, usually located in the small of the back. The pain can vary from mild discomfort to excruciating agony. Resolving a backache can be frustrating and relief can be slow. Unfortunately, most backaches are recur.

Causes:

Back pain can be related to using an overly hard or soft mattress, improper lifting, a slipped or herniated disc, muscle spasms, a blow or fall, arthritis, bone disease, curvature of the spine, menstrual cramps or other female pelvic disorders. In addition, kidney problems, bladder disorders, a duodenal ulcer, gout, or the presence of a tumor may result in chronic back pain. Most back pain is the result of a spasm of the large supportive muscles found to either side of the spine which go into a contraction, causing subsequent stiffness and pain. This type of backache usually heals naturally and is commonly linked to overexertion of some type. If back pain radiates into the legs, a ruptured or crushed disc may be indicated. Unfortunately only about a quarter of all back pain is found to have a specific cause.

Symptoms:

Physical: Lower back pain can develop gradually or can come on suddenly, usually when bending down. It can be completely disabling, rendering its victim totally immobile and paralyzed by pain. Back pain can be chronic or acute. Often a very small movement, such as leaning down to pick up a piece of paper, can cause excruciating pain, whereas in cases of heavy lifting, only minor soreness may result.

Psychological: Stress, including anger, grief, frustration or anxiety can precipitate a backache. Obviously, tense muscles, resulting from emotional stress, can predispose one to muscle spasms.

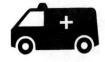

Medical alert:

Be sure to see your physician immediately if you have back pain that is accompanied by fever, vomiting, chest pain or difficult breathing; back pain that radiates down one leg to the knee or foot region; back pain that appears for no apparent reason; or chronic back pain that persists for longer than three days without relief.

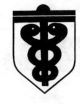

Standard medical treatments:

Backaches are hard to evaluate and can be difficult to treat. Medical doctors often disagree on what the exact causes of back pain are. The prescribing of muscle relaxants, such as flexoril or anti-inflammatories, such as naprosyn, are the most common conventional treatment for a backache. Over-the-counter analgesics, especially aspirin-based medications or ibuprofen drugs, are commonly recommended for pain.

Bed rest is also recommended by medical doctors, although staying off your feet for more than two days may actually promote a backache.

Surgical options: In cases where a herniated disc is causing severe and persistent back pain, surgical correction may be necessary. Today, back surgery has become simpler, requiring a smaller incision and a shorter hospital stay. Recovery involves the gradual increase of physical activity and the ability to sit, which places more stress on spinal discs than standing. Operations to correct herniated discs have a good success rate and can alleviate a great deal of misery.

SIDE-EFFECTS: Muscle relaxants can cause a significant amount of drowsiness, inability to concentrate, depression, confusion, restlessness, irritability, nausea, vomiting and dizziness. They should only be taken in cases of painful muscle spasms and should not be used as sleeping aids or tranquilizers. If you are pregnant or nursing do not take muscle relaxants or any other medication without your doctor's specific approval.

Success rating of standard medical treatment: fair. Unfortunately, except for pain killers or muscle relaxants, medical approaches are limited. Prevention is vital in avoiding back pain and injury. While medical evaluation of any backache is advised, there are several options that you can use to ease the pain of a backache and to prevent its return.

HOME SELF-CARE:

◆ Resting the affected muscles for at least 24 hours by lying flat on the back is very important.

◆ After bed rest, gradually increase physical activity.

◆ A program of exercising designed to strengthen certain back muscles is very beneficial. It is thought that improving your fitness and aerobic capacity enhances your recovery. Make sure to warm up and gently stretch your muscles before beginning exercises. Check with your doctor before staring such a program. Brisk walking while holding hand weights is highly recommended.

◆ Get a list of specific exercises designed to strengthen certain back muscles from your doctor or chiropractor. These can be invaluable in warding off future attacks.

◆ Sleeping without a pillow on a very firm mattress is recommended. A bed board can be placed under any mattress. Waterbeds are also beneficial in supporting back muscles, if the water pressure is not too low.

◆ If you have one specific tender spot in your back, lie on a soft ball such as a tennis ball or tightly balled up sock and roll your back on the ball to help decrease pain.

◆ Placing a rolled up towel or pillow in the small of the back may increase comfort.

◆ Many people have found relief through chiropractic adjustments. Before you go to a chiropractor, check with your physician and get recommendations.

◆ Swimming is especially beneficial for backaches. Stretching the back while in the water is easier and less risky. Jacuzzi or hot tub therapy can also alleviate discomfort.

◆ An ice pack may also help alleviate pain and should be applied to the area in short intervals. Ice therapy is good for the first couple of days after an injury, followed by the application of heat. Moist heat is preferable. Ice and heat treatments can be alternated with 30 minute intervals for each. You can use a conventional ice bag or make your own. Blue ice packs (soft ones) used for coolers also work well.

◆ If you sleep on your side, place a pillow between your legs. Don't sleep on your stomach, which puts stress on back muscles.

◆ Chinese medicine, in addition to the benefits of acupuncture, offers t'ai chi, which is comprised of a series of slow and fluid movements that can benefit anyone with back troubles.

◆ Yoga is also a good way to strengthen back muscles and promote flexibility, as well as ease backaches caused by mental stress

◆ Hot oil massage (eucalyptus, peppermint or wintergreen oil) can be very beneficial and pain-relieving. You can message yourself with electric back massagers or wood balls designed to roll over the spine. Several massage therapists have advocated using a hard rubber ball and placing it under the back in the tender area while lying on the floor. Rolling on the ball gently can produce the same beneficial results of message therapy.

◆ Wear shoes that fit well, are cushioned and have good support. Often, just standing for long periods of time in high heels or in very flat shoes can result in later back muscle spasms.

◆ Keep your elimination regular by following the recommended nutritional guidelines.

◆ Don't smoke. Smoking decreases oxygen to the spinal discs and can result in increased back pain.

NUTRITIONAL APPROACHES:

◆ Avoid meats and animal protein products if gout is suspected, due to the high uric acid content of these foods.

◆ Avoid steroids unless they're mandatory for treatment of a medical disorder, as bone loss can occur as a side-effect.

◆ Eat a diet rich in whole grains, fresh fruits and vegetables. Also eat foods rich in protein. Non-dairy based protein sources include; kelp, collard greens, kale, turnips, almonds, watercress, chickpeas, beans, sunflower seeds, and endive.

◆ *Calcium/magnesium:* Both essential for bone strength. Calcium citrate is recommended for its absorbability.

◆ *Silicon:* Improves the assimilation of calcium, needed for healthy bone and muscle.

◆ *Vitamin B12:* Increases the absorption of calcium and is vital to the production of healthy muscle fiber.

◆ *Vitamin C:* Essential for the production of new collagen and connective tissue. Vitamin C also acts as a natural anti-inflammatory.

HERBAL REMEDIES:

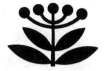

◆ *Willowbark:* A natural salicylate or pain-killer which also acts as an anti-inflammatory.
◆ *Comfrey:* Helps in building new tissue in the muscular-skeletal system.
◆ *Horsetail:* A good source of silicon, calcium and minerals
◆ *Slippery elm:* Rich in protein and healing properties
◆ *Hops:* A natural relaxant which is beneficial in easing the muscle spasms that accompany back pain. It also works to reduce stress, which may be a primary cause of back spasms.
◆ *Scullcap:*   Strengthen the nerves and alleviates pain.
◆ *Wild yam:* Relaxes muscle fibers and helps to relieve pain.
◆ *The following herbs in combination may be useful:* Capsicum, black cohosh, scullcap, myrrh gum, lobelia, skunk cabbage and valerian root.

PREVENTION:

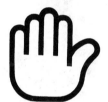

◆ Learning to lift correctly is of utmost value. Squatting down and lifting using the legs to bear the weight can avoid potential back injury.
◆ If you sit at a chair for long periods of time, make sure the chair has proper back support. Lumbar supports can be placed in car seats, etc.
◆ Wearing shoes that have the proper support and a comfortable heel height can decrease the incidence of back pain, especially if long periods of time are spent on foot. Check the height of your heels and purchase quality footwear.
◆ Make sure you don't slouch, and walk with good posture so as to not put unnecessary strain on back muscles.
◆ Don't sleep on your stomach.
◆ Avoid heavy shoulder bags or book bags, which can throw back alignment off.
◆ Keep yourself physically fit through a regular exercise program.
◆ Don't become overweight. Obesity can predispose one to recurring backaches.
◆ Use a vacuum with care. Movements associated with vacuuming can trigger a muscle spasm in the back.
◆ Avoid twisting the body abruptly.
◆ Don't smoke; smoking decreases the oxygenation of spinal discs.
◆ Keep your elimination regular by drinking plenty of water, exercising regularly and eating a high-fiber diet.

Bad Breath (halitosis)

DEFINITION:

Smellling good is right up there on most Americans' priority lists, and having bad breath is a definite no-no. Everyone seems to worry about this mouth malady, and as Mother Nature would have it, everyone has to occasionaly deal with it.

Bad breath, or halitosis, technically refers to an unpleasant smell which can originate from the mouth, throat or digestive system. It is a common disorder and can range from mild, stale-smelling breath to foul, fetid breath which usually accompanies some form of mouth or gum disease.

CAUSES:

Poor dental hygiene, food lodged between the teeth, gum disease, tooth decay, smoking, chewing tobacco, and drinking alcohol are responsible for most cases of bad breath in adults. The presence of disease such as sinusitis (mouth breathing), sore throats, or other conditions that may cause the tongue to become coated can also cause offensive breath.

Food particles that become trapped in dentures or certain foods (such as garlic) can also produce halitosis. In children, bad breath can be the result of diseases such as trench mouth or throat infections, especially chronically infected tonsils. Occasionally, a small child may insert a foreign object in the nose (such as Kleenex, cotton, etc.) which remains lodged there. A white or yellow discharge from the nose usually accompanies the bad breath in these situations.

More uncommon causes of bad breath are the presence of certain lung disorders such as bronchiectasis, some gastrointestinal disorders, tuberculosis and syphilis. There is also some speculation that intestinal gases from improper elimination can cause bad breath. Taking certain drugs, such as some antihistamines, some hormonal therapies, lithium, and penicillin may also create some degree of halitosis. Being very hungry or going without foods for a long period of time can induce a dry mouth which may produce "stale breath."

STANDARD MEDICAL TREATMENT:

The possibility of a serious cause for the bad breath will need to be ruled out. Your doctor will examine the mouth, throat and nose. A culture may be needed if a sore throat or mouth sores are present. Rarely will bad breath motivate one to make a visit to a physician unless it is persistent and unexplained. Over-the-counter mints, sprays, and mouthwashes offer only a temporary cure.

MEDICAL ALERT:

Persistent bad breath may be an indication of a serious disorder and should be checked out by your physician.

MEDICAL UPDATE:

◆ Pills are available now which act to control bad breath from the stomach rather than directly in the mouth. Ask your doctor about the effectiveness and availability of these pills.

HOME SELF-CARE:

◆ Good dental hygiene, including flossing, is the best preventative of bad breath. If your wear dentures, soak them nightly. A well-designed toothbrush, or water pick can also get to hard-to-reach areas of the mouth. Brushing the tongue is also recommended (the tongue has hairlike projections which can catch plaque).
◆ Use a mouthwash that contains zinc, which combats certain odors more efficiently (usually these are red in color).
◆ Use baking soda-based toothpastes or make your own paste with baking soda and water. Toothpastes are available now which have peroxide added to their baking soda formulas.
◆ Stop smoking.
 Note: You can check your breath by cupping your hands and steadily blowing out a stream of air.

NUTRITIONAL APPROACHES:

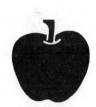

◆ A diet high in fiber will facilitate good elimination and help to prevent constipation.
◆ There is some indication that a diet high in fats can contribute to halitosis. Avoid dairy products and cured meats.
◆ Drink fresh lemon juice water every day.
◆ Chew whole cloves or fresh parsley, which are natural mouth deodorizers
◆ Chew gum or hard candy if you have trouble with a dry mouth or are taking a medication which causes the condition.
◆ Raw fruits and vegetables such as apples and carrots help to keep the mouth clean in between brushings.
◆ Raw oranges or other citrus fruits help combat a dry mouth.
Acidophilus: Helps keep the lower bowels functioning well and can reduce the formation of gases.
Liquid chlorophyll: Take two tablespoons of liquid chlorophyll with water or juice between meals.

Vitamin A, B complex, C with bioflavonoids and E help the body to eliminate toxins. *Zinc:* Some cases of bad breath are caused by a zinc deficiency

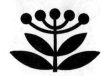

HERBAL REMEDIES:

◆ *Aloe vera gel:* Helps clean the digestive tract and contributes to the healing of mouth sores.
◆ *Cascara sagrada:* A natural laxative which can help to prevent constipation, which has been associated by some nutritionists with bad breath.
◆ *Cloves, fennel or anise:* Sweetens the breath and helps with digestion. Can be purchased in oil or tincture form.
◆ *Parsley:* Destroys odor. Chewing on fresh parsley can help eliminate garlic and onion breath.
◆ *Peppermint:* Can be taken in tea form; breath sweetener and digestive aid.
◆ *Myrrh:* Effective mouthwash but tastes unpleasant. Helps heal mouth sores and sore throats.
◆ Homemade gargles can be made with rosemary or peppermint oil. Use two drops to one cup of warm water.

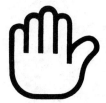

PREVENTION:

◆ Get regular dental checkups so as to avoid gum disease and tooth decay.
◆ Carry a toothbrush with you and brush after each meal.
◆ Drink water after you are done eating to remove food particles, and rinse your mouth out if you can.
◆ Keep your elimination regular by eating a high-fiber diet.
◆ Don't smoke or chew tobacco.
◆ Eat fresh parsley sprigs after a spicy meal.
◆ Eat plenty of fresh, crunchy vegetables to clean the teeth and stimulate the gums.

Bedwetting (enuresis)

Persistent bedwetting can be most frustrating for parents and extremely humiliating for the child involved. There are several myths that surround bedwetting, and getting your facts straight can be extremely important in handling a chronic bedwetter. Keep in mind that the problem is temporary and is experienced in numerous households. It usually has nothing to do with parenting skills and with some children, seems to be an inevitable part of growing up.

It is common for a child to wet the bed until four or five years old. The problem is so prevalent that it is not considered a disorder by some doctors unless it persists into puberty and beyond. However, repeated bedwetting after the age of five usually needs some kind of intervention. Bedwetting is a problem in a small percentage of adults.

It is important to realize that if a variety of treatments are tried and fail, most children outgrow the problem naturally, and they should be made aware of this fact. Bedwetting is considered an involuntary disorder, and runs in families. If one or both parents were bedwetters, the chances are good that their offspring will be also. Approximately one in every seven children experiences bedwetting. Boys are slightly more prone to bedwetting than girls.

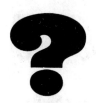

CAUSES:

It is difficult to determine whether bedwetting is a physical or psychological problem. Some recent studies have suggested that most bedwetting has some kind of psychological cause; however, this theory is firmly rejected by several professionals who believe that nothing more than a small bladder is responsible in the majority of cases. Bedwetting can also be the result of an immature nervous system, which controls bladder function, and is not usually connected to any other physical or emotional condition.

Very heavy sleepers appear prone to bedwetting, although some studies dispute this connection. Emotional upsets and extreme fatigue have also been linked to the disorder. Heredity, weak or small bladders, nutritional deficiencies and urinary tract infections have a relationship to bedwetting.

Allergies, especially food allergies, can cause a child to sleep less and affect deep sleep cycles, when bedwetting usually occurs. In a small number of cases, involuntary urination is present during the day and is usually linked to the presence of a physical abnormality or illness such as diabetes mellitus or spina bifida.

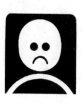

SYMPTOMS:

Physical: Bedwetting can occur once, or several times during the night. Once the habit of bedwetting is repeated it usually becomes consistent, although a dry night here and there is common. Sometimes a pattern can be detected as-far as how long a child will usually sleep before wetting. Bedwetting can begin shortly after potty training or occur several months later.

Psychological: Bedwetting may cause severe emotional stress, especially in an older child who may think of it as a sign that he is still a baby. Bedwetters over the age of three may feel shame, fear of sleeping in beds other than their own, and may experience a high degree of guilt. The way a parent reacts to chronic bedwetting is crucial in determining the child's perception of himself and the problem.

Bedwetting should be carefully explained to the child. There should be no scolding or reprimanding of any kind. Some psychotherapists have suggested that bedwetting is the result of repressed hostility or sexuality; however, the general consensus is that this does not appear to be the case in the majority of bedwetting situations.

The arrival of a new baby or some other threatening situation may also cause bedwetting. The most important thing to remember as the parent of a child who experiences this problem is to avoid any kind of negative response. Humiliating or punishing the child can actually aggravate the problem by causing more stress and by damaging the child's self-esteem.

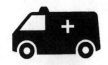

MEDICAL ALERT:

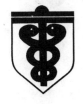

Always check with your physician to eliminate the possibility of a urinary disorder or a serious psychological problem.

STANDARD MEDICAL TREATMENT:

A physician will want to determine whether there is a specific physical cause for the problem. In older children, a cystometry, which requires catheterization, may be ordered to assess bladder function. If bedwetting persists, imipramine (Tofranil, janimine) may be prescribed. It helps to contract the sphincter muscle of the urethra. Imipramine is also an antidepressant, and should only be used if you and your doctor feel it is necessary. The benefits of this treatment are of questionable value. In cases where it has been used, it has rarely provided permanent relief. Your doctor may also recommend a bedwetting alarm system which can be effective, but usually takes several months of use.

SIDE-EFFECTS: *Imipramine:* (Tofranil, Tofranil PM, Janimine): Changes in blood pressure, abnormal heart rates, heart attack, confusion, anxiety, and restlessness are only a few of the side-effects listed.

Warning: Do not use Imipramine if there is a history of convulsive disorders in your family.

Success rating of standard medical treatment: fair. Using prescription medicines on a child with a bedwetting problem that is not physically caused is not advised unless the circumstances are extreme. Home self-care measures are usually as effective. In a large number of cases, patience is the key and the practice will usually cease after the age of five or six.

HOME SELF-CARE:

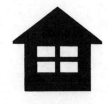

◆ Learning about chronic bedwetting for a parent is invaluable. Knowledge can help alleviate potentially embarrassing situations for the child. There are several good books available at local libraries on the subject.

◆ Use a felt-covered rubber pad under the sheeting.

◆ If the child is old enough, encourage him to change into clean clothes himself, if you have to do for him, do it quietly without comment.

◆ Give the child as much privacy and respect as possible, without referring to the problem as something to be ashamed of.

◆ Bedwetting alarms can be effective and function by sounding off when the child is wet. A moisture sensor is placed on the child's underclothing. The goal is to condition the child to awake when the bladder becomes distended. The method is slow and requires a great deal of patience. Allow at least two to four months for this type of approach. This is a negative feedback approach and does condition the child to associate urination with an unpleasant sensation. If your child is a heavy sleeper (and many bedwetters are), the alarm may wake up everyone but the child, therefore defeating its purpose.

◆ Some success has been found with setting an alarm at two different times during the night and waking the child to go to the bathroom. This takes a great deal of patience and can be stressful for all involved.

◆ Encourage the child not to drink any fluids after dinner, or for at least two hours before bedtime. (Some experts dispute the benefit of this practice and claim that the amount of liquid consumed has no bearing on the problem.) Common sense dictates that drinking less prior to bedtime could only help.

◆ A lack of sleep can actually worsen bedwetting. Consequently, children should retire early rather than be kept up late.

◆ Encourage the child to drink during the day and hold off urination as long as possible so as to condition the bladder.

◆ Reward your child by keeping a chart or book and letting him place a sticker or star for each morning he has risen without bedwetting. A reward system has proven beneficial in a large number of bedwetters.

NUTRITIONAL APPROACHES:

◆ If food allergies are present, avoid cow's milk, chocolate, and soda pop.

◆ Protein supplements: contribute to strengthening of bladder muscles. These are available at health food shops and can significantly improve physiological performance if the child is a poor eater lacks nutrients.

◆ *Potassium*: Helps to balance sodium and potassium in the system which affects kidney function.

◆ *Silicon, manganese and zinc:* Help to strengthen the bladder.

◆ *Vitamin A*: Also helps in facilitating bladder muscle function.

◆ *Cherry juice*: Can help to fight urinary tract infections and help in controlling urination.

Herbal remedies:

◆ Most herbs are bitter and children do not respond favorably to them. Try making herb tea solutions of any of the following herbs and mixing them in fruit juices. Making frozen fruit bars with herbal teas and fruit juices is also recommended. Most herbal preparations come in capsules, and many children can be taught to swallow them.
◆ *Buchu:* Helps to heal and strengthen the bladder.
◆ *Sweet sumach:* A traditional herbal treatment for bedwetting, considered a tonic for the urinary system.
◆ *Uva ursi:* Helps in keeping the urinary tract clear
◆ *Cornsilk:* Used to treat renal and cystic inflammations.
◆ *Parsley:* High in potassium; can also help improve bladder muscle tone.
◆ *The following herbs taken in combination may be useful:* Juniper berries, golden seal, marshmallow, watermelon seed, uva ursi, pan pien lien, ginger.

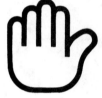

Prevention:

◆ There is no real way to prevent bedwetting. Many of the suggesstions made in the home self-care section could also be used as preventative measures, although with some children, bedwetting is inevitable.

Bladder Infections (cystitis)

Definition:

Unfortunately, most women will have one or more occasions to see their doctor for a bladder infection. The very nature of the female reproductive system and urinary tract puts women at risk for this particular type of infection. As a result, cystitis is one of the most common infections that physicians treat.

Medicaly speaking, a bladder infection is an inflammation of the urinary bladder. It can occur at any age and in either sex, although women are much more prone to them. Bladder infections are more common in women than in men because the female urethra, which leads from the bladder to the outside of the body is shorter; consequently, it is easier for bacteria to invade the female bladder. Approximately 50 percent of all women will experience a bladder infection at some time in their life and 20 percent will be reoccurring. Men over 50 with enlarged prostate glands are also susceptible to bladder infections.

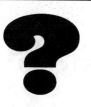

CAUSES:

Bladder infections are usually caused by a bacterial infection; however, in rare cases, a viral or fungal source is possible. Escherichia coli, a rod-shaped bacterium, is the most common cause and is found in the rectal area. Other bacteria which can travel from the ureters (tubes which come down from the kidneys) may also be responsible for cystitis. The gonococcus bacteria, which causes gonorrhea can also trigger a bladder infection.

"Honeymoon cystitis" refers to bladder infections brought on by frequent sexual intercourse. Childbirth can also increase your chances of getting a bladder infection. Some drugs and chemicals are capable of causing bladder inflammations. Occasionally, a structural abnormality can cause the urine to sit in the bladder too long, which can bring on an infection.

Excessive consumption of caffeine-containing beverages, especially coffee, is also connected to the incidence of bladder infections. In addition, alcohol addiction and cigarette smoking are considered aggravating factors in the disease. Using a diaphragm for contraception can also increase the incidence of bladder infections by interfering with the complete emptying out of the bladder.

The overuse of douches is also thought to increase the risk of infection. Bladder infections, while tiresome and annoying, are not usually considered dangerous. Prompt treatment is recommended to avoid chronic or disabling forms of the disease.

SYMPTOMS:

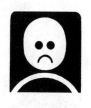

Physical: During a bladder infection, the lining of the bladder becomes inflamed and red. Consequently, pus or bleeding can result, which can become evident in the urine itself, which may appear cloudy or smell unpleasant. A continuous, dull pain, usually located in the lower abdomen, can be present and can intensify when urination occurs. A burning sensation during urination is also common, and the feeling that you need to frequently urinate persists, although the amount may be minimal. Chills, fever, loss of appetite, nausea and vomiting may also be present.

Psychological: In cases of "honeymoon cystitis," mis-understandings may result as to what exactly has caused the symptoms of a bladder infection. Knowing that bladder infections in newlywed women are normal can help dispel fears or remove any guilt experienced by the male involved. Concerning other psychological factors, some experts have linked the incidence of bladder infections to "nerves," or high anxiety states, mental or emotional stress, or fatigue.

MEDICAL ALERT:

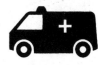

Always consult your doctor if you have any of the above symptoms. Painful urination may indicate the presence of a vaginal infection or other problem, and in

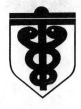

and of itself is not always indicative of a bladder infection.

STANDARD MEDICAL TREATMENT:

A urinalysis (MSU) will be done, along with an examination of the back and the abdomen. If there is a discharge present, a vaginal exam will be done and the discharge will be analyzed. Male urethral discharges will also be examined and a rectal exam will be performed if prostatitis is suspected. In children and men, a special X-ray may be ordered to rule out any physical abnormalities. This X-ray will either be a urogram, where an injection is administered prior to the X-ray, or a micturition cystography, which is only done under certain circumstances.

If a urinary tract infection is present, an antibiotic will be prescribed. Gantrisin, ampicillin, amoxicillin or the combination drugs bactrin or septra are commonly used. Tetracycline is also effective. If the infection is caused by a restricted urethra, surgery may be recommended. In addition, if the infections are especially problematic, some doctors will prescribe an antibiotic to be taken as a preventative measure. The most common of these is nitrofurantoin (macrodantin). This drug is considered perfect for bladder infections because it is excreted so quickly from the body that it does not affect other tissues.

NOTE: The routine use of an antibiotic as a preventive therapy is discouraged unless decided necessary by special circumstance.

Warning: Tetracycline should not be given to pregnant women or young children.

Success rating of standard medical treatment: very good. The cure rate with antibiotic therapy is around 85 percent.

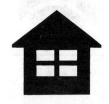

HOME SELF-CARE:

NOTE: A product called Dipstick can be purchased at any pharmacy and can indicate the presence of a bacterial infection, through a color change, when placed in the urine.

◆ Drink plenty of fluids (up to several gallons over the first 24-hour period. The abundant urination that follows such large fluid intake helps to flush the bacteria from the body. Fruit juices make the urine more acidic, which also facilitates relief. Cranberry juice is recommended because it is considered a natural antibiotic.

◆ Do not hold urine for long periods of time. Urinate every two to three hours.

◆ For women, after toilet use, wiping from front to back rather than vice versa can decrease the risk for a bladder infection. Most bacteria that cause these infections come from the rectal area.

◆ Hot sitz bathes can help alleviate the pain caused by cystitis.

◆ For women with recurring bladder infections, cotton underwear is recommended and the use of tampons is discouraged.

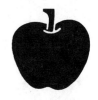

NUTRITIONAL APPROACHES:

◆ *Avoid* dairy products except yogurt, cottage cheese or buttermilk.
◆ *Avoid* alcohol and caffeine, coffee, soda pop, and high sugar foods. Bacteria thrive in high sugar environments.
◆ *Avoid* yeast products.
◆ *Drink large quantities of fluid.* Cranberry juice is considered very beneficial. Pure cranberry juice purchased from a health food store will not be sweetened with corn syrup. Drink at least three glasses per day. Recent evidence supports the presumption that women who routinely drink cranberry juice have fewer bladder infections than those who do not. Cherry juice is also recommended.
◆ *Fresh lemon juice* in water is excellent for its therapeutic value.
◆ *Drinking barely water* made by steeping barley in a small amount of water with lemon and honey can help to soothe the urinary tract.
◆ *Garlic and onions* are considered infection fighters.
◆ *Parsley juice:* Can be used as a natural diuretic.
◆ *Celery and watermelon:* Natural diuretics that also contribute to fluid intake.
◆ *Acidophilus tablets or liquid:* Important to counteract side-effects of antibiotics in replacing friendly bacteria. Balanced intestinal flora can help prevent subsequent infections.
◆ *Liquid chlorophyll:* Helps in purifying the blood and eliminating toxins thrown off by bacteria.
◆ *Vitamin B6, inositol and choline:* Can help to reduce fluid retention.
◆ *Vitamin C plus bioflavonoids:* Helps to make the urine more acidic, which fights the infection.
◆ *Magnesium and potassium:* Can be lost in the urine if diuretics are used.

HERBAL REMEDIES:

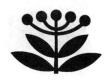

◆ *Uva ursi:* Promotes healing of the bladder, and is considered a bladder antiseptic. Use the tincture form in warm water.
◆ *Cornsilk:* Strengthens and helps in the healing of urinary tract infections.
◆ *Celery:* A urinary antiseptic which removes uric acid from system.
◆ *Hydrangea and flaxseed tea:* These are both natural diuretics.
◆ *Echinacea tincture in water:* Fights infection in the bladder.
◆ *Buchu:* Considered a urinary antiseptic and diuretic; can be used in tea form.
◆ *Dandelion root:* Helps the kidneys excrete waste products.
◆ *Watermelon seed tea:* Good for bladder and kidney ailments.
◆ *Goldenrod tea:* A natural urinary tract antiseptic.
◆ *Golden seal:* Cleans the urinary tract and is considered an herbal antibiotic

which has both antiviral and antibacterial properties.

- *Marshmallow tea:* Helps in strengthening and cleaning the bladder.
- Make a mixture of equal parts of fennel, burdock and slippery elm to make a tea and take before retiring. This combination is thought to help in cleansing the system.
- *The following herbs in combination may be useful:* Golden seal root, uva ursi, capsicum, juniper berries, parsley, queen of the meadow, watermelon, ginger and marshmallow.

PREVENTION:

- Use good hygiene after using the toilet.
- Women should empty the bladder before and after sexual intercourse.
- Always keep your system adequately hydrated by drinking plenty of fluids.
- Women should avoid using tampons, wear loose-fitting cotton underwear and take showers instead of baths.
- Choose another method of contraception other than a diaphragm, which can interfere with the complete emptying of the bladder and facilitate infection.
- Do not use douches or antibacterial soaps, which can change the normal balance of good bacteria, resulting in more susceptibility to infection.
- Avoid feminine hygiene sprays, douches, and bubble baths.
- Use meditative or relaxation exercises to alleviate the effects of stress.

Boils

DEFINITION:

Boils are both painful and unsightly, and can appear rather suddenly. The very nature of a boil demands your attention, and you'll want to treat it as soon as you can.

A boil is an infection usually caused by a bacteria that invades the skin through the hair follicle. A boil is referred to by the medical profession as a furuncle. Boils are tender, pus-filled areas of the skin and are usually round in shape. They may reoccur and persist for years and will often run in families. They may erupt in any part of the body, appearing as a single infection or in multiple groups. The staphylococcus aureus bacteria can usually be cultured from a boil or abscess. Boils are painful and unattractive and can leave scars. Unfortunately, they are also extremely common.

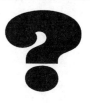

CAUSES:

Boils are usually caused by the bacterium staphylococcus aureus (staph) which invades a hair follicle or break in the skin. As a result, pus forms to fight the bacteria and inflammation occurs in the form of a tender, raised, red area. Boils should not be confused with acne. Other possible causes of boils include diabetes mellitus, which reduces resistance to bacterial infection, and poor hygiene. Boils can also be a sign of a weakened immune system.

SYMPTOMS:

Physical: Boils commonly cause itching, pain, redness, throbbing and swelling. In time, a yellowish tip may appear on the boil and it is common for swollen lymph glands to accompany boils. Boils usually heal within two to three weeks, by either coming to a head and bursting or by dispersing internally. They usually appear on the buttocks, scalp, face and in the armpits.

MEDICAL ALERT:

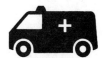

If a fever accompanies a boil, the boil appears on the face, has red streaks, or is fluid filled, see your doctor as soon as possible.

STANDARD MEDICAL TREATMENT:

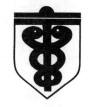

Treating a boil usually involves making a small incision in the center of the boil (lancing) to allow the pus to drain off. In addition, an antibiotic may be prescribed to fight the infection.

Success rating of standard medical treatment: fair. Like many stubborn types of recurring infections, boils can be difficult to cure. Often antibiotic therapy is temporary and can increase susceptibility to subsequent exposure to infections.

HOME SELF-CARE:

◆ *Warning:* It can be dangerous to squeeze a boil, especially around the lips and nose region, as the bacteria can invade the bloodstream and cause blood poisoning. Lancing the head of a small boil with a sterilized needle after a boil has come to a pronounced head is considered acceptable by most doctors, as long a there is no sign of spreading infection. Sterilize the head of a needle with a flame, and make a small nick in the head and gently encourage the pus to flow out. An antiseptic ointment such as neosporin can be used afterwards.
◆ Use warm compresses on the boil until it comes to a head and breaks on its own. Old traditional compresses include making a poultice of warm milk and bread or

using a clay pack. Denver mud is recommended for its drying properties and is believed to bring the boil to a head faster.

◆ Take showers instead of baths to reduce the chance of the infection spreading to another part of the body.

◆ After touching a boil, wash your hands thoroughly to prevent staph contamination of food, etc.

◆ Soaking the boil in an epsom salt solution is also beneficial in bringing the abscesses to a head.

NUTRITIONAL APPROACHES:

◆ Recurring boils can indicate that the immune system is weak. Various factors such as poor diet and food allergies may contribute to depressed immunity. Zinc and vitamin A are of particular importance in the treatment of boils.

◆ Avoid a diet high in sugars and fat, which can increase susceptibility to infection.

◆ Eat plenty of raw fruits and vegetables

◆ A juice fast may help to reduce toxins in the system.

◆ An onion poultice placed between two pieces of cloth and applied directly to the boil may help in expediting healing.

◆ Fresh hot figs applied directly to the boil also helps bring it to a head.

◆ *Chlorophyll:* Helps rid the bloodstream of toxins and should be supplemented in the diet daily.

◆ *Vitamin A and E:* Helps in strengthening the immune system. Vitamin E applied externally may also help to minimize scarring.

◆ *Vitamin C:* Fights infection and inflammation and helps with tissue regeneration.

◆ With any type of infection, it is recommended that the bowels move at least once a day. If constipation is a problem, a tea made from cascara sagrada works well as a mild laxative.

HERBAL REMEDIES:

◆ *Aloe vera gel:* Heals scar tissue when applied externally. It can also be taken in capsule form.

◆ *Garlic (capsules):* Natural antibiotic which boosts immune system; can also be applied externally in oil form. If skin is broken, irritation and pain can result.

◆ *Lian qiao:* An anti-inflammatory and antibacterial herb.

◆ Folk healers have long used herbal poultices in the treatment of boils, choosing burdock root, castor oil, chervil and licorice as being particularly well-suited for the task.

◆ Honey mixed with comfrey powder applied directly to a boil helps to bring it to a head.

◆ *Burdock leaf poultice:* Acts as a natural antibiotic and blood purifier.

◆ *Figwort:* Helps cleanse toxins and functions as an antiinflammatory and anti-bacterial agent.

◆ *Denver mudpack:* Brings the boil to a head. (Can be purchased in some pharmacies.)

◆ A bag of black tea used as a compress is an old folk remedy for boils.

◆ Steep one tablespoon of golden seal and one-half teaspoon of myrrh in pint of boiling water and use to wash the infected area.

◆ *Charcoal and water poultice:* Can help draw the boil to a head.

◆ *Slippery elm, black walnut and fenugreek poultice:* Mix herbal powders with aloe vera juice and apply to boils.

◆ *Dandelion:* Help clear toxins from the blood.

◆ *Echinacea:* Promotes healing and detoxifies the blood.

◆ *Golden seal:* An herbal antibiotic that helps in cleansing the lymph glands. Can be taken in capsule form or made into a paste and applied externally.

◆ *Pau d'arco:* Helps rid the body of toxins and infection.

◆ *The following herbs taken in combination may be useful:* Echinacea, myrrh gum and capsicum.

PREVENTION:

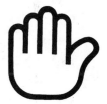

◆ Antiseptic soaps such as betadine are recommended to keep the population of staph down; however, there is some speculation that these chemicals may upset the natural balance of skin chemistry and increase susceptibility to infection.

◆ Keep the immune system healthy by avoiding prolonged use of antibiotics. If they are necessary, use acidophilus to replace friendly bacteria.

◆ Take essential fatty acids found in salmon and evening primrose oil to protect the immune system.

Bronchitis

DEFINITION:

An annoying tickly throat and stubborn hacking cough accurately describe bronchitis. Technically, bronchitis is an inflammation of the mucous membranes that line the bronchi, which make up the primary airways of the lungs. Bronchitis will usually clear up within a few days if the heart and lungs are healthy. This disorder commonly occurs during winter months and can appear more serious than it really is. Chronic bronchitis is a different, more serious disorder, usually resulting from prolonged smoking. Continual attacks of chronic bronchitis will cause the lungs to deteriorate.

CAUSES:

Bronchitis can develop as a secondary infection after any respiratory disorder such as a cold, flu, or even a sore throat. It is caused by a viral infection and does not respond to antibiotics. Some forms of bronchitis can also be caused by inhaling dust, pollution or chemical fumes. Allergies and asthma can predispose one to bronchitis. While the lungs are particularly resistant to bacterial invaders, they seem more susceptible to viral infections, which cause bronchitis.

SYMPTOMS:

Physical: A very deep cough that produces grayish or yellow phlegm or sputum is the most common symptom of bronchitis. The cough may initially be dry. Frequently, a sensation persists that phlegm needs to be coughed up when, in fact, there is nothing there. Other indicators of the disease are breathlessness, tightness in the chest, fever, chills, fatigue, wheezing, and pain in the upper chest which usually worsens upon coughing or deep breathing. While any cough that persists should be reported to your doctor, it is not unusual for coughing from bronchitis to drag out over several weeks.

MEDICAL ALERT:

Contact a physician immediately if you are breathless, cough up blood, have a temperature above 101 degrees or do not improve within 48 hours.

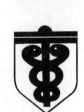

STANDARD MEDICAL TREATMENT:

Because bronchitis is usually caused by a virus, specific treatment is not possible. Treating the symptoms of the disease will be the primary concern of your doctor. He may prescribe a bronchodilator inhaler, and cough suppressants are also commonly recommended. Cough preparations containing codeine or hydrocodone are routinely used. If the cough produces yellow or greenish mucus, a secondary infection is usually present. In these cases an antibiotic will be prescribed.

Success rating of standard medical treatment: very poor. Bronchitis is usually virally caused. Unfortunately, antibiotics are routinely prescribed to treat the disorder, which have no effect on viruses.

NOTE: A new type of bronchitis is thought to exist which seems to target more women than men. It is especially stubborn and if it becomes bacterial, it can be treated with an antibiotic called Doryx.

HOME SELF CARE:

◆ Do not smoke or be around anyone that does. Tobacco smoke can irritate the bronchiole tubes.
◆ Over-the-counter cough medicines may be recommended by a physician. Those containing dextromethorphan are preferable if the cough is dry and unproductive. Frequently, if a cough is suppressed, bringing up mucus is also inhibited. Cough medicines should be used sparingly.
◆ Cough drops can help alleviate the tickly feeling that prompts coughing. Some wonderful herbal lozenges are available in health food shops.
◆ Stay home in a warm environment and get plenty of rest.
◆ A vaporizer or humidifier is recommended. Cool mist is preferable to hot. Staying in a closed shower stall with hot water running can substitute for a vaporizer if one is not available. A tent can be fashioned over a simmering pot of water and steam can be inhaled for at least 3 to 5 minutes.
◆ Use a heating pad or hot water bottle applied to the chest for 30 minutes.
◆ Drink plenty of fluids to help facilitate the removal of excess mucus and hydrate the system.
◆ Avoid caffeine due to its diuretic properties. Gaining fluid, rather than losing it, is desirable.
◆ Avoid alcoholic beverages, which can cause dehydration
◆ Eat hot, spicy foods such as red peppers. They not only cause the nose to run, but also the entire respiratory system secretes more fluid, which is beneficial in thinning out mucous.
◆ Hang the upper half of your body over the bed, placing your hands on the floor. Stay this way for 10 minutes. This position encourages expectoration and initiates more mucus drainage.

NUTRITIONAL APPROACHES:

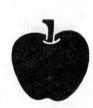

◆ Citrus juices are recommended, along with a diet high in raw fruits and vegetables.
◆ Barley water in combination with lemon juice can help relive bronchiole spasms.
◆ Hot lemon juice with ginger helps to relieve throat tickling which can provoke coughing and also works to expedite the movement of mucus.
◆ *Vitamin A or beta carotene*: Helps to protect lung tissue.
◆ *Vitamin C with bioflavonoids*: The earlier used the better. Vitamin C is considered an antiviral compound which has wonderful anti-inflammatory properties.
◆ *Vitamin E*: Needed to heal tissues and improve efficiency of breathing.
◆ *Cysteine*: An amino acid which can help build resistance to chronic bronchitis and other respiratory diseases.

HERBAL REMEDIES:

◆ Traditional botanical medicine has used herbs as expectorants for centuries. Most of these herbs also help to fight infection.
◆ *Garlic:* A powerful infection fighter that can be taken in capsule form.
◆ *Lobelia:* Helps to break of mucous congestion by relaxing the bronchi.
◆ *Mullein:* Helps to heal the lungs.
◆ *Elecampane:* A lung tonic and natural expectorant.
◆ *White horehound:* Can help relax the bronchiole tubes and ease congestion. *Note:* horehound candy is an excellent lozenge.
◆ *Cowslip:* Loosens phlegm and alleviates dry, hacking coughs.
◆ *Fenugreek:* Helps strengthen lungs and facilitates the movement of mucous.
◆ *Irish moss:* Helps lessen mucous congestion.
◆ Inhaling vapors made from eucalyptus leaves helps to relieve congestion; however, oil-based solutions should be avoided as they may cause irritation.
◆ Mustard poultices have been used for generations as a treatment for lung disorders. Mix one part dry mustard with three parts flour and add water to make a paste. Spread the paste on a cotton pillowcase or cheesecloth, fold it and place on the chest for up to 20 minutes. Check to make sure the skin is not becoming overly irritated.
◆ *The following herbs used in combination may be useful:* Garlic, fennel, comfrey, lobelia and mullein.

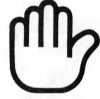

PREVENTION:

◆ Preventing bronchitis involves keeping the immune system strong by eating a nutritious diet and avoiding habits which contribute to lung disease, such a smoking.
◆ Do not smoke: Smoking irritates the bronchiole tubes and causes vessels to constrict.
◆ Eat a diet that is high in raw foods, which are natural sources of vitamins and minerals.
◆ Keep your lung capacity high by exercising every day.
◆ Treat a common cold or sore throat with care so that it does not progress into bronchitis.
◆ Take a vitamin C supplement daily and increase the dosage during a cold or sore throat. Taking garlic supplements has also been recommended if you have a tendency to contract respiratory ailments, especially during the winter months.

Bulimia

DEFINITION:

Sadly enough, eating disorders have become a way of life for a large number of young women in our country. Society's growing obsession with weight, combined with the lack of self-esteem we see so often in our young people, has set the stage for an epidemic of eating disorders.

Bulimia is one of these disorders and unfortunately, is growing in its number of victims. Bulimia literally means "an oxlike appetite," and is characterized by abnormally intense hunger, which can take the form of several eating binges over the course of a day, followed by induced vomiting or purging. Episodes of vomiting in bulimia can occur as rarely as once a month to several times a day, and are often hard to predict. Bulimics may also use large amounts of laxatives or diuretics to expel food as quickly as possible.

As previously mentioned, bulimia is on the increase and usually affects the adolescent or college-aged woman. Most victims of this disorder are between the ages of 15 and 30. It has been estimated that up to 20 percent of college coeds suffer from bulimia to some extent. The disorder has become so common among young women, it is considered normal behavior in some circles. Bulimia commonly affects young women who are well-educated and come from high-income families.

CAUSES:

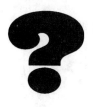

Bulimia is sometimes considered a form of anorexia nervosa, a psychiatric disorder. Both conditions are motivated by a morbid and profound fear of becoming fat. Some anorexics may eventually become bulimic. Dysfunctional family situations involving abuse, neglect, addictive behaviors, or unreasonable demands may predispose one to an eating disorder like bulimia. Some bulimics eat to relieve their feelings of depression and then induce vomiting to reduce their feelings of guilt.

SYMPTOMS:

Physical: Bulimics may have eroded tooth enamel from acid exposure due to repeated vomiting. As a result, the teeth may appear brownish in color. Swelling in the neck region, sore throats, weakness, cramps, dizziness, electrolyte imbalance, lack of menstrual periods, low pulse rate and blood pressure, underweight or overweight condition, and over-exercising are also common symptoms of bulimia.

Symptoms of bulimia are often found in conjunction with those of anorexia. Bulimics typically become very secretive and are usually very good at concealing their behavior.

In addition to the above physical symptoms, other indications of the behavior may include the following: leaving the house directly after a meal to enable vomiting; avoiding social situations where food is served; making excuses for not eating such as "I already ate" or "I'm not hungry"; the disappearance of large amounts of food; and a withdrawal from the social mainstream.

Psychological: Bulimia is a disorder surrounded by feelings of shame and guilt. Consequently, the bulimic may become withdrawn and isolated in order to ensure the privacy needed to binge and purge. Lying about activities, weight, etc. is also common. Bulimics are usually highly distressed about their compulsive behavior and may become depressed, withdrawn, or even suicidal. In addition, bulimics may suffer from low self-esteem, emotional stress, frustration, or obsessive perfectionism.

The ability to control weight, as in the case of the anorexic, may be a sign of a deep-seated need for approval or control. In some cases, just the sight of food for a bulimic can cause symptoms of physical stress such as a racing heart or sweaty palms. Other indications of bulimia or a prebulimic condition can be eating very fast, eating until the sensation of fullness is very uncomfortable, eating large amounts of food when hunger is really not present, eating alone, and feeling disgust or guilt while eating.

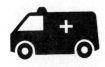

MEDICAL ALERT:

Bulimia can become life-threatening if electrolyte balance is sufficiently impaired. Left untreated, bulimia can cause serious metabolic problems. If you have induced vomiting in yourself, see a doctor immediately.

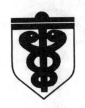

STANDARD MEDICAL TREATMENT:

Individual psychotherapy combined with family counseling can successfully treat bulimia. This therapy is usually designed to improve emotional maturity. Supervision and regulation of eating habits are also routinely recommended. Self-help groups and medical supervision are also commonly employed to treat the disorder. Antidepressant drugs such as Prozac are sometimes recommended. In severe cases, hospitalization is necessary and supervised treatment is administered over several weeks.

Success rating of standard medical treatment: good. Unfortunately, even after exhaustive psychiatric treatments, bulimics, like anorexics, may never return to normal eating patterns. In many victims, the risk of a relapse can exist weeks or even months after treatment is complete.

HOME SELF-CARE:

In the case of bulimia and anorexia, the caregiver may have to be the one to take the initiative in controlling the behavior. Ongoing professional counseling is required for both the victim and the caregiver or parent. It is vitally important that the bulimic feels total support from family and friends and that affection, encouragement and understanding are readily available. The power of love cannot be overstated. The continual outpouring of supportive statements, expressions of love and affection, and frequent hugging can help to motivate change in a bulimic who may feel unloved or unattractive. Often bulimics are withdrawn and can become aloof, making this type of relationship more difficult to promote. Don't give up even if your attempts to show love and affection are rejected.

Often bulimics are encouraged to record their feelings of anger or depression. The activity helps to release negative emotions that sometimes precipitate binge eating.

The bulimic should educate herself with the smartest ways to stay slim without compromising her health. This alternative is preferable to harmful habits which will eventually only serve to make her even more unattractive in the end.

Use hotline numbers when tempted to binge or purge (see numbers below). If you are involved with a self-help group, form your own hotline and call someone when you're tempted.

If you crave a particular food, wait at least 20 minutes before eating it. Often if the craving does not result from real hunger, it will pass.

Take a walk or arrange for another activity that is incompatible with eating

NUTRITIONAL APPROACH:

◆ Keep foods readily available that are visually appealing and healthy. Cut up fresh fruits and vegetables, almonds, dried fruits, active culture yogurt, etc.
◆ Keep healthy, low-fat foods around and if you crave a certain food, eat a very small amount rather than deny yourself totally, which may precipitate binging later.
◆ Eat three square meals per day. Skipping meals can promote binge eating.
◆ Avoid eating high-salt, high-sugar or high-fat foods as they can induce further food cravings.
◆ Take a strong multivitamin and mineral supplement: Because extreme vitamin and mineral depletion is common with bulimics, a strong vitamin and mineral supplement is recommended. Check with your physician on the amount and type needed. Liquid mineral formulas are quickly assimilated.
◆ *Protein supplements:* Liquid drinks are available and can be used as sources of calories and protein. Those free of amino acids are recommended.
◆ *Acidophilus:* Helps to stabilize intestinal bacteria and can be taken as a liquid or in capsules
◆ *B12 injections:* May be required to help promote cellular function and treat depression. The B vitamins are vital to a healthy mental outlook and if they are lacking in a bulimic, further mental deterioration can occur.
◆ *Brewer's yeast:* A good source of B vitamins. Do not take if allergic to yeasts.
◆ *Vitamin C:* Invaluable in its role in glandular and cellular repair and function.

- ◆ *Zinc:* Essential for the metabolism of protein and is quickly lost during periods of starvation
- ◆ *Potassium:* Needs to be replaced. Can be significantly lost if vomiting is a chronic behavior.
- ◆ *Iron:* Bulimics may become anemic and may need to build up their hemoglobin count.
- ◆ Germanium: Helps to supply oxygen to the cells.

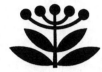

HERBAL REMEDIES:

- ◆ *Alfalfa:* This herb is considered a rich mineral source and blood purifier.
- ◆ *Black walnut:* Helps to balance minerals and hormones in the body.
- ◆ *Evening primrose oil:* Supplies vitamin A.
- ◆ *Catnip:* Considered a relaxant that can work to calm nerves and control feelings of stress and tension.
- ◆ *Hops:* Has a tranquilizing effect on the nervous system.
- ◆ *Chamomile:* Rich in calcium and can help calm the nerves. A cup of chamomile tea taken right before bed can help to induce relaxation and sleep.
- ◆ *Echinacea and ginger:* Both of these herbs calm the stomach and can quiet the stomach spasms that accompany vomiting.
- ◆ *Ginseng:* Strengthens the body and improves immunity.
- ◆ *Kelp:* A good source of essential minerals.

For more information on eating disorders contact:

American Anorexia/Bulimia Association
133 Cedar Lane
Teaneck, NJ 07666
201-836-1800

and

P.O. Box 7
Highland Park, IL 60035
312-831-3438

Center for the Study of Anorexia/Bulimia
1 West 91st Street
New York, NY 10024
212-595-3449

Burns

DEFINITION:

Every year in the United States, 2 million people are burned badly enough to require medical attention. Burns are categorized according to their severity. A first degree burn is superficial, and is characterized by redness. Most sunburns fit this type of burn category. A second-degree burn is deeper and results in blistering and splitting of skin layers. Scalding and severe sunburn usually belong to this type. Third-degree burns, in which the skin and underlying tissue and muscle are damaged, are usually painless because nerve endings have been destroyed, and the skin may be charred.

Burns are more common in children and the elderly, and are usually the result of home accidents which can be prevented.

CAUSES:

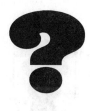

Burns can result from contact with hot water, radiation, sunlight, chemicals, electricity, fire or another heat source. They are often the result of carelessness in leaving children unattended in bath tubs, by fireplaces, stoves, campfires or with matches. Cigarettes can also cause fires when disposed of in trash receptacles or if left to burn after inadvertently falling asleep. Unprotected exposure to the sun can cause up to a second-degree burn.

SYMPTOMS:

Physical: First-degree burns cause a great deal of pain and result in skin redness but nothing more. They usually do not require medical treatment and will heal on their own. In the case of a sunburn, pain, restlessness, fever and headache can occur.

Second-degree burns are deeper and form blisters. Not all of the dermis is damaged; therefore, healing usually results without scarring unless the burn is extensive.

In third-degree burns, pain is usually absent. In addition, skin tissue and even muscle can be destroyed, with bones being visible in some cases. The area will look white or charred red. Loss of body fluids, pulmonary complications and infection are the primary dangers of third-degree burns. Scarring is common and skin grafting may be necessary.

In second or third-degree burns that affect more than 10 percent of the body, shock may occur. Shock is characterized by low blood pressure and rapid pulse caused by the loss of fluids and electrolytes from the burned area. Intravenous fluid must be administered in these cases.

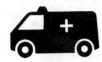

MEDICAL ALERT:

Any burn that is extensive or involves the face, hands, feet, eyes or pelvic area requires immediate medical attention. Third-degree burns must be treated by a physician immediately. Any burn that shows evidence of infection or doesn't heal within two weeks should be looked at by a physician.

FIRST AID:

◆ Apply cold water, not ice water, to the skin for at least five minutes.
◆ If the burn is chemical in nature, continue flushing the area with water.
◆ A cold water compress can also be used. Remove any watches, jewelry, rings, and constricting clothing from the area before swelling occurs.
◆ Dress the area with a clean non-fluffy material
◆ In the case of severe burns: Do not remove clothing that is stuck to the wound. Cover any exposed areas with a clean, dry, non-fluffy cloth and secure it until professional treatment is available.

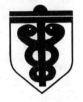

STANDARD MEDICAL TREATMENT:

A physician will determine the severity of the burn. Subsequent treatments include antibiotic therapy, skin grafting, antibacterial ointments, dressing, and hospitalization if burn is extensive enough for the administration of IV fluids to prevent dehydration and shock, and to guard against infection.

Success rate of standard medical treatment: good. Burn units for serious burns have the latest state-of-the-art equipment for treating burn victims. Good plastic surgeons can greatly repair severe burn damage through skin grafts.

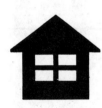

HOME SELF-CARE:

◆ Apply cold water, not ice water, to the burn site. Continue this treatment for at least five minutes.
◆ Using aloe vera gel after cold water treatment has been administered and the burn has started to heal is considered beneficial by some experts. Keeping a live plant nearby provides fresh juice which can be continually applied for days after the burn has occurred.
◆ Over-the-counter analgesics, including aspirin or acetaminophen, may help with pain.
◆ Do not break open blisters that appear with a second degree burn.
◆ Elevate the burned area to help prevent swelling and pain.
◆ Anesthetic creams or sprays are not recommended for burns, as they inhibit healing.

- The use of butter, Vaseline or other cream ointments is generally discouraged.
- In the case of minor burns, creams such as neosporin or bacitracin are not thought to be very helpful.
- Avoid cortisone-based creams or ointments. These can actually increase the risk of infection.
- For minor burns, a compress made from a milk-soaked cloth can promote healing.
- Keep the burn dry, clean and covered with a thick gauze pad. Change pad frequently.
- The use of Preparation H for first-or second-degree burns is advocated by some for its healing properties. It contains yeast, which apparently speeds up the healing process.

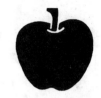

NUTRITIONAL APPROACHES:

- In the case of second-and third-degree burns, the diet should be high in protein for tissue regeneration. In addition, plenty of fluids should be consumed.
- Protein drinks can supplement a diet high in raw vegetables, fruits, cereal and nuts. Citrus fruits, potatoes and broccoli are good sources of vitamin C, which aids the healing process.
- *Potassium:* Potassium can be lost from burns and should be replaced.
- *Zinc:* Promotes tissue healing. Food highs in zinc include wheat germ, crab meat and low-fat dairy products.
- *Calcium and magnesium:* Help to expedite the healing of burns.
- *Selenium:* Helps with tissue elasticity.
- *Vitamin E:* Can be taken internally and used externally to minimize scarring if the burn is first or second-degree in its severity.
- *Vitamin A:* Required for the proper repairing of damaged tissue.
- *Vitamin C:* Helps in the healing process and can reduce inflammation.
- Using raw peeled potatoes on a minor burn is a traditional home remedy that has been used for generations

HERBAL REMEDIES:

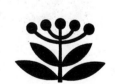

- *Myrrh or golden seal powder:* Can be used to dust a first-or second-degree burn.
- *White oak bark:* Contains tannic acid, which helps promote healing of skin. Can be used as a compress made from tea.
- A *comfrey leaf poultice* or salve for first-or second-degree burns helps to restore damaged tissue.
- *Marshmallow herbal compresses* can be applied to minor burns to promote healing and reduce pain.
- *Echinacea and chaparral:* Take internally for chemical burns helps to reduce the risk of infection.

- *Calendula tincture or cream:* Has antiseptic and antifungal properties.
- *Aloe vera:* Has healing properties and can reduce scarring.
- *Marshmallow:* Good for acid or fire burns. Apply directly to the burn in a wet compress and also take internally in capsule form.
- *Lavender oil:* Can be used directly on minor burns to relieve pain.
- *Yarrow:* An anti-inflammatory that can be used externally as a tincture.
- *St John's Wort oil:* Helps to heal first-or second-degree burns.
- *Tea tree oil:* Used externally for milder burns, this preparation helps to control pain and expedite healing.
- Ointments or lotions made from the following combination of herbs can be used for minor burns: Malva, chickweed, marigold, plantain, comfrey, marshmallow and mullein

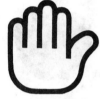

PREVENTION:

- If you have young children in the house, make sure stove controls cannot be reached.
- Turn pot and pan handles away from the edge of the stove so they cannot be grabbed by a child.
- Do not leave plugged-in curling irons, hot curlers, etc. where a child can reach up and grab them.
- Make sure a child is never left alone in the bathtub, where scalding can occur. Always check the temperature of the bath water yourself by immersing your wrist in the water before placing a child in the tub.
- Never leave a child unattended by a campfire or fireplace, and be sure to use fireplace screens to prevent sparks from flying.
- Keep electrical outlets covered and cords tucked away.
- Never leave matches or cigarette lighters within the reach of a child.
- Teach your child to stop, drop and roll if their clothes, hair, etc. is ever caught on fire, and practice this exercise.
- Have regular fire drills in the home and use fire safety guidelines provided by the fire department to design your own emergency fire strategy.
- Have a smoke alarm on each floor of your house.
- If you need to be outdoors for long periods of time, use a sun protectant lotion of at least factor 15. You don't have to feel hot to be getting a severe sunburn. Working near reflective surfaces such as water, bleachers, concrete, etc. can intensify the effects of the sun even on a cloudy day. Protect your skin.

Bursitis

Definition:

You played a round of tennis, and later that evening your elbow is sore and tender, and moving it is difficult and painful. Chances are you have a case of bursitis. Bursitis is an inflammation of the bursa, which is a fluid-filled sac located close to joints, and between tendons and bones. Bursitis usually clears up, then recurs. It commonly affects the hip, lower knee or shoulder. Bursitis can also be referred to as tennis elbow, and interestingly enough, has also gained a reputation for afflicting business professionals who routinely carry briefcases.

While bursitis may be miserable, the condition is not considered serious. There are as many as 78 bursae on each side of the body and when even one of them gets inflamed, the discomfort is substantial. If bursitis is severe and prolonged enough, some scar tissue can form and joint mobility may become impaired.

Causes:

Bursitis can result from friction, pressure or injury to the bursa membrane. Prepatellar bursitis, or "housemaid's knee," is caused by prolonged kneeling on a hard surface. Tibial tubercle bursitis, or "clergyman's knee," can result from long periods of kneeling and olecranon bursitis "student's elbow," results from periods of pressure exerted from a desk or table.

Shoulder bursitis may eventually cause the joint to become immobile. This type of bursitis can be a special problem for baseball pitchers. Bursitis has also been linked to calcium deposits, and some experts have associated the disorder with food or airborne allergies.

Symptoms:

Physical: Swollen, painful, tender joints are common in bursitis. The presence of pain will cause the joint to become immobile. People who suffer from bursitis are commonly seen trying to manually massage the painful area.

Medical alert:

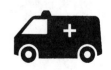

Symptoms of bursitis may be caused by gout or infection. Bursitis that persists should always be examined by a physician.

Standard medical treatment:

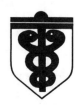

Rest is the primary treatment recommended. Ice packs may also be applied, and if infection is present, antibiotics and drainage of fluid may be necessary. A pressure bandage may also be used to stop fluid from reaccumulating. Anti-inflammatory drugs are also routinely prescribed. Injections of corticosteroids are used for severe cases.

Surgical options: In unusually persistent cases, a bursectomy may be recommended. This operation is minor and involves making a small incision in the skin where the contents of the bursal sac are permanently removed.

Success rating of medical treatment: fair to good. Medical science usually uses anti-inflammatory drugs or steroid injections to treat stubborn bursitis, which do provide some measure of relief. However, it is usually temporary and comes with side-effects.

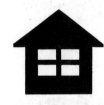

HOME SELF CARE:

◆ Use ice therapy by applying a soft ice bag to the joint and then removing it for five to ten minutes. Do not use heat if the joint feels hot or is swollen. Alternating heat with ice can also be beneficial, and experimenting with hot and cold temperatures is encouraged to see what works best for you. Frozen bags of vegetables work nicely as ice packs.

◆ Use a hot castor oil pack, which can be made by soaking several layers of flannel in castor oil, placing them over the affected area, and then covering these layers with a sheet of plastic on which a hot water bottle or heating pad is placed.

◆ Rest the joint until symptoms improve. Immobilizing it helps promote healing.

◆ Gentle exercise with your doctor's permission may help relieve pain in some cases. Stretching exercises are especially recommended.

◆ Physical therapy involving TENS (transcutaneous electrical nerve stimulation) may help with pain control.

◆ Ultrasound therapy: Helps control the formation of adhesions and scar tissue in joint injuries.

◆ DMSO (dimethyl sulfoxide) solution applied directly to the joint penetrates the skin and can help reduce inflammation. It is usually available in health food stores and should be diluted with water to 70 percent strength. When you dilute this chemical, it will heat up and should be used after it has cooled.

◆ Wrapping the joint with an elastic bandage may help alleviate discomfort.

◆ Time spent in a jacuzzi bath may also help with pain control.

◆ Over-the-counter anti-inflammatory drugs such as aspirin and ibuprofen may be used for pain but do not expedite the healing process.

◆ Alternative treatment considerations: Acupuncture can provide some relief from pain and is considered much safer than anti-inflammatory drugs and steroids.

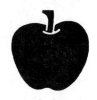

NUTRITIONAL APPROACHES:

◆ Stay away from animal meats, wine, and rich dairy products. Eat a diet high in fiber, whole grains, vegetables and fruits and drink plenty of pure water.
◆ *Calcium and magnesium:* Essential for bone and muscle function and collagen repair
◆ *Proteolytic enzymes:* Considered to be anti-inflammatory and will help reduce swelling and pain.
◆ *Vitamin A:* Promotes tissue repair. Beta carotene is a strong anti-inflammatory.
◆ *Vitamin C with bioflavonoids:* Promotes tissue healing and the regeneration of connective tissue, and counteracts inflammation.
◆ *Vitamin E:* Helps to reduce inflammation.
◆ *Vitamin B12:* Some studies indicate that injections of B12 can help control bursitis pain.
◆ *Germanium:* Reduces pain and inflammation in any inflammatory condition.
◆ *Quercetin:* Inhibits the release of histamine, which creates inflammation in bursitis.
◆ *Zinc:* Important in collagen synthesis.

HERBAL REMEDIES:

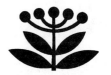

◆ A *chamomile poultice* applied directly to the inflamed area can help reduce pain and swelling in the joints.
◆ *Thyme oil* used as a hot compress or in a hot bath stimulates blood flow to damaged tissue and promotes healing.
◆ *Tumeric:* Has been used for centuries by Indian and Chinese traditional medicine for the treatment of inflammation. Make a paste of tumeric and water and apply to inflamed area.
◆ *Willow:* Contains salicylates for pain and inflammation, and can be taken internally as well as applied externally.
◆ *Bromelain:* An enzyme compound of pineapple which helps reduce swelling and inflammation. Bromelain is invaluable for its marvelous anti-inflammatory properties.
◆ *The following herbs taken in combination may be useful:* Yucca, burdock, redmond clay, pan pien lien and willow.
◆ *An herbal ointment containing the following herbs:* White oak bark, queen of the meadow, scullcap, lobelia and mullein.

PREVENTION:

◆ Staying limber seems to protect the joints from bursitis.
◆ Overuse of certain joints is usually the primary cause of the disorder, so "taking it easy" when playing tennis, pitching, etc. is recommended.

- ◆ Poor technique in playing racquetball, golfing, bowling etc. may also predispose one to bursitis. Professional coaching on proper form etc. may prevent the disorder. Don't use a metal tennis racquet if you have problems with bursitis. Metal tranfers more shock to the joints than wood.
- ◆ After an injury or a sprain, proper first aid is very important in preventing future bursitis. Rest the injured part, apply ice, use an elastic bandage to limit swelling, and elevate the injured area above heart level.

Cancer

DEFINITION:

Cancer has become a byword of the 20th century. Living in fear of contracting cancer is not uncommon due to the vast number of carcinogenic substances modern life exposes us to, not to mention harmful lifestyles which many of us choose to live.

Cancer is a term which refers to over 100 different diseases in which there is an unrestrained growth of cells, either within an organ or in the tissues. Benign tumors, unlike malignant ones, do not spread and infiltrate the surrounding tissue. Cells from a malignant tumor may spread (metastases) through the blood vessels and lymph system to other areas of the body, in which new tumors will begin to grow.

Areas in the body where malignant tumors most commonly develop are lungs, breasts, stomach, colon, skin, pancreas, liver, prostrate, uterus, ovaries, in the bone marrow, the lymphatic system, bones or muscles. Carcinomas are to cancers of the skin, mucous membranes, glands and organs. Leukemias are to blood cancers. Sarcomas refer to cancers of the muscles, connective tissues, and the bones. Lymphomas attack the lymphatic system.

Cancer ranks as the second most common cause of death in the United States, with heart disease as the first. Cancer has been known to exist from prehistoric times and can also affect animals.

CAUSES:

The exact cause of cancer remains a mystery. A breakdown according to percentage of cancers caused by agents is as follows: natural constituents of food 35 percent, tobacco: 30 percent, sexual and reproductive history, 7 percent, occupational hazards, 4 percent, alcohol: 3 percent, food additives: 1 percent, unknown: 20 percent. Other agents that have been linked with uncontrollable cell growth are ionizing radiation, chemicals in the air and diet, vitamin deficiencies, high-fat diets, stress, and environmental conditions.

The growth of cancer begins when oncogenes (genes which control cell growth) are transformed by an agent known as a carcinogen. Once this occurs, the change is transferred to the next generation of cells. Reproduction of these cells is more rapid than in normal cells, and the healthy cells' original function is lost. The clump of cells or tumors contribute nothing to the function of the body; rather, they deplete the body of nutrients.

The rate of growth in a cancerous tumor usually depends on its tissue of origin. Some tumors located in the lungs and the breasts may have been present for years before any symptoms appear. During this interval, cancerous cells may have spread to the liver, bones, brain, and elsewhere. Several types of cancers are considered hereditary.

SYMPTOMS:

Physical: Cancer can be responsible for a whole host of symptoms. Some of the more common ones include:
◆ a sore that does not heal
◆ nagging cough or chronic hoarseness
◆ coughing up bloody sputum
◆ a change in a wart or mole
◆ difficulty swallowing
◆ chronic indigestion
◆ a thickening or lump in the breast or any other area of the body
◆ bleeding or discharge, bleeding between menstrual periods
◆ obvious changes in bowel or bladder habits
◆ blood in the stool
◆ a persistent low-grade fever
◆ headaches accompanied by visual disturbances
◆ unusual fatigue
◆ excessive bruising
◆ repeated nosebleeds
◆ loss of appetite and weight loss
◆ persistent abdominal pain
◆ blood in the urine with no pain during urination
◆ change in size or shape of the testes
◆ continuous unexplained back pain

Psychological: Often, a person who is suffering from cancer will assume the worst. Unfortunately, a great portion of the public is unaware that the outlook for people with cancer has been steadily improving over the last twenty years. Statistics for cancer survival would appear even more encouraging if the incidence of lung cancer due to smoking had not gone up in women. Nearly half of all cancer patients can expect to be free of the disease within five years. Because of the widespread fear of cancer, often people will put off going to a doctor for troubling symptoms, which is the worst possible approach.

For the cancer patient undergoing treatment, support of family, friends and self-help groups is vital. Troubling hair loss can be managed quite well with wigs or attractive kerchiefs. Keeping oneself as attractive as possible is a tremendous plus and some believe may actually enhance getting well. Frequently, physicians employ meditation techniques through self-visualization to speed recovery. Find time to listen to good music, take walks, and keep your spirits up. Share and verbalize your fears and concerns. In regard to breast prosthesis, there are several good cosmetic options for those that have had breast removal, and these should be discussed with a plastic surgeon.

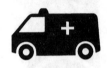

MEDICAL ALERT:

If you have any of the physical symptoms listed above, see your doctor immediately. Often the diagnosis is not cancer; however, if it is, early detection is crucial.

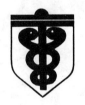

STANDARD MEDICAL TREATMENT:

The treatment of cancer can be divided into three categories: radiation, surgery and chemotherapy. Surgical removal of a malignant tumor and the tissue surrounding it is the most common form of cancer treatment. Estimates of 220,000 or more cases of cancer per year can be cured with surgery alone. A combination of treatments is used to improve the rate of cure. It is common to use radiation therapy prior to surgery to shrink the size of the operable tumor.

Biopsy: Used to diagnose tumor by removing cells surgically or through aspiration for microscopic examination.

Cytology test: Test that shows the shedding of abnormal cells, such as a pap smear. A urine cytology test is usually given to those who work in industries where bladder cancer is a known risk.

Imaging techniques: Low dose X-rays such as those used in a mammogram can detect early breast cancer. Ultrasound scanners can also produce images of organs and may screen for ovarian cancer.

Chemical tests: Blood in the feces or elevated levels of enzyme acid phosphates in the blood are detected through this means.

Direct examination: An endoscope, which is a tube with a lens, can be passed into the area in question and viewed. Cystoscopy, laparoscopy, colonoscopy and gastroscopy are of this type.

SIDE-EFFECTS: *Chemotherapy*: As in the case of radiation therapy, damage to normal tissue while attempting to destroy cancerous tissue is the main side-effect of chemotherapy. Loss of hair can result from chemotherapy as well as from radiation treatment, due to the damage to hair follicles. Hair loss is temporary, and hair sometimes grows back thicker and more healthy looking than before.

New drugs have been developed to help minimize the nausea and vomiting associated with chemotherapy and should be suggested by your doctor. Corticosteroids, tranquilizers, and tetrahydrocannabinol (THC) found in marijuana have been used to control nausea and vomiting. Other side-effects of chemotherapy may include fatigue, weakness, sterility, kidney and heart damage.

Success rate of standard medical treatment: Varies greatly according to the type of cancer.

MEDICAL UPDATE:

◆ The use of interleukin-2, a hormone which stimulates lymphocytes (immune cells) in hopes of destroying the tumors through the immune system is currently being tested.
◆ Interferon, a body chemical, is under study for the treatment of certain types of cancer.
◆ Genetic engineering, which can produce monclonal antibodies to attack certain types of cancer, is also in the research stage.
◆ A new ultrasound technique used after a mammogram can help reduce uncertainty about whether a breast mass is cancerous or not. This technique can reduce the number of biopsies performed. Using high-definition, digital ultrasound imaging.
◆ Biofeedback and self-visualization have also been used with some success as mental tools to help shrink tumors.
◆ Eating a diet high in fruits and vegetables has recently been found to help protect against lung cancer even in those exposed to cigarete smoke.

HOME SELF CARE:

◆ To minimize hair loss while taking radiation or chemotherapy, apply cold packs to the scalp.
◆ Keep yourself busy with things you love to do.
◆ Share your feelings with family, friends and self-help groups.
◆ Keep yourself looking attractive.
◆ Maintain a positive attitude.
◆ Make mild exercise such as walking a part of your daily routine.
◆ Use relaxation and self-hypnosis techniques to ease tension, and practice visualization therapy, which is considered a valid way of facilitating a cure for disease.

NUTRITIONAL APPROACH:

Some studies have suggested that if cells are deprived of oxygen, they may become prone to malignant growth. Consequently, because the blood provides all cells with oxygen, the condition of the bloodstream is important in the treatment and prevention of cancer. Vitamins, minerals and herbs which help in facilitating circulation and detoxification of the blood are thought to be of value.

The National Academy of Sciences has recently validated what several nutritionally oriented practitioners have said for years: that there is a link between diet and cancer. A high-fiber, low-fat diet is now accepted as a valid deterrent to some types of cancer. In addition, animal fats, high-sugar diets, caffeine and alcohol may increase your risk of several forms of cancer.

◆ Avoid the following foods: saturated fats, salt, sugar, alcohol, coffee, caffeine, and animal proteins. Restrict dairy foods.

◆ A macrobiotic diet has been used by some cancer patients, who claim good results. It involves eating brown rice and certain vegetables and should be investigated.

◆ Eat a diet high in fiber, raw fruits and vegetables, raw seeds and nuts, and drink plenty of freshly squeezed juices such as carrot, apple, spinach and kale.

◆ Keep the bowels active by eating soaked figs, prunes or raisins.

◆ *Beta carotene:* A strong antioxidant that can help to destroy free radicals in the body.

◆ *Garlic:* Take in capsule form for enhanced immune function. Also acts a natural antibiotic.

◆ *Germanium:* Helps to enhance cellular oxygenation and stimulates the immune system. Can also help to relieve pain.

◆ *Selenium:* Helps to properly digest proteins.

◆ If taking radiation or chemotherapy use vitamin B6 to minimize damage. Discuss dosage with your doctor.

◆ Take a strong vitamin and mineral supplement with each meal. Use vitamin injections when advised by your doctor. (Taking iron is not advised as some research suggests that excess iron levels may increase the risk of cancer and may also interfere with normal immune system functions.)

◆ *Vitamin A, E:* Important for proper immune function, which can be inhibited if taking radiation or chemotherapy. Both of these vitamins also participate in damaged tissue repair and regeneration.

◆ *Vitamin B complex:* Helps in maintaining normal cell division and cell function.

◆ *Vitamin C with bioflavonoids:* Considered an anticarcinogen by some professionals. Can help to detoxify the system.

◆ *Vitamin D:* Helps the body utilize calcium, vitamin A and essential minerals.

◆ *Calcium and magnesium supplement with silicon and zinc:* Important for the proper function of nerves and muscles.

◆ Chlorophyll obtained through wheatgrass juice is thought to help boost red blood cell development, which serves to oxygenate tissue.
◆ *Acidophilus:* Helps to replenish good bacteria, which is frequently killed with cancer therapies.
◆ *Germanium:* Studies indicate that a lack of germanium may increase the risk of contracting certain forms of cancer.

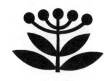

HERBAL REMEDIES:

◆ *Pau d'arco tea:* Helps to protect the liver and is especially recommended if taking chemotherapy or radiation treatments.
◆ *Burdock:* Helps to cleanse the blood and remove toxins, which can result from the cancer and from radiation and chemotherapy.
◆ *Chaparral:* Helps to eliminate toxins, and when used as a paste can help heal sores that may become malignant.
◆ *Dandelion:* Helps to clear the blood of toxins and is an excellent liver stimulant. The liver detoxifies the system of drugs, radiation effects etc., and must be kept as healthy as possible.
◆ *Echinacea:* Another herb that boosts blood purification.
◆ *Suma:* Works to help strengthen the entire system and helps to promote stamina.
◆ *Red clover:* Has been used as an anticancer agent since the 1930s.
◆ *Valerian root:* For external tumors, a valerian tincture may be beneficial.
◆ *The following herbs taken in combination may be useful:* Red clover, sheep sorrel, buckthorn bark, rosemary, barberry and prickly ash bark.

PREVENTION:

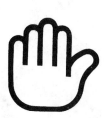

◆ Do not smoke. Smoking during pregnancy can increase the risk of cancer to the offspring. Also avoid breathing secondhand smoke.
◆ Do not drink alcohol heavily. Heavy drinkers are at greater risk for mouth, throat, esophagus, stomach and liver cancer.
◆ Eat a low-fat diet high in fiber and complex carbohydrates. Foods such as cabbage, broccoli, brussels sprouts, and cauliflower are thought by some to protect against cancer. Foods rich in potassium such as beans, sprouts, whole grains, almonds, sunflower seeds, sesame seeds, lentils, parsley, blueberries, coconut, endive, leaf lettuce, oats, potatoes with skin, carrots, and peaches are also suggested in designing an anticancer diet.
◆ Some studies have shown that germanium may be a factor in the prevention of cancer. A germanium supplement is recommended.
◆ Beta carotene has also been recently considered an anti-carcinogen, although research is on-going. Vitamin A may help protect against several chemically induced types of cancer.

◆ *Vitamin C:* May inhibit the formation of carcinogens in the body, therefore lowering the risk of certain kinds of cancer, especially stomach cancer.

◆ In some countries where breast cancer is low, iodine content in soils and foods is particularly high; therefore, an iodine deficiency may be linked to the incidence of breast cancer. Likewise, areas low in selenium have also been linked to a higher rate of cancer.

◆ Avoid eating fried foods, animal proteins, coffee, tea, caffeine, salt-cured or smoked foods, which contain nitrites or nitrates, such as bacon, sausage, lunch meats, hot dogs, and ham. In some cases, intestinal cancer may take as long as twenty years to finally develop. Some professionals recommend avoiding fluoride in the water or toothpaste. Use an air purifier in your home. Do not use artificial sweeteners. Do not eat charred or burned foods. Never eat moldy or rancid foods.

◆ Obesity has been linked to certain types of cancer, such as uterine or breast cancer. Stay at an optimum weight for your height and frame.

◆ Studies have found a higher incidence of prostrate cancer in males who have had a vasectomy.

◆ Avoid unnecessary X-rays.

◆ Avoid exposure to chemicals such as paint, garden pesticides (which are considered high-risk carcinogens), hair sprays, and excess sunlight. Get in the habit of using a strong sunscreen. Avoid exposure to asbestos, vinyl chloride, industrial dyes, and soot.

◆ Have your home checked for radon gas levels.

◆ Take screening tests for early detection of breast, cervical, colon and intestinal cancer.

◆ Exercise regularly. Exercise increases the efficiency of the immune system.

◆ Practice safe sex. Venereal disease has been linked to the development of cervical cancer, not to mention the danger of AIDS, which can itself lead to the contraction of cancer.

◆ Self-testing for colon cancer: Chemically treated strips of paper can be used after a bowel movement to detect the presence of blood. If the strip turns blue, retake the test in three days. If the result is positive, see a doctor immediately. The presence of blood in the feces does not always signal cancer and could be the result of a number of conditions.

◆ Self-testing for cancer of the testicles: Check for a lump after a shower or bath, when detection is easier. With fingers, of both hands, roll the testicles between the thumb and the fingers watching for a hard nodule or lump. If one is present, see your doctor right away.

◆ Self-testing for breast cancer: Stand in front of a mirror and raise your hands high over your head, pressing them together. Observe the shape of the breasts. Next, place your hands on your hips and press, watching for any dimpling of the skin on the breast or nipples that appear out of their normal positioning. Also look for any redness or thickening of the skin or nipples. Now raise one arm over your head, and with the other hand manually feel the breast, beginning at the outer edge, using a circular motion. Gradually move in toward the nipple. Make sure to completely feel the armpit area as well. Lymph nodes are found in this area and will move freely and feel soft. Look for lumps that are hard and not mobile. Repeat this process for the other side. Now lie on your back and perform the same self-exam. Gently squeeze each nipple, checking for a yellow or pink discharge. Doing a breast exam while in the shower and the skin is soapy is also recommended, as lumps are easier to detect on a soapy surface.

◆ If cancer runs in your family, get an annual checkup and watch for any warning signs of the disease.

Canker Sores (aphthous ulcers)

DEFINITION:

Having a bad canker sore can make you feel like you're all lip and that you'll never be quite the same. Canker sores, like the common cold, continue to baffle medical science. They afflict a large number of people, who are usually willing to try just about anything to get rid of them. Unfortunately, the cure for canker sores remains elusive, although shortening the duration of these annoying mouth ulcers is possible.

Canker sores are small lesions that usually occur on the inside of the cheek, tongue, inner lips and gums. There may be one or several sores present in an outbreak. While some doctors propose that they are viral in nature, this has not been conclusively proven.

Canker sores are painful and pesky, and usually heal within a week with or without any specific treatment. Approximately 20 percent of the population suffer from canker sores at any given time. Girls are more prone to them than boys, and they occur most frequently in school-aged children. The incidence of canker sores decreases with age. Why some people get them and some don't remains a medical mystery.

CAUSES:

Canker sores have afflicted mankind from the beginning of recorded history. While the cause of these sores remains unknown, in some people, physical or emotional stress seems to bring them on. In addition, they run in families so heredity may also play a role. For some women, canker sores occur more frequently during menstrual periods. Food allergies to walnuts, citrus fruits, chocolate, and shellfish have also been linked to the outbreak of canker sores.

Mouth injuries such as pricks or punctures, while in and of themselves are not a cause of cankers, can predispose one to their development. In some people, canker sores have been linked with nutritional deficiencies of iron, folic acid, vitamin B12, or just a poor diet in general. Victims of Crohn's disease have a higher incidence of canker sores.

Poor dental hygiene may also predispose one to canker sores. The presence of a fever commonly triggers the formation of canker sores. The ulcers may also be a hypersensitive reaction to the hemolytic streptococcus bacteria. These particular organisms have been isolated from canker sores. The occurrence of canker sores has also been associated with an abnormal immune response to the presence of normal mouth bacteria.

SYMPTOMS:

Physical: Canker sores look like oval white ulcers that are surrounded by an area of redness. They range in size from 1/8 inch to more than 1 inch in diameter. These sores can appear suddenly and disappear just as quickly. Prior to their outbreak, there may be a sensation of tingling or roughness in the mouth. Often canker sores can impede talking or eating. Canker sores may recur two to three times per year, and in some cases may be continuously present to some degree.

Psychological: Some people are prone to develop canker sores after periods of high emotional stress. Certain events such as divorce, death, change of employment etc. may decrease immunity and increase the chances of a canker sore forming.

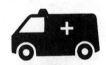

MEDICAL ALERT:

Any lesion or sore that does not heal within two weeks should be examined by a physician. If the sore becomes infected (grayish yellow color with a red ring around the base) see your doctor.

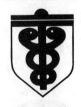

STANDARD MEDICAL TREATMENT:

Doctors don't really know the cause of canker sores; consequently, treatment does not involve curing them. Topical pain killers may be recommended. A waterproof ointment may be prescribed to protect the lesion, such as Zilactin™. If the sores become infected, an antibiotic such as tetracycline may be prescribed. In very severe cases, steroid drugs may be used to reduce inflammation.

Success rating of standard medical treatment: poor. Unfortunately, medical science offers no cure for canker sores. Treatment is purely symptomatic.

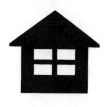

Home self-care:

◆ Drinking fluids from a straw minimize pain, especially for children suffering from canker sores.

◆ Sucking on ice can help decrease pain

◆ Orabase-B and Zilactin, both over-the-counter preparations, can be applied directly to the ulcers to stop pain and promote healing.

◆ Check ingredients of over-the-counter canker sore preparations, and use ones with benzocaine, menthol, eucalyptol, or camphor.

◆ Dab the sores with hydrogen peroxide or make a mouthwash of 1/2 teaspoon of hydrogen peroxide to 8 ounces of water. This can be used several times a day.

◆ Use 1 teaspoon of potassium chlorate in a cup of water as a mouth rinse.

◆ A dab of alum on the sore can help to prevent infection. Alum can be purchased in the spice section of a grocery store.

◆ Rinsing the mouth with an antacid like Milk of Magnesia can coat the ulcers and provide some relief from pain. Do not use this if sores are infected.

◆ Placing a wet tea bag which contains tannin, an astringent and pain-killer, directly on the sore can provide some relief.

◆ A paste of ground aspirin and water can create a covering on the canker sore and promote healing.

Nutritional approach:

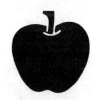

◆ A diet high in salads and raw onions is recommended. Apparently, onions contain sulfur and promote healing.

◆ Eat plenty of active culture yogurt every day. This approach also has some value in preventing the development of future canker sores.

◆ Avoid eating sugar, citrus fruits, coffee, nuts, fish or meat. Animal protein produces acid, which can aggravate the ulcers.

◆ Get vitamin C from foods such as broccoli, cantaloupe, bell peppers, and cranberry juice.

◆ *Raw potatoes:* Contain vitamin P, which helps to heal mouth sores. Place a raw potato directly on the lesion.

◆ *Cabbage juice:* Helps in healing ulcers.

◆ *Acidophilus:* Very important to promote friendly bacteria and is good for maintaining the proper chemical balance of mouth fluids.

◆ *L-lysine:* A deficiency in this amino acid can cause mouth ulcers.

◆ *Vitamin B complex with extra B12:* Good for healing and immune function. A lack of B vitamins has been linked to the outbreak of mouth sores

◆ *Vitamin C:* Can help to heal mouth ulcers and promotes tissue regeneration. Take internally and also make a paste out of vitamin C powder and liquid acidophilus. Taking a daily vitamin C supplement also helps to discourage the formation of new canker sores.

- *Vitamin E oil:* Can be applied directly to the sores to promote healing and relieve pain.
- *Folic acid:* Taken in a lozenge form, promotes healing of damaged mucosal tissue.
- *Pantothenic acid:* Antistress vitamin which may help to control precanker stress.
- *Vitamin A emulsion:* Use directly on the sores. Can help to promote healing of mucous membranes of the mouth.

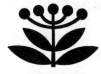

HERBAL REMEDIES:

- Golden seal or bay leaf tea may be used as a mouthwash. Straight golden seal powder from a broken capsule can be applied directly to the sores.
- *Myrrh:* Antimicrobial astringent that promotes lesion healing. Add drops of oil to warm water and use as a mouthwash.
- *Bistort:* An anti-inflammatory especially good for mouth irritations. Can be used in tincture form and added to water for a mouthwash.
- *Purple sage:* Good oral antiseptic and astringent which can be used in mouthwash form.
- Rosemary, thyme or juniper berry oils may be used in warm water as a gargle.
- *Lobelia:* Sores can be painted with a lobelia tincture several times a day to control pain and promote healing.
- *Myrrh gum:* Helps to heal mouth sores.

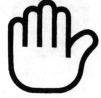

PREVENTION:

- Stay away from anything than can irritate or injure the lining of the mouth such as hard-bristled toothbrushes, sharp foods such as potato chips, nuts, and all salty or very spicy foods.
- In some cases, if the sore is caught early enough, drinking water every 10 minutes for an hour can inhibit further development.
- Body chemistry must remain in an acid/alkaline balance, which is maintained by a healthy diet high in raw foods and low in meat and fat.
- Taking vitamin C seems to prevent the onset of canker sores. Five hundred milligrams a day is recommended; however, always check with your physician first.
- Eat plain, active culture yogurt every day and take an acidophilus supplement.
- Eat a diet high in peas, lentils, and beans to prevent a deficiency in iron, folic acid and vitamin B which has been linked to canker sores.
- Keep your life as stress-free as possible. Get plenty of rest and exercise and use music, meditation or message therapy to reduce stress.

Carpal Tunnel Syndrome

DEFINITION:

In the age of the computer keyboard, carpal tunnel syndrome has become somewhat of a liability of fast typing for extended periods of time. This kind of stress on the wrist can create pressure on the nerve by overworking the tendons, which makes them swell.

Carpal tunnel syndrome develops over months or usually years, and is the result of continued repetition of movements of the hands or wrists. It involves damage to the nerve which carries brain signals between the brain and the hands. This median nerve, which passes through the carpal tunnel created by the wrist bones, can become crowded when tissues in the tunnel become inflamed. Carpal tunnel syndrome is a fairly common disorder, particularly for middle-aged women. It can affect one or both of the hands.

CAUSES:

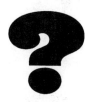

Carpal tunnel syndrome occurs when the median nerve, located in the wrist, is trapped and squeezed as it goes through a fibrous passage called the carpal tunnel. An excess of tissue can build up from repeated inflammation and make the condition worse. Common activities that can cause carpal tunnel to develop are; tennis, canoe paddling, typing, knitting or crocheting, extensive writing, small parts assembly, repeated blows to the front of the wrist, bone fracture or dislocation, and meat cutting.

In addition, playing certain musical instruments, extensive flexing or bending of the wrist in gymnastics, using a tool that requires the bending of the wrist over long periods of time, and decreased circulation during pregnancy are also thought to increase the chances of carpal tunnel syndrome.

There is some evidence to support the fact that a change in female sex hormone, which occurs during menopause, may cause an accumulation of fluid, with subsequent swelling in the wrists. Women who have just started using birth control pills may also experience symptoms of this disorder. In carpal tunnel syndrome, one or both hands may be affected.

SYMPTOMS:

Physical: Carpal tunnel syndrome can cause a tingling sensation in the thumb or other fingers; numbness of the thumb, middle or index finger; inability to perform tasks requiring dexterity; and shooting pains that go into the fingers or up into the forearm. If you have carpal tunnel syndrome, your little finger will not be affected.

Tapping the wrist may also cause you to feel a tingly feeling. The pain and tingling of this disorder may increase during the night, especially if the wrists are bent. Frequently, by simply shaking the hand or rubbing it, the symptoms of carpal tunnel syndrome may temporarily stop.

Warning: Chronic pain located in any joint could be a symptom of arthritis and should be examined by your doctor.

STANDARD MEDICAL TREATMENT:

Some cases of carpal tunnel syndrome clear up without medical intervention. Some physicians will prescribe a diuretic to reduce the amount of tissue fluid in the body. If the condition is severe enough, a steroid injection can be administered at the wrist to alleviate inflammation.

Surgery: If this condition persists and the pain is not manageable, surgery is recommended. In this procedure a neurologist or plastic surgeon will free the squeezed nerve by cutting through tough membrane of the carpal tunnel, thereby creating more space for the nerve passage. The success rate with this type of surgery is high. The operation requires a brief hospital stay, usually in a same-day surgery unit, and the procedure leaves a very tiny scar. If both hands are affected, it is usually recommended that each hand be done at separate times so dressing, bathing, etc. will not be too difficult during the recovery period.

Success rating of standard medical treatment: very good to excellent for surgical treatment. If contemplating the procedure, make sure you enlist the services of a neurologist or certified plastic surgeon who has expertise in this area.

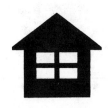

HOME REMEDIES:

- Very mild hand exercises such as rotating the wrists in circles helps to increase circulation and may alleviate some of the tingling. Exercise should be used with caution as resting the wrists is sometimes more effective to control symptoms.
- Over-the-counter medications such as aspirin and ibuprofen and non-steroidal anti-inflammatory anti-inflammatory medications can help to reduce pain. Acetaminophen is not effective in treating inflammation.
- A cold pack may help to relieve swelling.
- It is not uncommon for people to sleep with their wrists bent against the mattress, which can aggravate symptoms of carpal tunnel syndrome. Before going to bed, use a wrist splint to keep your wrist straight, which takes stress off the nerves. These splints, which are usually made of metal with Velcro fasteners, can be purchased at medical supply sources or can be especially made to fit your hand by a physical therapist.
- Change the position of your hands when crocheting, knitting, typing, holding

tools etc. to encourage better circulation.

◆ Use handles, pencils, pens, curling irons, scissors, etc. that are large and easy to operate.

NUTRITIONAL APPROACHES:

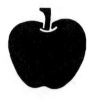

◆ A low-fat diet which inhibits fatty deposits is thought to be beneficial for carpal tunnel syndrome sufferers. Foods to emphasize are brown rice, whole grains, lentils, sunflower seeds, salmon, tuna, avocados, turkey, fresh fruits and vegetables.

◆ Avoid high-fat foods, smoking, stress, and caffeine.

◆ *Vitamin B6:* Recently more emphasis has been placed on the use of B6 to help relieve nerve-related disorders. There has been some conjecture that a lack of B6 can actually cause carpal tunnel syndrome. Dosages should be discussed with your doctor, as B6 can be toxic at high levels. Improvement is usually not seen for at least a month to six weeks.

◆ *Vitamin A, C, D and E:* Vital to tissue repair and healing, and can contribute to reducing inflammation. Vitamin C plays a significant role in connective tissue regeneration.

◆ *Calcium and magnesium:* Help calm the nerves and keep the nervous system healthy and functioning properly.

◆ *Potassium:* Important in proper nervous system function and in controlling the body's water balance.

◆ *Chromium and zinc:* Both facilitate tissue healing.

HERBAL REMEDIES:

◆ *Tumeric:* A natural anti-inflammatory which can be applied as a paste to the affected area to help control pain and swelling.

◆ *Ginkgo:* Improves circulation, which can help to decrease tendon and tissue swelling.

◆ *Hawthorne:* Helps clean the veins of unwanted deposits.

◆ *Bromelain:* Anyone who requires surgical intervention for carpal tunnel syndrome should take this enzyme for its ability to lessen swelling and inflammation.

PREVENTION:

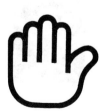

◆ Use a hand rest specifically designed for your typewriter or computer keyboard. This device keeps the hands level (rather than bent at the wrist) while typing.

◆ Use your whole hand when holding on to an object.

◆ If doing a manual job that involves a repetitive movement, take a break from the activity every 30 minutes.

◆ Avoid the excessive consumption of protein, which studies have linked to a predisposition to carpal tunnel syndrome.

Chicken Pox

DEFINITION:

Most adults can remember having chicken pox as children and may even have a few scars to show for it. Chicken pox is a normal part of childhood and can sometimes be harder on the parent than the sick child. Chicken pox is a common viral childhood disease which is characterized by a headache and a mild fever, followed by the eruption of small, red, itchy spots. The incubation period for chicken pox is between 14 to 17 days. Generally speaking, the older you are the worse your case of chicken pox will be. Chicken pox is usually contracted between the ages of five and nine, and is usually passed around through the classroom.

Rare complications from chicken pox include encephalitis and pneumonia. The risk of Reye's syndrome is also present when aspirin is given to a child up to the age of 21 when chicken pox is present (see chapter on Reye's syndrome).

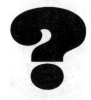

CAUSES:

Chicken pox is caused by a virus (varicella-zoster) that is spread from person to person through airborne droplets, or through contaminated bedding or clothing. A person with chicken pox is considered highly infectious from around two days before the rash appears until approximately a week later. Having had chicken pox provides lifelong immunity; however, the virus remains dormant within nerve tissue and may cause herpes zoster later on (see chapter on herpes). Chicken pox occurs more often in the winter and spring, in temperate regions, and is seen year round in warmer climates.

SYMPTOMS:

Physical: From 10 to 21 days after exposure, symptoms of chicken pox can occur. The severity of the disease is thought to be related to the extent of exposure. A rash, which initially resembles a flat red splotch, generally appears on the trunk, the armpits, on the upper arms and legs, on the scalp, inside the mouth and occasionally in the throat and bronchial tubes, which can cause a cough. The "spots" eventually become fluid-filled blisters within a few hours of eruption. After several days, they will dry out and form scabs. After the sores have formed crusts, the fever usually disappears.

The eruption of the pox continues in cycles which can last from three days to one week. These blisters are considered infectious. Children usually develop a slight fever with chicken pox; however, an adult with the virus typically experiences a high fever and can subsequently contract pneumonia. Adults can also experience flulike symptoms with the disease. The rash that accompanies chicken pox is extremely itchy and can be very miserable depending on the location of the sores. Once the scabs disappear, the child is no longer considered contagious.

MEDICAL ALERT:

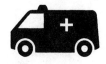

The older one is, the more severe chicken pox will be. In some cases, pneumonia and encephalitis can develop as secondary infections. Adults should avoid contact with exposed individuals. Women in their final stage of pregnancy who have never had the disease should avoid exposure to chicken pox. If they do catch the disease, the newborn may develop a severe case of the virus.

NOTE: Anyone who is taking cancer drugs or cortisone should immediately contact a physician if infected by chicken pox.

STANDARD MEDICAL TREATMENT:

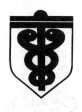

Complete recovery usually takes place without medical intervention within 10 days for children and somewhat longer for adults. Acetaminophen is usually suggested for fever and discomfort. Calamine lotion is the standard medication used to relieve itchiness and irritation. In very severe cases, or when the immune system is weak, an antiviral drug (acyclovir) may be prescribed, although there is some evidence that the drug is not effective unless administered immediately after the rash appears. If the sores become infected, an antibiotic ointment can be prescribed. No vaccine against chicken pox is available at this time; however, one is being developed.

Warning: Never give a child aspirin if a viral infection is suspected, as this can increase the risk of Reye's syndrome, a potentially fatal disorder.

SIDE EFFECTS: Acyclovir: (brand name Zovirax): Can be used as an ointment or taken internally. Capsules can cause dizziness, nausea, vomiting, headache, diarrhea, aching joints, loss of appetite, fatigue, fluid retention, swollen glands, leg pain.

Warning: Do not take this drug if pregnant or nursing without your doctor's consent.

MEDICAL UPDATE:

◆ Some studies have indicated that using acetaminophen (Tylenol) prolonged the illness and was not very effective in relieving symptoms. Some physicians believe that the general public are too quick to try to lower a fever. If a fever is not too high, it can actually speed the recovery process.

Success rating of standard medical treatment: poor. Most doctors will want to treat chicken pox without an office visit, unless complications arise.

HOME SELF-CARE:

◆ Keep the child's nails short and file them smooth to discourage scratching, which can lead to infection and scarring. Wash the hands often to prevent secondary infections. For very young children, soft gloves or socks over the hands are recommended.
◆ Sponge the affected areas with herbal tea preparations listed in herbal section.
◆ Make a warm bath using 1 cup of baking soda to 1/2 cup of apple cider vinegar.
◆ A cool bath can also help with itching, especially if pox are present in the genital area. Cornstarch may be added to the water.
◆ Clothing should be light and non-constrictive.
◆ Colloidal oatmeal baths have also been used with some success in controlling the itching. Aveeno brand of colloidal oatmeal can be purchased at a pharmacy.
◆ Do not use steroid-based ointments on the rash, which can increase the risk of infection.
◆ Dyprotex cream, an over-the-counter preparation, can be used in pad or lotion form. It helps to relieve itching and is less drying than calamine-based medications
◆ Using olive oil or castor oil on the dried-out scabs may cause them to drop off sooner.
◆ There is some evidence that antihistamines may help with itching. Consult your doctor about this option.

NUTRITIONAL APPROACH:

◆ Sores in the mouth may interfere with eating; therefore, nutritious cold milkshakes, popsicles etc., may be more appealing to the child. Oral numbing sprays can be used just prior to eating so ingesting food is easier. Check with your doctor or dentist for prescription varieties.
◆ Avoid salty or spicy foods and citrus fruits. Do not use sweets, chocolate, or meat. Offer the child mild foods that are easy to eat and digest, such as creamy mashed potatoes, rice pudding, scrambled eggs, and milkshakes.

◆ *Beta carotene:* Helps to enhance the immune system and aids in healing tissue.
◆ *Vitamin A:* Stimulates the immune system and also helps in tissue healing.
◆ *Vitamin C:* Helps to control fever and is thought to be a natural antiviral, which also helps to eliminate toxins created by viral infections.
◆ *Vitamin E:* Promotes healing and is considered a free radical.
◆ *Potassium, calcium, selenium and zinc:* Help to lower fever and replace electrolytes lost through sweating.
◆ *Liquid chlorophyll:* Helps to purify the blood of toxins released by viral invaders.
◆ Give plenty of liquids. Vegetable broths and mild fruit juices are recommended. Aloe vera juice is also suggested for its healing properties.

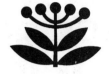

HERBAL REMEDIES:

◆ For itching, use an aloe vera or comfrey salve. A black walnut tincture can also be used.
◆ Use the following herbs in tea form:
◆ A combination tea made out of equal parts of yarrow, red raspberry chickweed and peppermint.
◆ *Catnip:* Acts as a natural sedative.
◆ *Chamomile:* Helps to calm the nerves and promote sleep.
◆ *Pau d'arco tea:* acts as a blood purifier.
◆ *Ginger and bayberry:* Work together to help protect against viruses.
◆ *Red clover:* Helps to cleanse the blood of impurities.
◆ *Yarrow:* helps in the healing of sores.
◆ *Golden seal:* a natural antibiotic that is also good for severe itching.
◆ Wet compresses can be applied to the pox using red raspberry, catnip, and peppermint powder mixed in a base of diluted apple cider vinegar.
◆ Hops can be used to promote sleep and calm the nerves.

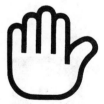

PREVENTION:

◆ It is recommended that young, healthy children be deliberately exposed to chicken pox so that the disease will not be contracted as an adolescent or adult. Those who have never had the disease and are pregnant, along with anyone who is taking immunosuppressant drugs, should avoid contact with groups of children.
◆ A chicken pox vaccine may be available in the near future.

Chronic Fatigue Syndrome

DEFINITION:

The words "chronic fatigue syndrome" have become quite familiar to most American households over the last two decades. This disorder, also called CFS. is a fairly new disease that causes a serious feeling of exhaustion for no obvious reason. CFS, also known as the yuppie flu, is persistent and quite resistant to treatment.

For unknown reasons, 80 percent of those who suffer from CFS are women, generally between the ages of 24 and 45. A cure or vaccine for this disease is not available. The symptoms of this condition are extremely hard to diagnose and specific causes of the disease are still under debate.

It has been estimated that thousands of people carry the Epstein-Barr virus, believed by most doctors to cause CFS, and have no apparent symptoms. Some health care professionals dispute the involvement of this virus and see this disorder as another disease resulting from Western life-style and diet. Chronic fatigue syndrome may persist for months or even years, and its occurrence is on the increase.

CAUSES:

The Epstein-Barr virus the same that causes mononucleosis is believed by many to cause CFS. It is contagious and can be transmitted by kissing, coughing, sharing food and through sexual contact. Some doctors question the involvement of this virus and regard the cause of CFS as an unsolved mystery.

Stress has been implicated as a possible cause in that highly motivated people seem more prone to develop the disease. Other causes that have been linked to this disorder are mercury poisoning, hypoglycemia, anemia, hypothyroidism and sleep apnea.

SYMPTOMS:

Physical: CFS usually causes persistent flulike symptoms such as a low-grade fever, sore throat, muscle aches and pains, extreme fatigue, excess sleeping, low stamina, swollen glands, and appetite loss. In addition, intestinal problems, anxiety, depression, irritability, sleep disturbances, mood swings, memory loss, and headaches may also develop. Sensitivity to light and heat, and recurring upper respiratory tract infections due to decreased efficiency of the immune system are also typical symptoms of CFS.

Psychological: People who suffer from this disease often feel that they are being patronized. Frequently, family members, friends and even physicians do not realize how incapacitating this disorder really is and may believe the victim is exaggerating or seeking attention. All parties involved need to educate themselves in order to fully appreciate the magnitude of this disease and its ability to disrupt daily routine. Marriages and other relationships can become very stressed by CFS. Avoid misinformation and never make assumptions that anyone suffering from CFS is just being lazy.

MEDICAL ALERT:

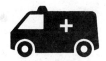

Anyone suffering from any or some of these symptoms should see a doctor immediately. No one should assume that they have CFS.

STANDARD MEDICAL TREATMENT:

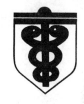

This disease is often misdiagnosed as hypochondria or depression. CFS symptoms are sometimes treated with antibiotics, which will have no effect on it if it is indeed caused by the Epstein-Barr virus. You can expect your doctor to run a battery of blood tests to check for elevated levels of antibodies to EBV and to rule out other diseases such as cancer, diabetes, AIDS, endocrine disorders, anemia, leukemia, etc.

If you have elevated antibodies and if several of the above symptoms are present, CFS will be suspected. Doctors will usually prescribe vitamin and mineral supplements and recommend rest. To date, the medical profession considers CFS to be incurable.

Success rating of standard medical treatment: poor. The medical profession offers little to people suffering from CFS.

Note: There have been several occasions when CFS was diagnosed and the real problem was clinical depression, which can be successfully treated.

HOME SELF-CARE:

◆ Very mild exercise has been suggested for CFS victims to increase stamina and oxygenate cells. Exercise also helps to improve sleep.
◆ Exercise and massage, in combination with elevation of the limbs, are believed to stimulate the lymphatic system which can, in turn, help strengthen the immune system.
◆ Stay away from allergens. CFS victims are often more prone to allergic reaction since their immune system is compromised.
◆ Try to get adequate amounts of sleep, including at least one daytime nap.
◆ Talk to others who suffer from the disease and share your feelings with your family and friends.
◆ Try to keep a positive attitude by setting and achieving small goals each day.

NUTRITIONAL APPROACH:

◆ As in any viral infection, the importance of susceptibility is often minimized by the medical profession. Strengthening the immune system is essential in building up resistance to infections from viruses like Epstein-Barr.

◆ Take a strong vitamin and mineral supplement daily. Those obtained from natural sources are recommended for better assimilation.

◆ A good protein supplement in liquid form is also recommended for tissue and organ repair and to increase stamina.

◆ Eat a diet that is at least half raw foods and drink plenty of freshly squeezed vegetable and fruit juices. Avoid eating sugar, white flour and fat.

◆ *Zinc:* Important in helping the body fight viral infections.

◆ *Magnesium:* Studies have suggested that those who suffer from CFS have unusually low levels of magnesium. Magnesium supplements are recommended along with an emphasis on magnesium-rich foods such as peas, nuts, whole grains, brown rice, and soybeans, and dark green leafy vegetables.

◆ Be sure to get extra selenium and zinc in your mineral supplementation.

◆ *Germanium:* Helps to enhance tissue oxygenation and boosts immune functions.

◆ *Vitamin B:* Injections are preferable and should be discussed with your doctor.

◆ *Vitamin C with bioflavonoids:* Has anti-viral properties.

◆ *Lecithin:* Helps boost energy and strengthens the immune system.

◆ *Vitamin A and E:* Considered powerful free-radical scavengers.

◆ *Chlorophyll in tablet or liquid form:* Helps to remove toxins from the blood and can increase stamina and resistance to disease.

◆ *Acidophilus:* Helps to replenish good bacteria that improve immunity.

HERBAL REMEDIES:

◆ *Burdock root:* Facilitates blood purification and removes toxins which are released by viral organisms.

◆ *Dandelion:* A nutritive herb with medicinal properties that also helps stimulate the liver and kidneys.

◆ *Echinacea:* Boosts immunity system and is a natural antiviral. Helps build up resistance to infections by stimulating the production of T lymphocytes.

◆ *Garlic:* Helps to fight viruses and promotes immunity and energy.

◆ *Golden seal:* A natural stimulant for spleen and liver function which boosts immunity and resistance.

◆ *Pau d'arco:* Helps to kill viruses and increases resistance to disease.

◆ *Poke weed:* Helps boost immune function, particularly in viral infections.

◆ *Licorice:* Has antiviral properties and functions as a natural anti-inflammatory.

◆ *Shitake mushroom:* A traditional Chinese treatment for increasing resistance to infection.

◆ *The following herbs in combination may be useful:* Echinacea, rutin, cloves, pau d'arco and golden seal.

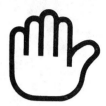

PREVENTION:

◆ There is some speculation that those who exercise regularly and are in good physical condition are more resistant to the Epstein-Barr virus.
◆ Keep the immune system healthy through proper diet, vitamin and mineral supplements and exercise.
◆ Make stress-reduction a part of your daily routine. Use counseling, relaxation techniques and exercise.
◆ Do not smoke, use alcohol or consume caffeine.

For more information contact:

The National Institute of Allergies and Infectious Diseases
9000 Rockville Pike, Niaid-OC, Building 31, Room 7A-32
Bethesda, MD 20892
1-301-496-5717

Colds and Flu

DEFINITION:

The American public spends an enormous amount of money every year on medications designed to relieve the miseries of colds and flu. Ironically, while medical science has managed to transplant hearts and clone genes, a cure for the common cold and influenza still remains out of reach. Both colds and influenza are caused by viruses that infect the upper respiratory tract. The word "cold" refers to a group of mild illnesses that are caused by over 200 different types of viruses. A cold is usually confined to the nose and throat, but can also affect the larynx (laryngitis). Most babies will get their first cold before they are 1. Susceptibility to colds and flu is at its greatest between the ages of 1 and 3. School children can get as many as 10 colds per year. Colds are more frequent during the winter months, when confinement makes the spread of the virus easier. The older one gets, the less his chances of catching a cold, due to increased immunity. An ordinary cold will usually clear up within three to five days.

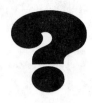

CAUSES:

The viruses that cause colds and flu are very hard to cure due to their ability to mutate into hundreds of different forms, making the formulation of a vaccine virtually impossible. We are more likely to catch a cold when our immune system has been weakened by allergies, poor diet, exhaustion, surgery or illness. In addition, stress or psychological shock is thought to make the system more susceptible to the viruses, which can remain dormant otherwise.

Exposure to drafts, going out with a wet head, and getting chilled are also associated with an increased risk for catching a cold or the flu. Apparently a sudden change in body temperature decreases the body's defenses against viruses that cause both of these ailments. Colds and flu are transmitted through airborne droplets and can be caught by kissing someone with a cold, sharing contaminated food or beverages, or being in a closed, hot, dry environment with someone who has a cold.

SYMPTOMS:

Physical: The exact symptoms of a cold or flu depend on the virus that is responsible. Major symptoms include nasal congestion, runny nose, coughing, sore throat, tickle in the throat, hoarseness, headache, fever, chills, restlessness, sneezing, watery eyes, and aches and pains. Initially, nasal discharge is runny and watery and will eventually become thick and greenish/yellow in color. The presence of a cold can reactivate the herpes simplex virus, which can remain dormant in the body, resulting in the formation of a cold sore.

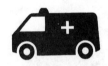

MEDICAL ALERT:

See your doctor if you have chest congestion, a fever higher than 102 degrees F., white or yellow lesions in the throat, shortness of breath, swollen glands, extreme pain in the sinus, ears or chest, difficulty swallowing, wheezing, or excessive loss of appetite.

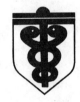

STANDARD MEDICAL TREATMENT:

After your doctor has examined your ears, nose, throat and chest, they may order a chest x-ray to rule out the possibility of pneumonia. Frequently, a throat culture will be performed to check for the presence of strep. If a bacterial infection is present, antibiotics will be prescribed. Doctors treat at least 50,000 patients per year for colds and flu. They usually recommend analgesics, decongestants, and cough syrups, which are most often purchased at a pharmacy without a prescription. Drugs containing pseudoephedrine found in cold tablets and nasal decongestants, and hydrocodone which controls coughing and loosens phlegm may also be recommended.

Warning: Pregnant or nursing mothers should not take any cold or flu medications without the approval of their doctors. Certain antihistamine preparations have been associated with birth defects.

Success rating of standard medical treatment: very poor. The common cold has baffled doctors for years. Treatment is purely symptomatic and can usually be administered with over-the-counter or herbal preparations at home. Very often, people with upper respiratory tract infections do not believe they can recover without an antibiotic, which some doctors will prescribe for a cold or flu. Antibiotics have no effect against the viruses that cause colds and flu.

MEDICAL UPDATE:

◆ The two most promising possibilities for curing the cold are the drug interferon and the use of synthetic antigens. To date, both of these alternatives are still in the experimental stage.
◆ A new drug called rimantadine HCL (Flumadine) has recently been approved for preventing and treating illness caused by various strains of influenza A virus in adults.

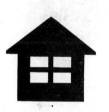

HOME SELF-CARE:

◆ Drink lots of liquid. While this remedy seems overemphasized, it has real merit. Fluids help to keep mucus secretions more liquid, which can prevent secondary infections.
◆ Use a cold mist vaporizer to keep the nose and bronchiole tubes from drying out, which can aggravate coughs associated with colds.
◆ Get plenty of rest.
◆ The healing properties of chicken soup are considered valid in the scientific world. For one thing, the salt content of the soup can help alleviate dizziness associated with colds and flu. Sip hot soup slowly over a period of time.
◆ Make a eucalyptus oil inhalant by putting some oil or tincture in 2 cups of boiling water and inhale. This can also be used in a hot bath to alleviate congestion.
◆ Take a hot shower or use a sauna to help clear congestion.
◆ Avoid nasal sprays that shrink swollen membranes. They can actually aggravate congestion and can become habit-forming. To open the nose naturally, eat some food flavored with hot pepper sauce, horseradish or hot mustard. These are virtually guaranteed to make your nose run.
◆ Saline preparations available in sprays can help soothe sore noses.
◆ Use a dab of mentholatum or petroleum jelly around the sore part of the nostrils.
◆ The value of antihistamines, which unnaturally dry up mucous membranes, is debated. Histamine, which is a problem in allergic reactions is not associated

with colds or flu. Overly dry membranes can become even more irritated. There is some evidence that suppressing the symptoms of a cold can prolong it. Runny noses, coughs, etc., help to move infected secretions out of the body. Antihistamines can also cause significant depression in some individuals.

◆ Over-the-counter cough syrups which contain dexthromethorphan can be as strong as some prescription medications.

◆ For headaches, ibuprofen is recommended. Do not give aspirin to children. Reye's syndrome is associated with the ingestion of aspirin by children with viral infections.

◆ Acetaminophen and aspirin are believed to increase nasal blockage in some people and may actually inhibit antibodies that fight viruses.

◆ An old home remedy for colds and flu is the footbath, which is made by dissolving 1 tablespoon of mustard powder in a quart of hot water. Soak both feet in this solution for up to 10 minutes.

◆ Walking every day for 20 to 30 minutes can help to increase circulation, which may lessen the duration of a cold by boosting the body's defense mechanisms. Very strenuous exercise is not recommended.

Nutritional approach:

The idea of feeding a cold is not advised by everyone. It is believed that by not eating, the body is able to fight infection and rid itself of toxins more efficiently. For this reason, going off of solid food is suggested by some who believe that a liquid diet has more merit. Drink plenty of citrus fruit juices such as orange, pineapple, grapefruit or tomato juice. Hot soups are also wonderful and can provide both nutrients and liquid. Sipping pure water all day is also recommended. One of the best ways to quiet a coughing spell is to drink a glass of water.

◆ Avoid sugar consumption: Some studies show that vitamin C and sugar compete for transport into white blood cells.

◆ *Acidophilus:* Helps to replenish friendly bacteria that help fight infection, which can be destroyed by antibiotics.

◆ *Vitamin A and beta carotene:* Help to lessen inflammation of mucous membranes and are immune system boosters.

◆ *Vitamin C:* Some studies suggest that vitamin C destroys the cold virus. Check with your doctor to approve a large dose. Drink at least 5 to 6 glasses of citrus juice per day. Taking 500 milligrams of vitamin C four times per day seems to dramatically eliminate common cold and flu symptoms.

◆ *Zinc gluconate lozenges:* Can be dissolved under the tongue and should be taken at the first sign of a cold or flu. Zinc has been found to cut down, not only on cold and flu symptoms, but also on the duration of these infections. Do not take more than the recommended dose, as zinc can be toxic in large amounts.

◆ *Monolaurian:* A fatty acid which is believed to have an antiviral effect. It can be taken in capsule form.

◆ *Potassium, selenium, calcium and magnesium:* Boost the body's ability to fight infection. If a fever is present, these can be lost through excessive sweating.
◆ *Aloe vera juice and liquid chlorophyll:* Help to eliminate toxins from the blood.
◆ *Barley water:* Can be made by steeping barley in water and adding lemon peel and honey.

HERBAL REMEDIES

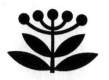

The advantage of using herbal remedies over antibiotics is that herbs generally do not destroy the body's friendly bacteria, which are essential for good health. Herbs will not compromise the immune system, and if used prudently can be of great value in treating both bacterial and viral infections.
◆ *Boneset:* Promotes sweating and can help to reduce fever. Is also a good expectorant and helps alleviate muscle pain.
◆ *Catnip:* Helps to bring down a fever and break up mucus congestion.
◆ *Chamomile tea:* An old traditional comforting treatment for colds.
◆ *Comfrey and fenugreek:* Helps control coughs and hoarseness.
◆ *Garlic:* An antimicrobial which is good for a variety of infections. Garlic can be purchased in odorless capsules.
◆ *Hops or valerian tea:* Both of these herbs have a natural tranquilizing effect and can help promote restful sleeping.
◆ *White horehound:* A natural expectorant that eases congestion.
◆ *Licorice cough drops or tea:* Helps to soothe irritated throats and helps to relieve coughs.
◆ *Echinacea:* Helps to fight any viral infection and can be purchased as an extract.
◆ *Slippery elm tea:* Excellent for sore throats.
◆ *Ginger tea:* A good remedy for the treatment of chills.
◆ Jade screen powder available at Chinese pharmacies is used for anyone plagued with frequent colds.
◆ *Astragalus membranaceous:* Used by the Chinese to reduce the incidence and length of a cold.
◆ *The following herbs taken in combination may be useful:* Bayberry, cloves, willow, and white pine.

PREVENTION:

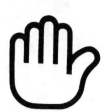

◆ Don't smoke
◆ Taking a massive dose of vitamin C upon the first symptom of a cold or flu is believed by some professionals to prevent the onset of either ailment.
◆ Daily doses of vitamin C are also thought to help prevent colds and flu.
◆ Don't eat a diet high in sugar.
◆ Taking garlic capsules may lower one's chances of catching a cold.

- If a family member has a cold, flush used tissues away so that the virus is less likely to spread. The use of paper plates, cups and plastic utensils can also lower the possibility of further contamination to others.
- The best way to keep a cold from spreading is to wash hands frequently.
- Keep your home humidified, especially in the winter. Do not keep your home too hot, as dried out mucous membranes seem more prone to catching colds and flu.
- Keep stress levels down with regular exercise, relaxation, and meditation.
- Don't get chilled by sitting in a draft or by overdressing and then sweating.

Colic

DEFINITION:

Anyone who has had a baby with colic has gained an entirely new appreciation for the notion of patience and long-suffering. A colicky baby is usually unhappy and as a result, the whole family can be placed under stress. The heart-wrenching cries that usually accompany colic can be quite disturbing, especially for new parents who need to understand that colic is a common disorder and in no way reflects negatively on their parenting skills.

Colic refers to spasmodic intestinal pain experienced by an infant that can come in waves of varying intensity and cause significant physical distress. It most commonly appears around three to four weeks of age and usually disappears at twelve weeks.

CAUSES:

The incidence of infantile colic is high and occurs in one out of ten babies. The exact cause of colic is unknown. Some studies suggest that the incidence of colic is higher among bottle-fed babies, although breast-fed babies can get colic too. If you are nursing, some foods you eat may cause colic in the infant. Foods to avoid are cabbage, onions, garlic, spicy foods, and chocolate.

There is also evidence that cow's milk can cause colic, not only in formula products but in breast milk itself, when the mother eats dairy products. It is recommended that nursing mothers avoid drinking cow's milk. Some studies have suggested that colic is an allergic reaction to certain kinds of protein. Changing your baby to a protein-treated formula may help you to assess whether this is indeed the cause of the colic. Eating too rapidly, excessive swallowing of air, and constipation have also been cited as possible causes of colic.

SYMPTOMS:

Physical: Episodes of colic are characterized by irritable screams or cries of the infant accompanied by a drawing up of the legs and clenching of the fists. Your baby's face may become red and the baby may audibly pass gas. Intervals of quiet between cries is also typical of colicky babies. Colic tends to worsen in the evening and can be difficult to deal with if prolonged.

Babies with colic will often try to frantically feed, then pull away. Some theories have speculated that exposure to stressful situations or even to wind may induce colic. Babies who experience colic are usually healthy otherwise. For some babies, having a bowel movement brings some relief.

Psychological: Frequently, the caretaker of a colicky infant needs support from other family members so fatigue and exhaustion do not become overwhelming. Often new mothers believe that their fussy baby is an indication of their own inadequate mothering. Colic has nothing to do with successful mothering and will disappear within the first few months of infancy.

MEDICAL ALERT:

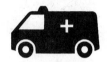

If your baby is experiencing diarrhea, fever, constipation or acts sick, see your physician immediately.

STANDARD MEDICAL TREATMENT:

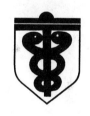

Typically, medical treatment is minimal. In very severe cases an antispasmodic drug such as phenobarbital may be prescribed, although this form of treatment is not recommended for infants under the age of 6 months.

SIDE-EFFECTS: Phenobarbital: (Barbit, Solfoton): Drowsiness, lethargy, difficulty in breathing, skin rash, allergic symptoms, nausea, vomiting, diarrhea. Keep out of reach of children. Can be lethal if overdosed.

Success rating of standard medical treatment: poor. Doctors seem at a loss to provide a successful treatment for colic. Other than strong anti-spasmodics or sedatives, treatment is minimal and not very effective.

HOME SELF-CARE:

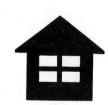

◆ Taking the baby for a ride in the car can often help to bring about sleep.
◆ Make sure that your baby has been adequately burped after a feeding. Burp him more than once during a feeding and keep the baby's head supported in a comfortable position while feeding.
◆ Placing the infant securely on its stomach on top of a running dryer or washer (carefully supervise this activity) can help to soothe stomach pain and facilitate the

movement of gas.

◆ Place the baby on its stomach on your lap and gently swing the baby back and forth on your knees.

◆ Use a heating pad or hot water bottle on a comfortable setting under the infant's stomach. Caution: watch for overheating or leaky hot water bottles.

◆ A mechanized baby swing may help to soothe the infant and provide a break for the parents also.

◆ If the baby must be held, carry the infant in a front sling or pouch so you still have your hands free. An activity like vacuuming may help get the baby to sleep while in the sling.

◆ The use of a pacifier may be helpful.

◆ Play music or try a soft noise in the nursery, such as a fan, radio static, or an aquarium filter.

◆ Don't overfeed the baby. While the infant may appear hungry and take more breast milk or formula, this usually only serves to worsen the problem. Using certain weak herbal teas in pure water may help pacify the baby and treat the spasms.

◆ Give the baby a warm bath in the evenings, when the colic is at its worst.

◆ Don't let your baby oversleep in the day. If naps go for longer than three hours, wake the baby.

◆ Keep the baby's feet warm. Traditionally it has been believed that cold feet may cause abdominal pain in infants. Some traditional home remedies suggest putting the baby's feet in warm water.

◆ Never smoke around an infant. Studies indicate that colic dramatically increases when infants are exposed to cigarette smoke.

◆ Avoid formulas that have been iron-fortified. Excess iron in an infant's diet can cause intestinal problems.

◆ If mixing a formula with water make sure it is not too concentrated, as it may cause intestinal irritation.

NUTRITIONAL APPROACH:

◆ Breast feeding is generally recommended over bottle feeding and should optimally last for the first six months of the infant's life.

◆ If breast feeding, do not eat dairy products. Avoid onions, garlic, caffeine, cabbage, broccoli, ham, bacon, shellfish, bananas, nuts, chocolate, strawberries, oranges, tobacco and alcohol.

◆ If using a formula, try one that has been protein-treated or is not synthesized from cow's milk.

◆ Try 2 oz. of warm water in a bottle to reduce the symptoms of colic and fill the baby's need to suck.

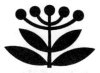

Herbal remedies:

◆ *Catnip, peppermint, fennel, anise, chamomile tea.* Make tea as usual and administer 1 tablespoon at a time to the baby. Tea may also be given in a bottle as long as it is not too concentrated.

◆ *The following herbs taken in combination may be useful:* Peppermint, fennel, papaya, ginger, catnip, wild yam, cramp bark and spearmint. Weak teas can be made with these herbs and administered with a dropper or through a bottle. Check with your doctor before giving your baby medication of any kind.

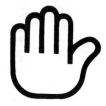

Prevention:

◆ Feed your baby in a relaxed atmosphere in an upright position.
◆ Don't leave the baby with a bottle propped in his or her mouth.
◆ Breast feed if possible and avoid eating foods which may cause problems.
◆ Try to keep feeding time as regularly scheduled.
◆ Make sure if you mix powdered formula with water that the mixture is not too rich or concentrated. Use pure water for mixing.

Colitis

Definition:

Unfortunately, colitis is one of many disorders linked with the Western lifestyle and diet. Victims of colitis usually struggle to find the reason for a flair-up of the disease and in most cases, have to modify their diet to control occurances.

Technically speaking, colitis is an inflammation of the colon or large intestine which brings on episodes of diarrhea or constipation. Anyone who has experienced colitis doesn't want to be located too far from a bathroom facility. The disorder can be quite inconvenient and can create anxiety about eating for fear of its possible consequences. Colitis can be sporadic or can exist as a chronic disorder. It is unpredictable and may be linked to several factors, both physiological and psychological.

Causes:

Colitis has a number of causes. A viral, bacterial or parasitic infection may cause colitis. Prolonged use of an antibiotic may also provoke colitis. In the elderly, an impaired blood supply to the intestinal wall may also cause the disorder. Ulcerative

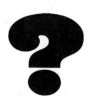

colitis usually begins in adolescence and has an unknown origin. Faulty diet, constipation, eating too rapidly, drinking too much liquid with meals, ingesting excessive cathartics, and stress have all been linked to colitis.

SYMPTOMS:

Physical: Colitis usually causes diarrhea or constipation, with hard, dry, pelletlike feces and the passage of stringy mucous in the stool. In addition, the following symptoms may also accompany the disease: pain during a bowel movement, weakness, fatigue, cold sweats, stomach cramps, headache, fever, nausea, loss of appetite, bloating and gas, and, in severe cases, rectal bleeding (bloody, watery stools may be a symptom of ulcerative colitis).

Psychological: Some physicians have found a correlation between episodes of colitis and stressful situations. Periods of emotional anxiety can initiate a flair-up of the disease.

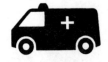

MEDICAL ALERT:

Any of the above physical symptoms may indicate colon cancer and should be checked out by your doctor immediately.

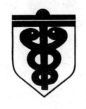

STANDARD MEDICAL TREATMENT:

Often an infection that causes colitis will resolve itself without treatment. For bacteria-caused colitis, the type of antibiotic used depends upon the type of bacteria involved. Antibiotics such as erythromycin are routinely used to treat campylobacter infections. Metronidazole is used to treat amoebic infections and metronidazole or vancomycin are prescribed for clostridium infections. If the diagnosis is ulcerative colitis, corticosteroid therapy is recommended either by mouth or by enema. Diet modifications and vitamin therapy are also routine.

If constipation is present a mild, non-irritating laxative and stool softener may be prescribed. For cases with severe abdominal pain, an antispasmodic may be recommended. When nervous tension is seen as a precipitating factor, a mild sedative or tranquilizer may be suggested.

SIDE-EFFECTS: Erythromycin: (E-base, E-mycin, Eramycin Eryc, Erypar, Erythrocin): Nausea, vomiting, stomach cramps, diarrhea, itching, hairy tongue, vaginal or anal irritation, yellowing of skin and eyes (if this symptom appears, discontinue usage immediately). There is no restriction on using this drug if pregnant or nursing.

Metronidazole: (Femazole, Flagyl, Protostat): Nausea, loss of appetite, occasional vomiting, diarrhea, upset stomach, cramping and constipation, metallic taste, dizziness, inability to sleep, irritability, depression, sense of pelvic pressure.

Warning: Do not use this drug if pregnant or nursing without your doctor's consent.

Success rating of standard medical treatment: fair to good. Often the use of antibiotics in treating certain forms of colitis can create more intestinal irritation. In most cases, medical treatment can provide some level of relief; however, colitis can sometimes evade conventional medical approaches and modification of diet, personality and lifestyle may prove more beneficial.

HOME SELF-CARE:

◆ *Warning:* If diarrhea is severe, avoid overusing Imodium and Lomitil. See your doctor. If ulcerative colitis is present, do not use aspirin, ibuprofen, naprosyn, voltaren or feldene. These can cause further damage to the intestinal lining. Check with your doctor before taking any medication.
◆ Have regular screenings for colon cancer. Chronic colitis can increase your risk.
◆ Learn to use relaxation techniques such as yoga, biofeedback, controlled breathing, self-hypnosis, etc.; to reduce daily tension and control stress.
◆ Incorporate a regular exercise program into your routine to help relieve stress.

NUTRITIONAL APPROACH:

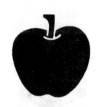

◆ It is important when experiencing a loss of appetite, characteristic of colitis, to eat the right foods and take vitamin supplements daily.
◆ In some cases of colitis, where diarrhea is severe, a liquid diet is suggested for a short time. Carrot or cabbage juice and herb teas are excellent.
◆ When eating solid food, chew thoroughly and do not drink with meals.
◆ During a flare-up, avoid high-roughage foods which contain skins and seeds, especially popcorn. Interestingly, for some people, the inclusion of fibrous foods is not irritating and seems to promote healing. For example, some colitis sufferers cannot tolerate fresh peas, while others find them perfectly digestible. Check with your physician and then experiment with certain foods.
◆ Puree cooked vegetables until a flair-up of the condition quiets down.
◆ Emphasize the following foods: yellow fruits, cantaloupe, pears, watermelon, kelp, agar, and cucumbers. Fruits with pectin, such as apples and pears, seem especially beneficial. You might do better if you peel all fruits and remove all fibrous parts. Avoid fruits that have been canned in sugar and dried fruits.
◆ Do not eat dairy foods. A lactose intolerance may be part of the problem.
◆ Use soups, especially vegetable broths. However, do not take them too hot.
◆ Make it a habit to eat fruit at the end of a meal. If fruit juices are too irritating, dilute them with pure water.
◆ Zwieback toast and other mild foods such as rice cereal are recommended.
◆ Do not eat fried foods or any other foods that seem to aggravate the disorder.

Keep a list of offending foods. Foods to avoid are coffee, dairy foods, eggs, wheat gluten and generally, raw vegetables.

◆ Remove the skin from turkey or chicken before eating.

◆ Do not smoke or drink alcohol.

◆ Take an acidophilus supplement (milk-free) to replenish friendly bacteria which are destroyed by antibiotics.

◆ The use of folate or folic acid, which is B vitamin, is considered very beneficial for colon-related disorders and is highly recommended.

◆ *Vitamin A:* Helps to heal mucous membranes. A deficiency of vitamins A, E and K have been noted in some cases of colitis. These vitamins are important for the proper metabolism of the intestinal mucosa.

◆ *Vitamin D:* A vitamin D deficiency is common in people that suffer from chronic colon disorders, and should be supplemented.

◆ *Vitamin E:* Promotes tissue healing.

◆ *Pancreatin:* Helps to promote digestive function.

◆ *Salmon oil and primrose oil:* can provide essential fatty acids, which the body may be lacking when colitis is present.

◆ Magnesium deficiencies have been found in people suffering from inflammatory bowel diseases.

◆ *Potassium and calcium:* These minerals can be quickly lost if chronic diarrhea is present.

◆ *Cabbage powder:* Has the ability to help in healing gastrointestinal ulcers.

HERBAL REMEDIES:

◆ *Golden seal and myrrh tea:* Should be taken several times a day for their anti-inflammatory properties. Golden seal is considered a natural antibiotic.

◆ A bayberry bark enema made from 1 tablespoon of bayberry bark to one quart of water is recommended for its healing properties.

◆ *Slippery elm:* Helps to control diarrhea and soothes inflamed and irritated tissue in the colon.

◆ *Comfrey root:* Helps in fighting bacterial infections and aids in healing of bleeding ulcers.

◆ *Mullein:* Soothes inflammation in the digestive tract.

◆ *Roman chamomile:* An anti-inflammatory herb which helps with digestion.

◆ *Mexican wild yam:* Anti-spasmodic and stimulates bile.

◆ *Hops:* A digestive stimulant and natural tranquilizer for the nerves.

◆ Use peppermint or fresh ginger tincture for bloating and gas.

◆ *Use bistort drops for diarrhea:* Bistort acts as an anti-inflammatory in the colon.

◆ *Aloe vera gel:* A healing herb.

◆ *Poke root:* Helps in the healing of digestive tract ulcers.

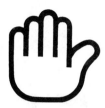

PREVENTION:

◆ A low-fat, high-fiber diet can help minimize colitis in some cases.
◆ Keeping the colon active by eating foods that promote proper elimination is suggested.
◆ Avoiding irritating foods, such as heavy, rich junk foods, salt, sugar, and fried foods, etc. can help to prevent colon irritations.
◆ Don't eat under high-stress situations, when anxious or hurried. Chew food thoroughly.
◆ Don't overuse over-the-counter laxatives, which can irritate the colon.
◆ Stay away from smoking, fumes, chemical sprays and food additives.

Constipation

DEFINITION:

Here is the mystery question of the day: How often should a person have a bowel movement to be considered healthy? This question will usually spawn a variety of answers ranging from after every meal to four times per week. Generally speaking, if you have a bowel movement less than three times per week, and if those movements are sometimes difficult, then you can consider yourself constipated.

Technically, constipation refers to a decrease in bowel movements or difficulty in the formation or passage of the stool. While most Americans feel that at least one bowel movement per day is optimal, there is no real medical evidence to support this. Individual bowel patterns can range from three movements per day to only three per week. It is the consensus of many health care professionals, however, that having one bowel movement per day is preferable.

More women suffer from constipation than men. Most cases of constipation can be remedied with some simple life style changes.

CAUSES:

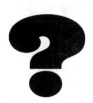

Constipation can be caused by a number of factors such as lack of physical exercise, being confined to bed, decreased liquid intake, diet low in fiber, and lack of fruits and vegetables. In addition, pregnancy, abnormal contractions of the bowel due to colitis, neurological and endocrine disorders, diabetes, and an underactive thyroid gland can also contribute to constipation.

Some medications, including codeine, antacids with aluminum, iron tablets and some narcotics and antidepressants are associated with a decrease in bowel movements. Stress and anxiety are also linked to constipation. Physical obstructions in the bowel caused by a stricture, tumors or diverticulosis may result in constipation as well. An enlarged prostrate or the presence of endometriosis may put pressure on the rectum, subsequently decreasing bowel activity.

SYMPTOMS:

Physical: Symptoms which may accompany constipation include painful bowel movements due to the hardness of the stool, inability to have a complete bowel movement, bloating, gas, and a feeling of sluggishness. Chronic or severe constipation can lead to hemorrhoids, insomnia, indigestion, and diverticulitis. There is some belief that the prolonged constipation can increase the risk of colon cancer.

MEDICAL ALERT:

See a doctor if constipation symptoms are severe and last for over two weeks, if there is blood in the stool, or if a distended abdomen accompanies constipation.

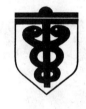

STANDARD MEDICAL TREATMENT:

If constipation is severe, your physician will perform an abdominal and rectal exam. The stool will be checked for blood and in some cases a sigmoidoscopy, barium enema and colonoscopy may be advised. Cancer, colitis, or an intestinal obstruction will have to be ruled out. Customary medical treatment involves increasing dietary fiber intake with Metamucil or Konsyl, which contain bran in the form of psyllium. A stool softener (Colace) is sometimes prescribed and laxatives such as Milk of Magnesia, senna, dulcolax, castor oil or fleets enemas may be recommended especially for the elderly. Certain laxatives have a specific effect on the colon and include contact stimulants, lubricants, increasing the bulk of intestinal contents, increasing secretions of intestinal mucosa, and softening the stool.

SIDE-EFFECTS: With most laxatives and stool softeners, repeated use may inhibit the ability of the colon to contract normally and result in dependence. Pregnant women should always consult their doctor before taking a laxative of any kind. Milk of Magnesia should not be taken by those on a low-salt diet or those suffering from kidney disease. Commercial laxatives are recommended only as a last resort. Laxaties that contain castor oil can damage the intestinal lining and those containing mineral oil can inhibit the body's absorbtion of minerals and vitamins. The safest laxatives are those that are vegetable-based such as Metamucil, Perdiem and Citrucel. Psyllium-based laxatives can be effective.

Success rating of standard medical treatment: fair. Physicians will generally prescribe a laxative preparation. Such preparations are usually effective but can become habit forming. Most health care professionals agree that when an individual is otherwise healthy, dietary and life-style changes should remedy most cases of constipation.

HOME SELF-CARE:

◆ Exercise regularly. If pregnant, take a 20 minute walk per day to lower the risk of constipation

◆ Repeatedly postponing a bowel movement when the urge is present can lead to constipation. Try to have a movement after a large meal by sitting on the toilet for at least 10 minutes. With this method the bowel may be encouraged to eventually move on its own. Read while you're waiting to help relax the system. Don't try to force a bowel movement.

◆ Sit on the toilet every morning, preferably after exercising or breakfast, even if the urge to have a bowel movement is not present. This activity can help to retrain the bowels.

◆ Create a relaxation regimen to counteract the effects of eating under stress or time constraints.

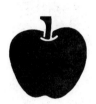

NUTRITIONAL APPROACH:

Several disorders are attributed to chronic constipation and colon toxicity. A lack of fiber in the diet causes food to remain in the colon too long. Thus causes water to be absorbed, which results in dry, hard stool. When this occurs, the natural mucus which lines the colon and keeps waste material moving at a regular pace is impaired. The longer the waste is retained in the colon, the more toxic it can be to the system. The American diet is notorious for being deplorably low in fiber and in fresh fruits and vegetables. The American Dietetic Association recommends 20 to 35 grams of dietary fiber for adults per day. It is best to try to manage constipation through diet and life-style changes and to get off of laxatives altogether.

NOTE: Whenever increasing fiber intake, drink plenty of fluid.

◆ Upon arising, drink a glass of fresh lemon juice in warm water.

◆ Avoid all junk foods, white flour, fried foods, sugar, coffee, alcohol and emphasize high-fiber foods and vegetable juices. Peas, apples, bran cereals, cooked dried beans, oatmeal, and nuts are highly recommended. Soaked figs, prunes or raisins are also an excellent source of fiber. Fresh rhubarb can act as a powerful natural laxative but should not be eaten by people who have a history of calcium kidney stones.

◆ Chew food completely and don't overeat. Eating too much can overload the system and cause a sluggish colon.

◆ Eating directly before going to bed is discouraged.

◆ Drink plenty of water and avoid coffee, tea and alcohol, which can actually dehydrate the system by acting as diuretics.
◆ *Vitamin B complex:* Facilitates proper digestion and colon health.
◆ *Vitamin E:* Can help heal an irritated colon.
◆ *Aloe vera juice:* Helps in forming a soft stool.
◆ *Linseed oil:* Helps to soften a hard stool.
◆ *Folic acid:* Some studies have shown that women with chronic constipation were also deficient in folic acid.
◆ *Apple pectin:* A good source of fiber that can be purchased in health food stores.
◆ Drinking weak molasses water is an old traditional remedy for constipation.
◆ Use psyllium as a bulk laxative. Powdered psyllium can be purchased at a health food store and must be taken with plenty of water or the accumulation of fiber can actually aggravate constipation. Metamucil and Effer-syllium contain ingredients that have been synthesized from psyllium. Use a shaker and mix these according to their instructions with fruit juice.
◆ Avoid caffeine. Caffeine stimulates the nerves that control intestinal contraction and can prevent the bowel from functioning normally on its own.
◆ Do not smoke: Nicotine affects the bowel the same way as caffeine. Other drugs such as ephedrine and phenylpropanolamine can cause constipation if used regularly.
◆ Avoid over-the-counter laxatives that contain phenophthalein, which is too irritating to the bowel. Avoid laxatives that contain mineral oil, which can interfere with the absorption of vitamins and certain fats
◆ If using a stool softener, use one that contains docusate such as Colace or Dialose.
◆ Learn to relax using breathing, biofeedback, or yoga. Stress and anxiety can cause constipation.
◆ For some people, ingesting milk products, such as cheese, can cause constipation. Watch your diet for culprit foods.
◆ *Acidophilus:* Good for the proper functioning of the digestive tract. Can be obtained by eating yogurt with active cultures or by taking a liquid supplement, which provides a higher dose of the bacteria.

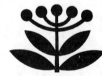

Herbal remedies:

◆ Steep raspberry leaves and flaxseed to make a tea and drink it first thing in the morning.
◆ *Cascara sagrada:* Take in capsule form before retiring. This herb increases peristalsis of the colon and has been used for generations as a remedy for constipation.
◆ *Cassia senna:* The leaves of this herb have a natural laxative effect.
◆ Aloe vera: Another traditional treatment for constipation, although, not considered as effective as cascara sagrada and cassia senna.

- *Burdock and alfalfa:* Both help to loosen hard material from the bowel.
- *Barberry:* Has a cleansing effect on the colon.
- *Slippery elm:* Helps to heal the lower intestinal tract.
- *Licorice:* Add licorice to herbal teas to enhance laxative action.
- *The following herbs in combination may be useful:* Psyllium, fennel, senna and buckthorn.

PREVENTION:

- Drinking plenty of water, exercising and eating a diet high in fiber seems to be the magic formula to avoid constipation. Try not to become dependent on stool softeners and laxatives. Eating a diet high in oat bran, leaving skins on fruits and vegetables and using psyllium can help to prevent constipation.
- Raise children on high-fiber cookies and treats and get them used to drinking adequate amounts of water every day.

Croup

DEFINITION:

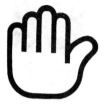

If you are a new parent and have never seen a croupy baby, the symptoms of croup may scare you to death. Rest easy. Croup sounds awful, but is usually not serious.

Croup refers to a common respiratory condition that typically afflicts young children between the ages of three months and four years. Croup causes the voice box and the windpipe to become inflamed, which produces its characteristic and alarming bark-like cough. Croup is usually worse at night and is characterized by difficult, noisy breathing accompanied by a harsh, hoarse cough.

Croup can be a recurring problem for some children and will eventually be outgrown as airways enlarge. It is rarely found after the age of seven. The symptoms of croup are quite frightening; however, croup is rarely fatal. Croup outbreaks tend to occur is the late fall and winter.

CAUSES:

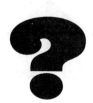

Croup is a viral infection, although a severe form of croup may be bacterial. Several different viruses can be responsible for the disease. Secretions which dry in the larynx, trachea and bronchi cause difficult breathing and coughing. Croup can be caused by the same viruses that cause colds and often runs in families. The

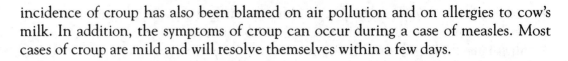

incidence of croup has also been blamed on air pollution and on allergies to cow's milk. In addition, the symptoms of croup can occur during a case of measles. Most cases of croup are mild and will resolve themselves within a few days.

SYMPTOMS:

Physical: Croup typically causes rapid or difficult breathing, gasping, wheezing or grunting when breathing in (stridor), harsh coughing which resembles a seal bark, a pulling in of the breastbone, and tightness in the lungs. Vomiting, spasms in airway passages, sore throat, and fever can also occur with croup. In cases of bacterial croup, the airway may swell and close off, and immediate medical attention is required.

Psychological: The symptoms of croup can be frightening for both parents and child. Reassure your child that the disease is not serious. Frequently, children end up in emergency rooms because the harsh cough and audible breathing which characterize croup appear serious in nature.

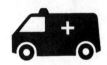

MEDICAL ALERT:

If your child is drooling, has a high fever or has signs of insufficient oxygen (bluish lips or nails), or if breathing is very labored, characterized by forward leaning when sitting, see a doctor immediately. A more serious respiratory obstruction called epiglottitis can be confused with simple croup and requires immediate medical attention.

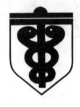

STANDARD MEDICAL TREATMENT:

Treatment for croup focuses on dissolving dried mucus secretions in the larynx. Your doctor will recommend using a humidifier, and if a bacterial infection is present, antibiotics will be administered. If the child is not getting enough oxygen admission to the hospital is recommended, where using an oxygen tent or performing a tracheostomy may be necessary.

Success rating of standard medical treatment: fair. Simple croup can be treated at home and does not require antibiotics unless complications are present. Most doctors will recommend a common-sense approach to treating the disease.

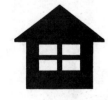

HOME SELF-CARE:

CAUTION: To avoid the risk of Reye's syndrome, do not give children with a viral infection aspirin (see chapter on Reye's syndrome).
◆ Humidifying the air is the best treatment for croup. Use a cool mist vaporizer and make sure it blows close enough to the child so the moist air is readily

inhaled. If a vaporizer is not available, close the bathroom and run the shower on hot to create steam. Do not put the child in the shower. Because steam rises, it is best not to place the child on the floor. Stay in this environment for at least 20 minutes.

◆ A croup tent may be fashioned by draping sheets over the rails of the crib and directing the humidifier steam under the sheets. This should not be done without constant supervision and for only 15 to 20 minute intervals.

◆ An attack of croup can sometimes be relieved by briefly taking the child out in the cold night air. A brief ride in the car with the windows down may be helpful.

◆ An old remedy for an attack of croup is to place a cold compress on the throat.

◆ Encourage the child to sleep in a slightly upright position, using pillows to prop up the head.

◆ A child suffering from croup should never be exposed to cigarette smoke.

NUTRITIONAL APPROACH:

◆ Avoid milk and other dairy products, which can cause more mucus to form. Use citrus juices, vegetable broths and herbal teas to supplement fluid intake, which should be greatly increased with croup. Avoid cold fluids, as they may induce more spasms. Adequate drinking is vital to controlling the cough and should be strongly encouraged throughout the day.

◆ Do not be too concerned if your child turns down solid food. Concentrate on a nutritious liquid diet offered in small amounts, several times a day.

◆ Pitted dates crushed and made into a syrup can help if throat is sore.

◆ *Vitamin C with bioflavonoids:* Helps to fight infection and strengthens the immune system.

◆ *Zinc lozenges:* Promotes immune function and helps in healing. Do not use these for prolonged periods of time.

◆ *Vitamin A:* Helps to restore normal mucous membranes.

◆ *Vitamin E:* Helps to oxygenate cells and repair tissue.

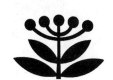

HERBAL REMEDIES:

◆ The Chinese use essential oils, which are rubbed on the chest and neck. Check with your health food store for various types.

◆ Give the child a hot ginger bath and then wrap the child to encourage sweating. Make sure the child does not become chilled. Use strong ginger tea that is added to bath water.

◆ Old-fashioned poultices can be made by slicing onions and garlic, placing them between light cloths and then applying a heating pad on top of the poultice which is placed on the chest. This old remedy helps to open the pores and can relieve congestion.

◆ Eucalyptus oil rubs can be used; however, placing oils in a vaporizer is not recommended as further irritation of the lungs may occur.

- ◆ *Marshmallow:* Soothes inflamed mucous membranes and can be taken internally in the form of a capsule.
- ◆ *Hyssop:* An antispasmodic expectorant that helps quiet coughing spasms.
- ◆ *Garlic:* Can be taken in capsules or liquid; a good antiviral agent that fights infection.
- ◆ *Anise:* Helps to calm irritated, dry coughs.
- ◆ *Wild cherry:* Acts as a natural cough suppressant.
- ◆ *Echinacea tincture:* Especially good if a fever is present, and helps to fight bacterial and viral infections.
- ◆ *Licorice or horehound lozenges:* Help to soothe and heal inflamed throats.
- ◆ A tea made from sage and thyme in equal parts with a pinch of ginger, cardamon and cloves can help control coughs.
- ◆ *Mullein:* Helps in controlling coughs.
- ◆ *Comfrey:* Helps to promote healing of respiratory tract.
- ◆ *Fenugreek:* Prevents the excess formation of mucous and is good for the respiratory tract.
- ◆ *Red raspberry, slippery elm and rose hips:* Help to control coughing. Use in tea form.
- ◆ Lobelia drops in extract form used according to direction can help control coughing spasms
- ◆ *The following herbs in combination may be useful:* Chickweed, comfrey mullein, lobelia, and marshmallow.

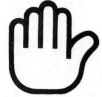

PREVENTION:

- ◆ Frequently, with small children croup is inevitable even if precautions are taken to prevent it.
- ◆ Keeping small children from getting chilled or catching colds can help to avoid croup.
- ◆ Using a humidifier all winter long may be helpful. Giving children a daily dose of vitamin C has been advocated for years as a way to help protect against viral infections. Do not give small infants any supplements without your doctor's consent.
- ◆ Keep your child's immune system strong by breast feeding if possible and avoiding the introduction of cow's milk, citrus juices, wheat, etc., until the latter part of the first year. Food allergies, which can develop early in life, can be responsible for a variety of respiratory ailments which stress the lungs and the immune system.

Dandruff

DEFINITION:

Television and magazine commercials have made most of us acutely aware of the embarrassment that comes from those "tell-tale flakes." Thank goodness dandruff is not the social disaster they would have us believe. It is perfectly normal for everyone to experience some degree of dandruff as the scalp periodically sheds dead skin cells to make room for new ones. Severe dandruff, on the other hand, may require some special treatment. However, it in no way deserves the social stigma Madison Avenue has attached to it.

True dandruff refers to a scalp disorder characterized by extreme shedding of small flakes of dead skin. Dandruff does not affect the hair, poses no danger to health and has nothing to do with going bald.

CAUSES:

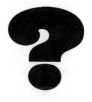

Dandruff is caused either by a mild form of seborrheic eczema or by psoriasis of the scalp. It has also been associated with yeast infections and impaired sebaceous or oil glands in the scalp. An overly dry scalp can sometimes cause flaky skin; however, technically this is not true dandruff.

SYMPTOMS:

Physical: Dandruff typically causes an itchy, scaly rash on the scalp, which leads to the continual shedding of small flakes of dead skin. These flakes can become trapped in the hair and fall to the collar or shoulders.

MEDICAL ALERT:

Consult a doctor for the following symptoms: Severe flaking, persistent itching of the scalp, redness, particularly along the neckline, or crusting of the scalp.

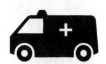

STANDARD MEDICAL TREATMENT:

If over-the-counter shampoos are not effective, your doctor may prescribe a lotion which contains a steroid. Sometimes, physicians will prescribe antifungal creams even though dandruff is not caused by a fungus. Lotions containing salicylic acid or tar help to loosen dead skin that is difficult to remove and may be recommended by your doctor. A dermatologist may also prescribe a lotion which contains sulfur and resorcin (deprosone) to act as a drying agent. In some cases of

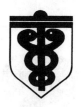

dandruff, your physician may recommend antibiotic therapy.

SIDE-EFFECTS: There is some controversy over the safety of shampoos or lotions that contain coal tar, which may be carcinogenic.

Caution: When using a dandruff shampoo or lotion use special care to protect your eyes.

Success rating of standard medical treatment: good to fair. Most people rarely see a physician for dandruff unless it is particularly severe. Many over-the-counter shampoos can help with mild cases of dandruff. Whenever significant crusting of the scalp is present, a dermatologist should be seen.

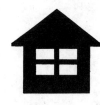

HOME SELF-CARE:

◆ Don't pick, scrape or scratch the scalp.

◆ Avoid the use of irritating, drying shampoos and rotate dandruff shampoo with regular shampoo to avoid a residue buildup.

◆ Wash your hair frequently using a non-oily shampoo. Some antidandruff compounds to look for are zinc pyrithione compounds and selenium sulfide, (Selsum Blue). Stay away from shampoos that contain coal tar as it may be carcinogenic. Sebulex, Sebucare, Ionil, and DHS are effective antidandruff shampoos and should be used strictly according to directions.

◆ When using a dandruff shampoo, leave it on the scalp for at least five minutes to achieve maximum effectiveness. If the dandruff is especially stubborn, cover your head with a shower cap and leave the preparation on for an hour.

◆ Massage the scalp with olive and rosemary oil, and leave on for 20 minutes. Brush out any loose flakes and then shampoo. Wheat germ oil is also thought to be beneficial. When using an oil treatment, put hot towels over the scalp and take a sauna or steam bath

◆ Alternate hot and cold water on the scalp.

◆ Avoid hair products such as moose, gels or hair sprays, which can cause additional flakiness.

◆ P&S liquid, an over-the-counter preparation, can help to remove stubborn crusts and can be used occasionally.

◆ Avoid rinsing your hair with beer or any other alcohol-based liquid as these can further dry out the scalp.

NUTRITIONAL APPROACH:

◆ Avoid a diet high in fats and fried foods

◆ *Zinc:* Important for the synthesis of protein, which comprises the scalp.

◆ *Lecithin:* Strengthens scalp membranes.

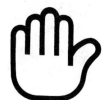

HERBAL REMEDIES:

◆ *Yucca:* Contains natural steroid saponins and can be purchased in health food stores as a soap or shampoo.
◆ *Kelp tablets:* Promote hair growth and help to keep the scalp healthy.
◆ *Soap bark:* Good for cleansing the scalp due to its saponin and anti-inflammatory properties.
◆ *Rosemary:* Helps to control dandruff, especially if psoriasis is the cause.
◆ *Thyme and rosemary rinse:* Make thyme/rosemary tea by steeping 1 heaping tablespoon of dried thyme and dried rosemary in 2 cups of water to which is added 1 tablespoon of apple cider vinegar. Strain the solution, pour it over shampooed hair and do not rinse out. After shampooing rinse.
◆ Shampoos with tea tree oil are also thought to help heal the scalp and promote normal functioning of hair follicles.

PREVENTION:

Taking good care of your scalp by washing the hair often with non-drying shampoos and avoiding hair supplements that contain alcohol can help prevent dandruff.
◆ Don't injure the scalp with excessive scratching or brushing.
◆ Eat a well-balanced diet and avoid saturated fats.

Depression

DEFINITION:

During the first part of the 20th century, depression was considered a rather shameful psychiatric ailment that was placed on the back burner and badly neglected and misunderstood. It has only been recently that depression has been recognized as a legitimate disorder with both psychological and physical components.

Technically, depression is characterized by feelings of sadness, pessimism, a general loss of interest in life, and a sense of worthlessness. If it is severe enough, it becomes a psychiatric illness. The symptoms of depression are perfectly normal responses to certain situations, such as the death of a loved one, a divorce, the loss of a job, etc. Depression becomes a clinical disorder when it persists without an apparent cause and becomes incapacitating.

Depression is more common in women, which suggests that hormonal factors may be of significance. Eighty percent of all suicides are related to depression. The highest rate is among elderly men who have become lonely and isolated, although the rate is increasing in younger segments of the population. Fifteen percent of the population will experience a bout with depression serious enough to require medical attention. According to the DSM-III, a depressed state must persist for at least one month to be technically called depression. Be assured that depression is not a hopeless condition, and can be successfully treated.

CAUSES:

In many cases of depression, there is no identifiable cause. Depression can be triggered by certain physical conditions such as stroke, hepatitis, chronic fatigue syndrome, and post-surgical recoveries. Hypothyroidism, postpartum adjustments, adrenal misfunctions, menopause and in some cases, the use of birth control pills can also cause depression.

Recently a connection between antihistamines and depression has been found. Many depressed patients suffer from a deficiency of norepinephrine or serotonin in their brain chemistry, which can create negative feelings.

In addition, lack of light, especially common in certain work environments and during the winter months, can also create feelings of depression. Social and psychological factors such as dysfunctional families, lack of maternal nurturing, abrupt changes in life-style, the death of a loved one, divorce, and financial struggle can also contribute to depressive illness. Studies suggest that allergies, endometriosis and eating too much sugar may also be linked to depression, although there is no conclusive evidence to support these connections. Elderly people commonly suffer from depression which may be caused by loneliness, isolation or over-medication. There is some evidence to suggest that chemical pollutants are linked to depression. Heredity is a strong factor in predicting depression. Approximately half of all people who suffer from depression have one or both parents who experienced the disorder.

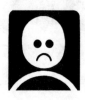

SYMPTOMS:

Physical and psychological: The intensity of symptoms depends on the severity of the depression. Mild depression involves feelings of anxiety or changeable moods and crying for no apparent reason. In more severe cases, one might experience a loss of appetite, colon disorders, difficulty sleeping, loss of interest in what were enjoyable activities, fatigue, lethargy, slow movement and thought or extreme agitation and nervousness.

In severe cases of depression, thoughts or attempts at suicide are common, and delusions or hallucinations can occur. The intensity of symptoms associated with depression can vary with the time of day. Typically, the worst time is the morning. However, as the disease progresses there is no one better time.

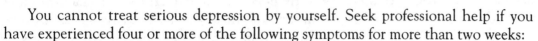

NOTE: Manic-depressive disease is characterized by alternating periods of high elation, and frantic bursts of energy with periods of deep melancholia and lethargy. This particular disorder requires medical attention.

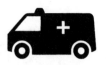

MEDICAL ALERT:

You cannot treat serious depression by yourself. Seek professional help if you have experienced four or more of the following symptoms for more than two weeks:

◆ Persistent sorrow, anxiousness or empty feeling
◆ Feelings of hopelessness or pessimism
◆ Feeling of worthlessness, helplessness or guilt
◆ Lost interest or pleasure in ordinary activities, including sex
◆ Sleep disturbances such as insomnia, oversleeping or waking up too early
◆ Changes in eating patterns-either overeating, or loss of appetite with a weight gain or loss
◆ Fatigue, malaise
◆ Thoughts of suicide or death, or suicide attempt
◆ Restlessness or irritability
◆ Difficulty making decisions, concentrating or remembering facts

NOTE: If you feel suicidal and need support look under "suicide prevention service" or "mental health services" in the phone book for a 24-hour hotline and use it.

STANDARD MEDICAL TREATMENT:

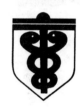

There are three primary forms of treatment for depression:

1. Psychotherapy: This method involves either the individual or a group meeting together for mutual sharing and counseling. This treatment lends itself to depression that is caused by personality adjustments and the inability to cope with life-style challenges. Cognitive therapy, group therapy, and psychoanalysis fall under this category. Often this type of treatment is used in combination with drug therapy.

2. Drug therapy: This treatment involves the use of antidepressant drugs and is recommended for people who are experiencing physical symptoms of depression. Prozac has become the most widely prescribed drug for depression and is the subject of some controversy, although the FDA has concluded that its benefits far outweigh its possible liabilities.

Tricyclic antidepressants such as Sinequan, Ttoranil and Norpramin are also used. Monoamine oxidase (MAO) inhibitors increase the action of certain neurotransmitters (such as Parnate and Nardil). Lithium is used for manic depressive disorders, and chlorpromazine is another antipsychotic drug used to control mood swings.

3. ECT or electroconvulsive therapy involves the administering of mild electrical shock under anesthesia. This treatment is usually reserved for only those suffering from serious depression that have failed to respond to other alternatives. It is considered a safe and effective option. Improvement after a treatment can begin right away. Some physicians feel that ECT is safer and even better than drug therapy. ECT has had a bad reputation in the past; however, its methods of administration and control have greatly improved and it should be investigated. The value of shock therapy in a suicidal individual should not be underestimated.

SIDE-EFFECTS: Prozac (fluoxetine hydrochloride): Anxiety, nervousness, sleeplessness, drowsiness, weakness, tremors, sweating, dizziness, dry mouth, upset stomach, appetite loss, nausea, vomiting, diarrhea, gas, rash, changes in sex drive, increased appetite, acne, hair loss. In addition, virtually every body system has been affected by side-effects too numerous to list here. The most recent and controversial of these have been unexplained acts of aggression, suicidal tendencies and abnormal psychological behavior. The FDA has found Prozac to be safe regardless of the controversy surrounding its widespread use.

SIDE-EFFECTS: ECT: A temporary loss of memory. Anyone who has recently suffered a heart attack should not undergo ECT.

Success rating of standard medical treatment: good. With proper psychological therapy in conjunction with drugs, chances of recovery are good.

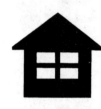

HOME SELF-CARE:

◆ Regular exercise is a very good way to counteract depression. During exercise, the brain releases endorphins, which can help promote a sense of well-being. Studies suggest that depression is more common in less active people. Taking a regular brisk walk can be extremely helpful for people suffering from depression.

◆ Get plenty of rest. Just being tired or fatigued can create feelings of depression.

◆ Share your feelings with friends, a counselor or a self-help group. Force yourself to get involved no matter how much you might resist. Make sure you place yourself in environments where you will make friends.

◆ If confronted with a seemingly impossible dilemma, share it with someone who can give you a fresh and objective point of view.

◆ Try meditating through yoga or biofeedback, and use relaxation techniques such as music tapes or rhythmic breathing to alleviate tension and stress.

◆ Avoid eating or shopping binges, which will only serve to compound the problem.

◆ Pursue an artistic endeavor such as painting, sculpting, crafts, etc.

◆ Read an uplifting book.

◆ Learn to laugh and don't take yourself or others too seriously. Life is too short to waste on negative thinking. There are places to go and people to see!

◆ Don't listen to depressing music, which can intensify feelings of sadness or loneliness. Get out of the house and let the therapeutic beauties of nature lift your spirits.

◆ Join a church. Spiritual food can provide sustenance for a heavy heart. A famous author once said that human beings can never be truly happy until they have discovered their spirituality and their relationship with a loving God.

◆ Take a vacation.

◆ Sign up to volunteer in some service-related activity such as tutoring children in math or teaching adults to read. Make it a personal goal to try to do something good for someone at least once a day no matter how insignificant that act may be, and then give yourself credit for accomplishing the task.

◆ Make sure you have adequate exposure to sunlight. Open your blinds, and go for walks. Improve the artificial lighting of your environment if natural light is unavailable.

◆ Treat yourself to a regular professional massage. A good massage can create a sense of well-being and invigoration.

◆ Get off any unnecessary medication. Some drugs that can cause depression are corticosteroids, high blood pressure medications, sedatives such as Valium, oral contraceptives, glaucoma drugs and some antihistamines.

NUTRITIONAL APPROACH:

Recently, there has been more emphasis placed on the connection between state of mind and diet. Some organic factors can create depression such as hypoglycemia, alcohol, caffeine, and nicotine, etc. and should be considered in designing a strategy for treating the disease. There is no question that the foods we eat greatly influence the chemistry of the brain. Carbohydrates have been found to calm the brain, while protein can increase levels of alertness. Complex carbohydrates raise the level of tryptophan in the brain, which can produce relaxation. Make sure your diet is adequate in complex carbohydrates. A diet too low in these can cause a depletion of serotonin levels, which may increase depression

◆ Emphasize foods such as whole grains, turkey breast, fish, beans, fresh fruits and vegetables.

◆ Avoid empty calories that can produce drastic sugar swings in the bloodstream and stay away from caffeine, which artificially induces energy, followed by a let-down.

◆ B complex is essential to proper brain function, especially vitamin B12. Check with your doctor for dosages and look into vitamin B injections if necessary.

◆ Don't smoke or drink. Alcohol is a sedative and can create feelings of depression rather than mask them.

◆ *Vitamin C:* Involved in the synthesis of neurotransmitters in the brain.

◆ *L-tyrosine:* Combined with vitamin B6 can promote positive moods and create motivation. Amino acid dosages should be determined by a physician.

◆ *Choline, inositol and lecithin:* Important for the normal functioning of the brain.

◆ *Niacin:* Promotes good circulation in the blood vessels of the brain.

◆ *Pyridoxine, Vitamin B6:* Some people using oral contraceptives as well as experiencing depression have been lacking in this compound.

◆ *Calcium and magnesium:* Have a calming effect on the system. Studies have discovered that magnesium levels are low in depressed individuals and rise after recovery.

◆ *Folic acid*: Studies have indicated that a lack of folic acid may predispose one to mental illness.

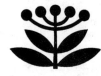

Herbal remedies:

◆ *Oats*: Considered a natural antidepressant.
◆ *Ginkgo*: Stimulates brain function.
◆ *Gotu kola*: Considered brain food and helps to combat mental fatigue associated with depression.
◆ *Dong quai*: Helps to tranquilize the nerves.
◆ *Borage*: Helps restore the adrenal cortex and has antidepressant properties.
◆ *Basil*: A traditional herbal antidepressant.
◆ *Skullcap and hops*: Have a natural sedating effect without the side-effecta of prescription drugs.
◆ *Suma*: Increases oxygen supply to brain cells.
◆ *St John's Wort*: Historically used as a mood elevator and can help to relieve insomnia.
◆ *Damiana*: Stimulates the nervous system, which helps to elevate moods.
◆ *The following herbs in combination may be useful*: Valerian, mistletoe, wood betony, black cohosh, ginger and capsicum.

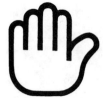

Prevention:

◆ Depression is a normal part of living and cannot be altogether avoided, however certain life-styles seem to lessen the chance of depression becoming a full-blown psychiatric illness.
◆ Exercising regularly seems to be the most important factor. Exercise, in conjunction with a nutritious diet cannot be overestimated in its importance as a deterrent to depression.
◆ Keeping busy, joining community groups, and clubs, involvement in creative hobbies, and sharing feelings can also help avoid a depressed state.
◆ Avoiding alcohol, caffeine and nicotine is crucial to keeping mentally healthy.
◆ Do not use antihistamines or any other unnecessary drugs. Often, depression is linked to certain medications, both prescription and over-the-counter. Review what you are taking into your body and consult your physician to see what can be eliminated or decreased.
◆ Keep yourself spiritually focused. Find meaning in your life that transcends the physical world. Surround yourself with good music, good books, uplifting art and learn to glean joy from the beauties of nature.
◆ Involve yourself in serving others. Uplifting someone else can work as a marvelous antidepressant.

Diabetes

DEFINITION:

It's hard to believe that a sweet, seemingly harmless substance like sugar could act as a poison to thousands of people. To anyone suffering from diabetes, elevated sugar levels in the blood means trouble. The disease called diabetes mellitus results from insufficient levels of insulin produced by the pancreas, which causes high blood sugar levels. Insulin enables cells to absorb sugar; consequently, when it is low, sugar remains in the bloodstream, causing the symptoms of diabetes. Excess sugar in the bloodstream can cause all kinds of problems such as nerve damage, vision loss, infections, kidney and heart aliments.

Diabetes is an ancient disease and was described in Egyptian writings as early as 1500 BC. Diabetes is the most common endocrine disease and affects approximately 11 million Americans.

There are two types of diabetes mellitus: insulin dependent (type I), also called juvenile diabetes, which is the more severe; and non-insulin dependent (type II), also called adult-onset diabetes. Type I usually appears in people under 35, most commonly between the ages of 10 and 16. It affects young boys and men in particular. Its onset is rapid and is due to the destruction of the insulin-producing cells of the pancreas. It will often appear after some kind of trauma to the body, such as a fracture.

Type II diabetes affects an estimated 5.5 million Americans. In type II diabetes, the pancreas produces insulin; however, a lack of chemical receptors located on the cells causes sugar to remain in the bloodstream. People who suffer from this type of diabetes are usually overweight. Middle-aged and elderly women are particularly susceptible. Two out of five people that suffer from type II diabetes are unaware they have the disease. Frequently, just losing weight in type II diabetes can resolve the problem.

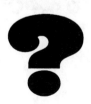

CAUSES:

Heredity plays a major role in the incidence of type I and type II diabetes. Not everyone who carries the genes responsible for type I diabetes will develop it. Another possible cause of diabetes is an immune response following a viral infection, such as the flu, chicken pox, or a bad cold, which results in the destruction of pancreatic cells. A small percentage of pregnant women develop diabetes.

Type II diabetes is directly related to obesity. Lack of insulin is not the problem in type II diabetes, but rather a lack of insulin receptors. Often with a weight loss as low as 10 to 15 pounds, the symptoms of type II diabetes can be controlled. Either

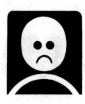

form of diabetes can be brought on by other diseases such as acromegaly, hyperthyroidism, Cushing's syndrome and pancreatitis. One form of diabetes is directly related to stress and can disappear once the stress is resolved.

SYMPTOMS:

Physical: Symptoms of type I diabetes, which usually develop rapidly, are: frequent urination (white spots may appear on underpants indicting dried splashes of glucose filled urine), excessive thirst and appetite (drinking sweetened fluids increases urination and makes symptoms worse); dry mouth; blurred vision; and reduced resistance to infection. In addition, urinary infections, impotence, the absence of menstrual periods, boils, and tingling in hands and feet may occur. Weight loss, fatigue, apathy, leg cramps and mood swings are also common.

A fruity sweet, acidic smelling breath indicates a condition known as ketosis. If untreated at this point, a diabetic coma and death can occur.

In type II diabetes a lack of symptoms is common. The symptoms of type II diabetes may not develop until years after the onset of the disease. Frequently, people suffering from type II diabetes are unaware of any unusual symptoms.

Psychological: Because type I diabetes is a lifelong incurable disease, it carries with it the potential for serious emotional effects on not only the patient, but on close family and friends as well. Feelings of anger, depression, anxiety, and frustration are common reactions to the day-to-day stress of diabetes. In addition, poorly controlled sugar levels can produce negative responses such as mood swings and irritability. Once again, avoiding drastic changes in blood sugar levels helps to counteract these psychological problems. Family and friends should be aware of the profound emotional impact that diabetes can have.

COMPLICATIONS OF DIABETES:

MEDICAL ALERT:

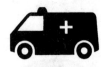

There are three complications that can be potentially dangerous for a diabetic. They are hyperglycemia (too much blood sugar), hypoglycemia (too little blood sugar), and the higher risk of infection with wounds.

Warning: Any diabetic who is experiencing the following symptoms requires immediate medical attention:

- ◆ Blood sugar levels above 200 milligrams
- ◆ Temperature above 101
- ◆ Vomiting or abdominal cramps
- ◆ Large amounts of sugar and acetone in the urine

Symptoms of hyperglycemia: This condition indicates that there is too much sugar in the blood and insulin is needed. It is characterized by excessive urination, blurred vision, dizziness, excess thirst or increased appetite. Often blood glucose can be high and no symptoms will be noticeable. More severe symptoms include stomach cramps, loss of appetite, nausea, vomiting, fatigue, deep, rapid breathing, acidic sweet breath, dehydration and unconsciousness. Seek medical attention immediately.

Symptoms of hypoglycemia: This condition occurs when there is not enough sugar in the blood and insulin levels are too high. If severe enough it can produce insulin shock. Symptoms include headache, confusion, aggressive behavior, cold clammy feeling, excessive sweating, paleness, impaired vision, trembling, rapid heartbeat, drowsiness, and possible unconsciousness. This condition requires immediate medical attention. If you feel only mild symptoms of low blood sugar follow the suggestions listed in the self-help section to raise blood sugar levels quickly. If this condition occurs frequently, your insulin levels may need adjusting. Contact your doctor.

Another complication of diabetes is the risk of wound infection, particularly if located on the feet and legs. Any wound needs immediate medical attention.

Note: If you have diabetes it is crucial that you take very good care of yourself so as to avoid complications of the disease, which are difficult to manage medically.

Other complications of diabetes include: Uurinary tract infections, vaginal yeast infections, thrush, skin infections, vision impairment, increased risk for heart disease, high blood pressure and stroke, and special pregnancy considerations. Any illness may increase the amount of insulin needed.

STANDARD MEDICAL TREATMENT:

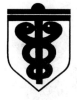

The goal of medical treatment in diabetes is to relieve symptoms, prevent complications and prolong life. The main objective sought by your doctor is to keep the level of blood glucose as near to normal as possible. Usually a glucose tolerance test is administered to measure the body's reaction to sugar. If diabetes is diagnosed, the maintenance of an optimal level of blood sugar will be the goal. This is achieved through weight control, regular exercise, and good dietary management.

For those suffering from type I diabetes, regular self-administered injections of insulin one to four times a day is required. Some patients wear insulin pumps. These are portable computerized units that administer constant amounts of insulin into the blood-stream via a needle and catheter. Not everyone can use this device and its potential should be discussed with your physician.

The development of inhalable insulin and oral insulin is still in the experimental stage. Insulin is available in a variety of types and strengths. It is obtained from either an animal source, or a human type is genetically engineered.

Your physician will help you to plan a diet in which carbohydrate intake is regulated to avoid marked levels of glucose fluctuations. You may also be encouraged to check your sugar level with a blood test obtained by pricking your finger, rather than a urine test. Your doctor will want to check your blood glucose at regular intervals and you will be given a urine-testing kit. In type II diabetes, hypoglycemic tablets may be indicated which lower blood sugar levels. These fall into two categories: sulfonylureal agents and diguanides (Phenformin).

NOTE: A positive glucose tolerance test does not always mean that diabetes is present.

SIDE-EFFECTS: Insulin injections for type I diabetes: humulin, novolin, velosulin, lente iletin, ultralente, semilente, isophane, mixtard, protamine. Insulin injections must be administered as prescribed. Possible side-effects are an allergic reaction, drug interactions with a number of medications, and hypoglycemia.

SIDE-EFFECTS: Oral hypoglycemic drugs used in typeII diabetes.

Acetohexamide: (Dymelor) chlropropamide; (Diabinese) glipizide; (Glucotrol), glyburide; (Micronase) tolazamide; (Tolinase) tolbutamide; (Oorinase): Loss of appetite, nausea, vomiting, weakness, heartburn and tingling hands and feet. For an overweight diabetic it is far better to lose weight than to try to maintain normal blood sugar through the above drugs.

Warning: None of the above drugs should be taken by pregnant or nursing women. These drugs can also interact with a number of other drugs. Always check with your doctor taking any other medication.

Success rating of standard medical treatment: very good. While diabetes is currently incurable, medical science offers the diabetic the promise of a fairly normal life. Avoiding complications of diabetes is vital. Medical treatment for complications is much less effective.

MEDICAL UPDATE:

◆ Insulin injections may soon be a thing of the past. Recent studies of aerosol doses of insulin administered with a nebulizer have had very encouraging results. The April 28th issue of the Journal of the American Medical Association reported that insulin levels rose faster with the aerosol than by injection. This new product is scheduled for release in approximately five years and opens up new possibilities for a variety of other disease treatments.

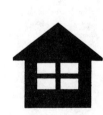

HOME SELF CARE:

◆ Treatment for mild hypoglycemia: This condition requires the ingesting of a simple sugar as quickly as possible. Take some orange juice, sugared soda pop, candy or fruit. In the case of severe hypoglycemia or insulin shock, an injection of glucagon is required. If unconsciousness results and glucagon is not available, put honey, sugar, or any kind of sweetened syrup under the person's tongue.

◆ Check your blood sugar with chemically treated strips available at any pharmacy through a finger prick test. A new device called a glucometer from Miles Laboratories makes this test easier and gives immediate results.

◆ An exercise program is vitally important for anyone suffering from diabetes. Diabetics who are physically fit seem to increase their sensitivity to insulin and therefore require less. A physician should be consulted in planning what is an appropriate level of exercise. A 45-minute walk per day is usually recommended and can significantly cut your insulin requirement. After getting your doctor's approval, make that walk a routine and try to do it at the same time each day.

◆ Be very attentive to your feet and legs. Often foot injury may not be noticed because of nerve damage resulting from diabetes. Even a small sore requires medical attention. Wear shoes that are designed to fit your foot with good support and socks that are well-cushioned. Do not cut your toenails too short.

◆ Take immaculate care of your mouth and teeth. Brush often, floss and visit your dentist regularly. Diabetics are more prone to gum infections.

◆ Protect your eyes: One of the most serious complications of diabetes is eye disease, where small blood vessels in the eye rupture and leak. Sometimes, these vessels migrate in front of the retina and can cause of impaired vision. Detecting the first signs of this damage is crucial. Diabetics should have their eyes examined at least once a year. Laser treatments may help to minimize retinal damage from these vessels.

◆ Protect your kidneys: Watch for protein in the urine which may indicate that kidney malfunction is present. Monitor your urine for protein and see your doctor if any is present.

◆ Avoid the use of oral contraceptives unless recommended by your doctor. Because diabetes increases the risk of coronary artery disease, oral contraceptives are discouraged.

◆ Avoid over-the-counter drugs which contain sugar and other ingredients that interfere with blood sugar levels such as aspirin in large doses, caffeine, ephedrine or epinephrine and phenylephrine, commonly found in cold preparations and nasal sprays.

◆ Do not smoke: Smoking increases the risk of heart disease.

◆ Wear a medical alert ID bracelet and keep a diabetic ID card with you at all times.

◆ Rotate your injection sites.

◆ Make sure to inform your dentist and other heath care professionals that you are a diabetic.

◆ If you have suffered any other illness, your need for insulin may increase, even if you have stopped eating. Contact your doctor whenever you get sick and monitor your sugar levels carefully.

NUTRITIONAL FACTORS:

Diabetes has been linked to life-style habits typical of Western culture. While a hereditary predisposition to diabetes is important in determining susceptibility, environment and diet are significant factors in its development. The typical

American diet, which is high in refined carbohydrates and notoriously low in fiber, is believed to contribute to the incidence of diabetes.

Obesity is another factor that increases the chances of developing the disease. The proper management of diet is crucial for the diabetic. The American Diabetic Association recommends that anyone with type II diabetes eat a diet that is up to 60 percent carbohydrates.

◆ Avoid an excess consumption of animal protein. Try to get your protein from vegetable sources like beans.

◆ Avoid alcohol, which can significantly raise blood sugar.

◆ Avoid all refined sugars. If you have a sweet tooth, eat fruit instead.

◆ Eat a diet low in fats and high in complex carbohydrates and fiber. The ADA recommends 40 grams of fiber per day. Fiber can be found in whole grains, legumes, vegetables and fruits. Fiber also lowers cholesterol levels, which is very desirable for diabetics. Research has shown that fiber plays a vital role in regulating blood sugar levels and glucose tolerance.

◆ Keep your weight down. For overweight diabetics, weight loss is a high priority. Obesity is the number one cause of type II diabetes. Obesity can decrease the number of insulin receptors in the body, aggravating diabetes. Frequently, just by losing weight, type II diabetes will be resolved.

◆ Eating smaller meals throughout the day may be preferable to three large meals. Experiment and see what works to keep blood sugar as stable as possible.

◆ Watch your carbohydrate intake at breakfast. Some studies have shown that insulin resistance is greater in the morning. Whole wheat toast, cottage cheese and poached eggs (in moderation) are recommended.

◆ If you plan to engage in a strenuous activity, your doctor may recommend that you eat an extra large meal beforehand to avoid a drastic drop in blood sugar.

◆ *Acidophilus:* Also helps to decrease risk for yeast infections by keeping intestinal flora at normal levels.

◆ *Chromium:* Significant evidence supports the fact that chromium levels can help determine insulin sensitivity. Chromium can be taken as a supplement. There is some evidence that chromium may actually help prevent type II diabetes. The American diet is notoriously low in chromium.

◆ *Pyridoxine:* Important in preventing complications arising from diabetes.

◆ *Thiamine:* Plays an important role in sugar metabolism.

◆ *Vitamin C:* Because the transport of vitamin C into cells is linked with insulin levels, it is assumed that some diabetics may suffer from a vitamin C deficiency.

◆ *Vitamin E:* Important in helping prevent future complications from diabetes. Diabetics appear to have an increased requirement for this vitamin

◆ *Manganese:* Diabetics sometimes show lower than normal levels of this mineral, which can further complicate diabetic symptoms.

◆ *Magnesium:* This supplement is extremely important to diabetics, due to its possible prevention of retinopathy.

- *Onion and garlic:* Both of these in specific studies have significantly reduced blood sugar.
- *Carnatine:* Studies have indicated that carnatine supplementation can result in the improved breakdown of fatty acids, which may play a role in preventing diabetic ketoacidosis.
- *Zinc:* Some research suggests that a zinc deficiency may play a role in the development of diabetes. Zinc is important to insulin metabolism. Additional studies indicate that diabetics lose too much zinc through the urine.
- *Potassium:* Helps promote insulin sensitivity. Artificial insulin can result in a potassium deficiency.
- *Biotin:* A B vitamin that can help improve glucose metabolism.
- *Calcium:* Important in maintaining proper pH balance.
- Avoid using fish oils, salt, and white flour products. Ingesting these causes an elevation of blood sugar.

Note: Do not take abnormally high dosages of vitamin C or B1, as these can inhibit the action of insulin

HERBAL REMEDIES:

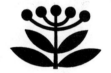

Note: Insulin-dependent diabetics are unlikely to be able to get off insulin completely. The following herbal recommendations may help to reduce their insulin requirement.

- *Pterocarpus marsupium:* Used in India for centuries for the treatment of diabetes, this herb is believed to directly benefit damaged pancreatic cells.
- *Huckleberry:* Helps promote insulin production.
- *Bilberry:* Can help to increase insulin production.
- *Cinnamon and tumeric:* Are used in Pakistan and China to boost the ability of insulin to metabolize glucose.
- *Garlic:* Helps to fight yeast infections. Diabetics are especially prone to Candida due to the high sugar environment of their blood.
- *Ginseng tea:* Is believed to help lower blood sugar levels.
- *Fenugreek:* Helps to reduce blood levels of glucose.
- *Blueberry leaves:* Used as traditional folk medicine for diabetes. Acts like a mild form of insulin and can significantly lower blood sugar levels under certain conditions. Anthocyanic acid, which is blueberry extract, can be purchased at some health food stores.
- *Goats's rue:* Boosts cells in the pancreas responsible for insulin production
- *The following herbs in combination may be useful:* Licorice root, golden seal, mullein, uva ursi, cedar berries and capsicum.

PREVENTION:

- Don't become overweight. Any overweight adult is susceptible to type II diabetes. Eat a diet low in fat and high in fiber and exercise regularly. Stay away from refined white flour and white sugar products and avoid alcohol.

◆ Do not consume large amounts of unrefined sugars. Studies suggest that people suffering from adult-onset diabetes have a dulled sense of what is sweet and therefore require more sugar.

◆ Supplement your diet with chromium, which is believed to help prevent the onset of type II diabetes.

◆ Harvard University researchers have found that vigorous exercise can significantly reduce the risk of adult-onset diabetes by about one-third. Exercise is considered the most effective preventative measure for adult or non-insulin dependent diabetes.

American Diabetes Association
1660 Duke Street
Alexandria, VA 22314
703-549-1500

Juvenile Diabetes Foundation
60 Madison Avenue
New York, NY 10010-1550
212-889-7575

Diarrhea

DEFINITION:

Diarrhea can often strike without warning and gives the notion of "nature calling" a whole new meaning. Getting a bad case of "the runs" can make you do just that—for the nearest bathroom facility. Having diarrhea can also make you feel just plain lousy, and while it's of little comfort during your seige, diarrhea will usually resolve itself.

Diarrhea is a common ailment characterized by the increased frequency, or fluidity of bowel movements. Diarrhea is not considered a disorder in itself but is, rather, a symptom of another physiological problem. Diarrhea affects everyone occasionally and usually clears up within a couple of days without treatment. Chronic diarrhea may indicate the presence of a serious intestinal condition. Diarrhea in babies, small children and the elderly is more serious than in adults due to the risk of dehydration.

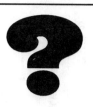

CAUSES:

Diarrhea occurs when too much water is passed along with the stool during a bowel movement due to decreased absorption in the intestinal tract walls. The most common cause of diarrhea is eating contaminated food or drinking impure water. Food poisoning causes diarrhea to begin within six hours of eating and usually indicates the presence of staphylococcus or clostridium bacteria in the food. When diarrhea occurs 12 to 48 hours after eating, salmonella or campylobacer bacteria may be involved.

The presence of the Norwalk virus can also cause diarrhea. Gastroenteritis, food allergies, typhoid, drug toxicity, ameobic dysentery and shigellosis can also cause cases of acute diarrhea. Chronic diarrhea, which commonly occurs as random attacks of loose stools, can be brought on by Crohn's disease, colitis, diverticulosis, colon cancer, irritable bowel syndrome and emotional anxiety.

Diarrhea can also be the result of the incomplete digestion of certain foods, overuse of laxatives, antacids, intolerance to caffeine, excessive consumption of fruit or of green fruit or rancid foods. Infant diarrhea commonly results from viral infections. Breast-fed babies are less likely to contract these infections. A intolerance to cow's milk may also cause infant diarrhea.

SYMPTOMS:

Physical: Adult diarrhea is characterized by runny stools, cramping, gas, nausea, weakness, cold sweats, increased frequency of bowel movements, thirst, abdominal pain, vomiting and sometimes a fever. The unusual loss of fluids through the bowel can lead to dehydration and loss of electrolytes (minerals).

Psychological: Nervous diarrhea is brought on during periods of high emotional stress. Psychological counseling centered on biofeedback or relaxation techniques may help to control this type of diarrhea.

MEDICAL ALERT:

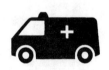

See your doctor immediately if there is blood in the stools, the stool appears unusually dark(some medications which contain bismuth subsalicylate such as Pepto-Bismol or iron may turn the stool black), severe abdominal or rectal pain, if urination has stopped, if you have a fever above 101 or if the diarrhea lasts more than two days. If an infant shows any of the following signs of dehydration, seek medical attention immediately: glazed eyes, sunken eyes, unresponsiveness, dry, sticky tongue, depressed fontanelle at upper front part of the head, loose skin, or drowsiness. Any infant diarrhea that does not stop within 48 hours should be investigated by a doctor.

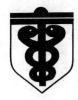

STANDARD MEDICAL TREATMENT:

Water and minerals lost during severe diarrhea need to be replenished. Your doctor may suggest a product such as Pedialyte, Resol, or Lytren for infants and small children. For adults, electrolyte mixtures such as Gatorade may be recommended. Antidiarrheal drugs may be required; however, they should not be taken to treat diarrhea that results from infection, as these medications may prolong the illness.

If the diarrhea persists, your physician may require a stool culture, a barium x-ray, sigmoidoscopy or biopsy of the rectum. Your physician may recommend over-the counter remedies such as Imodium which causes the bowel to tighten up. Other products such as Pepto-Bismol and Kaopectate may be effective if the diarrhea is not too severe.

Dyphenoxylate may be used by your doctor if symptoms are more persistent. Narcotic preparations such as Paregoric, Parepectolin or Parelixir may be prescribed for adults. Lomotil, a narcotic-like preparation, may also decrease the frequency of bowel movements in adults. If dehydration is severe enough, intravenous fluids may be administered either at the doctor's office or in the hospital.

SIDE-EFFECTS: Iimmodium (loperamide): Side-effects with Immodium are few. Some known side-effects are abdominal pain, bloating, constipation, dryness of mouth, dizziness, and rash. An inability to concentrate and fatigue are also associated with this drug.

Do not take this drug without your doctor's approval if pregnant or nursing.

SIDE-EFFECTS: Difenoxin (motofen): Nausea, vomiting, dry mouth, dizziness, light-headedness, drowsiness, fatigue, headache.

Warning: Nursing mothers should not nurse while taking this drug. Pregnant women should only take this with their doctor's approval.

SIDE-EFFECTS: Lomotil: Dryness of skin, mouth, nose, redness of the face, fever, unusual heart rates, drowsiness, inability to urinate. Less common symptoms: abdominal discomforts, swollen gums, numbness in the extremities, nausea, vomiting, and dizziness.

Do not take this drug without your doctor's approval if pregnant or nursing.

SIDE-EFFECTS: Paregoric: The incidence of side-effects is low. Known side-effects are nausea, upset stomach, light-headedness, dizziness, sedation. Paregoric is a narcotic drug that should not be taken with sleeping pills, alcohol, or tranquilizers.

Pregnant women and nursing mothers should only take this with their doctor's approval. Addiction and withdrawal are possible side-effects.

Success rating of standard medical treatment: good. Most of the above preparations can significantly help to control diarrhea. Intravenous fluid administration can prevent dehydration in small children and infants, a common fatal complication of diarrhea at the turn of the century.

HOME SELF-CARE:

◆ If an electrolyte fluid is not available, sugar and salt can be added to water. (One teaspoon of sugar and a pinch of salt to 1 quart of water). Measure the salt accurately. An excess of salt can cause additional dehydration.

◆ Another good fluid replacement can be made from mixing 1/2 teaspoon of honey and a pinch of salt in 8 ounces of a clear fruit juice.

◆ Over-the-counter drugs such as antacids, antibiotics, and quinidine can cause diarrhea. In addition, some non-steroidal anti-inflammatory drugs such as Meclomen, some blood pressure medications, gold compounds and digitalis may also cause diarrhea. If you are undergoing cancer treatment, diarrhea can ba a common side-effect. Check with your physician to see if anything you might be taking could be the cause.

◆ Adding a teaspoon of sugar to juice or water enables the intestines to absorb more of the water content.

◆ Antidiarrhea medications like Pepto-Bismol can actully prolong certain types of food poisoning like salmonella by slowing the speed in which the food moves through the intestines. The general rule is if you have a fever, don't take the pink stuff.

NUTRITIONAL APPROACH:

◆ Avoid all dairy products, and limit intake of fats and wheat. Do not consume alcohol, caffeine, or artificial sweeteners.

◆ A traditional remedy for diarrhea is to sip a drink made from equal parts of tomato and sauerkraut juice.

◆ Cabbage juice has been used for generations to help in the healing of intestinal lesions.

◆ Rice water made by steeping rice helps to form the stool and supplies B vitamins. Brown rice is preferable. Blackberry juice may be added to the strained rice water.

◆ A clear diet which consists of broths, apple juice, Jello, etc. is recommended to give the bowel a rest. Avoid carbonated beverages or make them go flat by shaking them. Drink plenty of fluid. Use popsicles, iced fruit bars, or flat sodas to encourage children to increase their fluid intake.

◆ Avoid citrus juice, which is too pulpy and irritating.

◆ Foods which can be consumed by children or adults suffering from diarrhea are rice cereal, bananas, applesauce, mashed cooked carrots, active culture yogurt, plain dry crackers, and steamed chicken without the skin.

◆ Carrot soup is an old remedy especially good for children suffering from diarrhea.

◆ *Potassium:* potassium is lost in watery stools and needs to be replaced. Calcium, magnesium and zinc should also be replenished.

◆ *Acidophilus:* Replaces friendly bacteria in the intestinal flora, which helps to solidify stool and fight infection.
◆ *Guar gum:* Helps in forming stool.
◆ *Pectin:* Forms a gel when mixed with water and helps in forming the stool
◆ *Carob powder:* Helps to normalize the bowels.

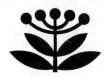

HERBAL REMEDIES:

◆ *Slippery elm:* May be taken by capsule or mixed into mashed bananas or applesauce.
◆ *Red raspberry tea:* Another old traditional treatment for diarrhea.
◆ *Garlic:* Can help kill any bacterial or viral infection that may be causing diarrhea.
◆ *Golden seal:* Contains berberine, which helps to control acute diarrhea brought on by intestinal bacterial infections.
◆ *Marshmallow root:* Soothes the mucous membranes of the lower intestinal tract
◆ *Dill:* A favorite herb among American folk healers. Dill water inhibits the growth of intestinal bacteria.
◆ *Ginger:* Weak ginger tea helps to settle the stomach and soothe the bowels.
◆ *Agrimony:* Helps heal the intestinal tract and soothes inflammation.
◆ *Echinacea:* An antibacterial herb that also boosts the immune system.
◆ *Comfrey:* Has anti-inflammatory properties which help promote tissue healing.
◆ *Poke root:* Helps to heal ulcers found in the intestinal mucosa.
◆ *Catnip tea:* Herbal remedy recommended for children due to its mildness.
   The following herbs in combination may be useful: Comfrey, marshmallow, slippery elm, ginger, wild yam and lobelia.

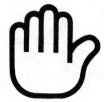

PREVENTION:

When traveling drink only bottle or canned beverages. Don't use ice unless you make it yourself from bottled water. Stay away from raw food. Cook all foods thoroughly and peel all local fruits. Don't drink out of any mountain stream or natural water supply no matter how clean it looks. Often pure looking water supplies are contaminated by bacteria.
◆ Use good hygiene when preparing food. Wash hands frequently; keep dishes, glasses and silverware well cleaned. Disinfect areas where bacteria can grow.
◆ Avoid using wood cutting boards, which can harbor bacteria.
◆ Refrigerate foods immediately after eating. Don't let leftovers sit out, especially foods containing dairy products.
◆ Make sure that hamburger, poultry, and pork are cooked all the way through.
◆ Do not let foods such as salad greens become contaminated by coming in contact with raw poultry, pork or other meats.

- Eating dill has long been accepted in folk medicine as a way to prevent diarrhea. It is believed to kill intestinal bacteria that cause diarrhea.

To prevent infant diarrhea:

- Breast feed instead of bottle feed your baby if possible.
- Do not introduce dairy products, citrus fruits or wheat into you baby's diet too early.
- Wash your hands with soap and water after each diaper change.
- Try not to overuse antibiotics, as these can cause chronic diarrhea .

Earache

DEFINITION:

Having an earache is a miserable experience, and for children it can cause a significant amount of pain and distress, especially during the nighttime hours. Typical earaches result when the eustachian tube, which runs from the back of the throat to the eardrum, becomes congested.

Middle ear infections, also known as otitis media, are the most common kind of earache. Earaches affect 20 to 40 percent of children under the age of 6 and are the most frequently diagnosed childhood disorder. An estimated 30 million doctor's office visits per year are for middle ear infections. Most children will outgrow their tendency for ear infections by age 3.

An earache can be characterized by a dull, throbbing or stabbing pain in the ear. Middle ear infections can cause the eardrum to burst, which causes a discharge of fluid and an immediate sense of relief caused by fluid pressure. A perforated eardrum should always be examined by a doctor, although it will usually heal on its own. Higher altitudes and cold climates seem to increase the risk of ear infections.

CAUSES:

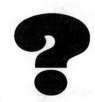

There are three main conditions which can cause an earache: infections of the external ear, referring to the canal which leads to the eardrum; infections of the middle ear, which is the area beyond the eardrum; and a blockage of the eustachian tube, which usually causes both ears to hurt.

Middle ear infections, which constitute the most common kind of earache, are usually brought on by abnormal eustachian tube function. This tube clears fluid from the middle ear and regulates pressure. In infants and small children, it is much smaller in diameter and can easily become blocked. Once an obstruction is present, fluid will build up in the tube, providing an excellent environment for bacterial growth.

The organisms most commonly responsible for ear infections are the streptococcus pneumonia and the hemophilus influenza. Occasionally, a viral infection may be present in the inner ear. Conditions that can cause a blockage of the eustachian tube are weak tissue support around the tube causing it to collapse, an abnormal opening to the tube, and chronic allergies or infections.

Bottle feeding has been linked to the incidence of ear infections in babies, which illustrates the advantage of the built in immunity contained in breast milk. Allergies to cow's milk can be avoided by breast feeding.

Swimmer's ear, which only affects the canal in front of the ear drum is caused when water becomes trapped in the ear canal and breaks down the skin lining. As a result, bacterial infection can breed. The decompression that can occur in air travel can also trigger an earache. In addition, childhood diseases such as measles, chicken pox, and throat infections can also cause earaches. Contamination of the middle ear can also occur during vigorous nose blowing, sneezing, or when the nose is plugged. Earaches usually clear up within three to five days.

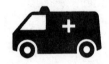

SYMPTOMS:

Physical: External ear infections can cause itching, burning pain, and discharge. Middle ear infections can cause earache (sharp, dull, throbbing or stabbing pain), fever, chills, irritability, red, swollen eardrum, hearing loss, vertigo, nausea, buzzing or ringing sounds and a blocked sensation. In babies, agitation, pulling at the ear and sleeplessness may be present.

MEDICAL ALERT:

An ear infection can be a serious medical condition. Anyone with the above symptoms should see their physician immediately. An untreated middle ear infection can lead to hearing loss or deafness, mastoiditis (an infection of the bone behind the ear), or a brain abscess. Treatment with antibiotics makes these complications rare. A viral infection of the inner ear may lead to labyrinthitis, which causes severe vertigo and sudden hearing loss.

Note: Permanent hearing loss is a rare occurrence with common ear infections.

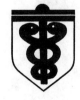

STANDARD MEDICAL TREATMENT:

Oral antibiotics are the primary method used by physicians to treat an earache. Amoxicillin is usually the drug chosen because it specifically targets the bacteria commonly involved. Amoxicillin is a form of penicillin. If an allergy to penicillin exists, trimethoprim-sulfamethoxazole (Bactrim, Septra) can be prescribed.

Antibiotic therapy usually lasts for 10 to 14 days.

Occasionally some doctors recommend a decongestant, assuming that it may help relieve any congestion which has blocked the eustachian tube. When the pain of an earache is particularly severe, anesthetic eardrops may also be prescribed. Antibiotic eardrops are used to treat infections of the external ear. Frequently, this type of ear infection will clear up with drops only; however, oral antibiotics are usually prescribed anyway. Pain killers like Tylenol are also commonly recommended by doctors for earaches.

A myringotomy, which involves placing tiny tubes through the eardrum to increase fluid drainage from the eustachian tube, has become a popular form of treatment for children with chronic ear infections. Recently this procedure has created some controversy in that some investigation has disclosed that up to 50 percent of myringotomies are unnecessary. Furthermore, controversy exists as to whether the existence of these tubes may, increase susceptibility to ear infection.

Success rating of standard medical treatment: fair to good. While the use of antibiotics has been very effective in clearing up the majority of ear infections, new strains of bacteria that appear to be resistant to present antibiotics require new antibiotics like Augementin, designed to destroy the b-cat bacterium. Some studies suggest that the majority of earaches will resolve themselves within three days. The incidence of chronic middle ear disease in children has actually increased since the advent of antibiotics. While antibiotics may be required, they should be used judiciously. The effectiveness of putting tubes in the ears should also be discussed with your doctor.

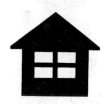

HOME SELF-CARE:

Warning: No type of eardrop should be used if a ruptured eardrum is suspected. See your physician.

◆ Apply heat locally as a hot moist pack to the outer ear. A warm towel soaked in chamomile tea and placed behind the ear can help with pain. Resoak and use as often as needed.

◆ A hot water bottle wrapped in a towel can also be used on the ear. Heating pads can also be used.

◆ Placing hygroscopic anhydrous glycerine into the ear can help draw out fluids and reduce pressure.

◆ Ear drops can be warmed prior to using by placing the bottle in a cup of hot water.

◆ Garlic oil drops placed in the ear can help to fight any infection present. Use an eyedropper to apply oil.

◆ If you have swimmer's ear, don't scratch your ear. Make a solution of one part white vinegar to one part rubbing alcohol and place one to two drops in the ear three times a day. Some studies have indicated that this solution can cure up to 75 percent of external ear infections.

◆ An old remedy consists of roasting a lemon in the oven and using the juice as eardrops.

◆ Don't blow your nose during an earache; if you must, do it very gently.

◆ Keep the ear canal dry by placing cotton plugs in the ears when showering or washing your hair.

◆ Use acetaminophen for pain. Do not give aspirin to anyone under 21 because of the risk of Reye's syndrome.

◆ Prop your head up when sleeping, which helps promote drainage of the eustachian tubes.

◆ For adults who suffer from chronic ear infections, a decongestant nasal spray or an over-the-counter oral decongestant may help dry up any fluid present. Note: Do not overuse nasal sprays as they can become habit forming and can cause a rebound effect, where congestion is actually increased.

◆ Homemade nasal spray made out of 1 teaspoon of glycerine in 1 pint of warm water can also be used.

◆ Using salt water gargles at the first sign of an earache can help to bring more blood to the eustachian tube and help to fight infection.

NUTRITIONAL APPROACH:

If you have a child that suffers from recurring ear infections, it is important to concentrate on building up his or her immune system. Incorporate plenty of fresh fruits, vegetables, and whole grains into the diet.

◆ Avoid dairy products, which encourage the production of mucus. Avoid foods high in empty calories, junk foods, fats and meats.

◆ Drink the juice of orange or lemon diluted with 25 percent water. Some pure maple syrup may be added.

◆ Emphasize fresh juices, both fruit and vegetable.

◆ *Beta carotene:* Helps in controlling infection.

◆ *Vitamin C:* A natural anti-inflammatory which helps to heal tissue and strengthen capillaries.

◆ *Zinc picolinate:* Boosts immune response and helps to reduce infection.

◆ *Manganese:* Some studies have linked a deficiency of manganese to the incidence of ear disorders.

◆ *Acidophilus:* Take liberally in active culture yogurts, especially if on any kind of antibiotic. Antibiotics kill friendly bacteria, which in turn increases susceptibility to future infections.

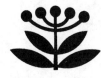

HERBAL REMEDIES:

◆ Oil of lobelia can be used as an eardrop if the infection is external.

- A warm wintergreen and rosemary oil rub around the ear may help to alleviate pain.
- *Pasque flower:* Works as an analgesic directly on the ear. Use as eardrops made out of a tincture
- Mullein oil warmed can be soothing and help to control pain. If a perforation of the eardrum is suspected do not use this remedy.
- *Echinacea:* Considered a natural antibiotic. Taken internally is good for fighting viral and bacterial infections.
- *Fenugreek:* Helps to loosen mucous and promote drainage.
- *Golden seal:* A powerful astringent that reduces mucus production and fights infection.
- At the start of an earache, an eardrop mixture made from equal parts of golden seal tincture, eucalyptus oil, pasque flower, myrrh tincture and almond oil may be used to stem the infection.

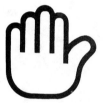

PREVENTION:

Breast feeding your baby may be the most effective way to prevent the incidence of ear infections. Breast milk provides the baby with antibodies for the first six months, has anti-inflammatory properties and protects the child from allergies to certain foods, especially cow's milk. The role of food allergies as a major cause of earaches is strongly documented in medical publications. Any allergic reaction will cause swelling and inflammation of the eustachian tube and nose which can encourage infection.

- If you bottle feed your baby, do not prop the bottle. This can cause a regurgitation of the fluid into the middle ear and may increase the risk of infection.
- Do not introduce foods such as citrus fruits, wheat or cow's milk into your baby's diet too early, which could increase the risk of food allergies.
- Try to protect your baby or small child from exposure to colds and flu.
- When swimming, wear earplugs to avoid trapping water in the ear.
- After swimming, shake your head to remove any excess water and dry the ear as thoroughly as possible. A preventative home remedy for those prone to swimmer's ear is to insert one or two drops of a solution made from one part white vinegar and one part rubbing alcohol in each ear. This helps to dry out the canal and maintains the normal acid balance of the area.
- Do not smoke. Even second-hand smoke can irritate mucus-secreting canals.
- If you have trouble with earaches, cover your ears when it's windy or wear earplugs.
- When flying, chew on gum or candy, which helps keep the eustachian tube open during changes in air pressure

Eczema (atopic dermatitis)

DEFINITION

Victims of eczema are often frustrated by the persistence and unpredictability of this bothersome skin rash. For someone with eczema, it can seem that coming in contact with just about anything can cause a flair-up of the disease.

Eczema, also known as dermatitis, is a chronic skin disorder characterized by dry, itchy skin. Persistent scratching of these affected areas causes weepy, infected irritated patches of skin to form. As areas of eczema dry they produce crusts. Prolonged scratching and infection will eventually produce areas of skin that are rough and thickened.

The first sign of eczema in a small child may be the presence of red, chapped cheeks. Tiny red pimples may appear on the child's buttocks, inner creases of the elbows or behind the knees. With time, eczema can spread and is commonly found on the backs of legs, fronts of arms and especially on the hands.

Fifty percent of infant eczema cases clear up by 18 months of age. Adult eczema is usually persistent and often resists treatment. Eczema is an inflammatory disease of the skin that is associated with asthma and is considered, at least to some extent, an allergic disorder. Eczema affects between 2 to 7 percent of the population.

CAUSES:

Like many allergic disorders, eczema runs in families. Two-thirds of people who suffer from eczema have family members with the same condition. The following factors can produce a flair-up of eczema: emotional stress, food allergy, excessive sweating, continual contact with water or detergent agents, certain chemicals and contact allergens such as wool, or nickel.

PHYSICAL SYMPTOMS:

Eczema produces oozing, red scaly, itchy patches of skin. Blistering is common. In severe cases lesions may form and can become so irritated that they bleed. Eczema causes the water-holding capacity of the skin to decrease. In several cases of eczema, the skin seemed to be more susceptible to bacterial growth, especially the staphylococcus aureus bacteria.

Frequently, intense itching can occur before any irritation is visible. Continual scratching can cause the visible symptoms of eczema to appear.

Psychological: Emotional stress can provoke eczema and increase the intensity of its symptoms. Some studies have shown that people who suffer from this condition manifested higher than normal levels of anxiety, hostility and psychological neurosis than the general public.

Medical alert:

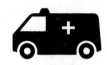

For severe infections, where skin is weeping, antibiotics may be required. See your physician as soon as possible.

Standard medical treatment:

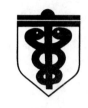

Your doctor will probably treat eczema with topical steroid ointments and lotions. If the infection is severe, antibiotics will be prescribed. For severe night itching, an antihistamine may be recommended.

SIDE-EFFECTS: *Corticosteroid ointments*: Cortisone can dramatically decrease inflammation and itching; however, it also suppresses cell activity and growth. If cortisone is used over a long period of time, the skin can become fragile and weak, which increases its susceptibility to infection and damage. The risks of prolonged use of these preparations is particularly risky when facial skin is involved, due to its delicate nature.

Success rating of standard medical treatment: fair to good. Physicians often ask a person suffering from eczema not to scratch, which is a totally unrealistic request. The best therapy medical science can offer the victim of eczema is the use of corticosteroid preparations and antibiotics if the infection is severe enough.

Home self-care:

◆ Keep short fingernails on small children and put gloves or socks on their hands at night.
◆ Avoid the use of soap, which has a tendency to dry out the skin. Use non-lipid containing cleansers. Cetyl alcohol preparations such as Cetaphil lotion may be beneficial. Moisturel is another non-irritating skin cleanser. If you must use soap, purchase a very mild type of soap bar such as Dove.
◆ Some physicians recommend using petroleum jelly to keep drying and scaling in control. Petroleum jelly helps to trap moisture on the skin.
◆ Use skin emollients that contain urea or lactic acid such as Ultra Mild 25 and Lac-Hydrin five.
◆ Avoid wearing wool, silk or synthetics, which may aggravate itching.
◆ Bath and shower quickly and not too often. Dry yourself totally and use a cream to moisten your skin.
◆ Make sure to rinse yourself thoroughly after using a hot tub or pool. Chlorine residue on the skin may cause or aggravate eczema.
◆ Clothing that comes in direct contact with the skin should be cotton only, especially in the case of infants and children.

- Do not overdress children. Becoming too hot causes sweating, which aggravates eczema.
- Antihistamines reduce itching but should be used with caution.
- The use of a non-oily zinc ointment can be used to control severe itching.
- Oatmeal baths can help relive the itching associated with eczema. An oatmeal bath can be made by using a powder such as Aveeno in the bath water.
- Use baking soda as an after-bath powder to help dry the skin.
- Ensure that your detergent or fabric softener sheets are not causing an allergic skin reaction. Rinse your sheets and towels twice. Avoid bleach or fabric softeners.
- Never handle substances such as insulation which is made of fiberglass, household cleaners, or any caustic chemical without proper skin protection. If you suffer from hand eczema don't wash the dishes without protection. Use rubber gloves worn over cotton gloves.
- Keep your environment moist. Use a cool mist vaporizer or attach a humidifier to your furnace system.
- Buy and use cosmetics judiciously. Experiment with hypoallergenic varieties and use as little as possible. Usually, high-priced cosmetics are no more or less likely to cause an allergic reaction. Unfortunately, a product that you have used for years with no problem can become an irritant. Often ingredients are revised or fragrances added and eczema can result.

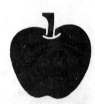

NUTRITIONAL APPROACHES:

- Do not consume dairy products. This is particularly important for young children. Allergies to cow's milk can severely aggravate eczema.
- If you know you are allergic to wheat avoid foods from the same family which will probably also cause eczema, such as, rice, rye, millet and barley. Experiment and see if you can find a correlation between your diet and outbreaks of eczema. Keep a journal of your food intake and when eczema occurs.
- Emphasize the following foods: parsley, green leafy vegetables, sprouts, celery, pineapples, grapes, melons, kelp, unsalted seeds, onions, papayas, and pears.
- Studies indicate that those with eczema appear to suffer from an essential fatty acid deficiency. Using primrose oil can help to correct this condition.
- Increase your intake of fish oils which have excellent anti-inflammatory and anti-allergic properties.
- Apply powdered calcium for relief from itching.
- *Vitamin A:* This vitamin is vital to the development and proper functioning of the skin. In vitamin A deficiencies, the skin becomes susceptible to the same kind of thickening found in eczema.
- *Bioflavonoids:* Very useful in all allergic conditions. Considered anti-inflammatory agents. They also increase the body's utilization of vitamin C.

◆ *Zinc:* Zinc supplements have been found to be particularly beneficial for victims of eczema.

HERBAL REMEDIES:

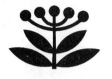

◆ Echinacea tincture taken internally facilitates the purification of toxins from the blood.
◆ Kochia oil is used medicinally in China for a variety of disorders and applied externally can help to minimize eczema. It might have to be special-ordered through health food stores or herbal distributors.
◆ Black current oil taken internally has proven beneficial for some cases of eczema.
◆ St. John's Wort oil is an old, traditional herbal remedy for skin irritations of all kinds.
◆ Make a chaparral bath by adding chaparral tea to a small amount of bath water.
◆ *Burdock:* Especially good for scaling eczema if taken internally. This herb has a long history of use in treating eczema. It has an anti-inflammatory effect and also helps to control staph infections, which commonly accompany eczema. Can be used in powdered form directly on the affected areas.
◆ *Chickweed:* Acts as a soothing astringent that helps to heal lesions.
◆ *Heartsease:* Particularly beneficial for weeping eczema if used externally as an ointment or cream. A wet compress can also be made by soaking a towel in Heartsease tea and applying it to affected areas of skin.
◆ Blueberry leaf, hawthorne berry and licorice all reduce the production and secretion of histamine, which causes inflammation and itching. These can be taken internally, used externally, or both.

PREVENTION:

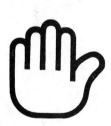

◆ Do not introduce foods such as citrus fruits, cow's milk and wheat into your baby's diet too soon. This may increase the child's susceptibility to allergic disorders.
◆ If you are prone to skin rashes and allergic reactions, avoid baby lotions or any skin preparation that contains lanolin or fragrance. Look for the hypo-allergenic label.
◆ Stay away from metallic jewelry. Nickel allergies can cause severe eczema. Use stainless steel or gold posts on pierced earrings, cloth watch bands, and make sure rings and necklaces are not made of nickel.
◆ Cats and dogs that are kept in the house may aggravate eczema.
◆ Artificial fingernails or eyelashes may cause an allergic skin reaction.
◆ Switch from antiperspirants to deodorants. An antiperspirant contains aluminum chloride, aluminum sulfate and zirconium chlorohydrates which can irritate sensitive skin. Watch out for strong deodorant soaps also.

◆ Try to wash your hands in cold water rather than hot; hot water is much more drying.
◆ Do not use colored toilet paper or tissue.
◆ Humidify your environment, especially during the winter months.

Endometriosis

DEFINITION:

Menstrual discomfort, in and of itself is usually bad enough. Unfortunately, endometriosis makes monthly matters worse. Endometriosis occurs when fragments of the uterine lining that become engorged with blood every month become implanted in other areas such as the ovaries, fallopian tubes, or uterine muscles. Endometrium tissue can also form in the vagina, the pelvic floor, the bowel, or in scar tissue that has grown in the abdominal wall after surgery. A recent study disclosed that the most common site of endometriosis is in the deep peritoneal cavity of the pelvis.

During each menstrual cycle, in response to the presence of estrogen, these tissue fragments bleed in the same way that the uterine lining does. Because blood cannot escape these abnormal locations, blisters can form that cause irritation and scarring of surrounding tissue. Consequently, a fibrous cyst may develop around each blister. These cysts can burst, causing abnormal bleeding of dark, brown blood accompanied by pain.

Because endometriosis is connected with the menstrual cycle it commonly occurs between the ages of 25 and 40. Endometriosis is more frequent in women who have not had children. It is estimated that 40 to 60 percent of women who undergo hysterectomies have had some form of endometriosis. Endometriosis affects approximately 12 million American females. In its mild form, it is considered a common disorder.

CAUSES:

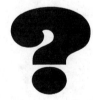

The exact causes of endometriosis are not fully understood. How the uterine tissue escapes remains somewhat of a mystery. One theory called reflux menstruation suggests that uterine contractions during heavy periods may force the lining upward through the fallopian tubes. Another theory proposes that endometrial tissue can form independently from undifferentiated cells located in the abdomen.

Spreading endometrial cells through the blood and lymph channels is also considered a possible cause of the disorder. Other possible causes of endometriosis are cauterization of the cervix, the use of IUD's and possibly as a complication of a laparoscopy. A relatively new theory suggests that endometriosis is a congenital birth defect resulting from the migration of endometrial cells to other areas.

SYMPTOMS:

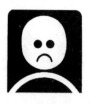

Physical: In the majority of cases, endometriosis causes no perceivable symptoms or symptoms so mild, they are dismissed. More severe symptoms include abdominal pain and back pain, especially during or after menstrual periods, heavy periods (including the passage of clots and tissue), irregular periods, painful sexual intercourse, nausea, vomiting, and constipation.

There is some controversy over whether endometriosis causes infertility, although it is generally accepted as a possible cause. In cases of endometriosis where periods are particularly heavy, an iron deficiency can occur.

Note: In some cases, pregnancy and breast feeding can decrease the symptoms of endometriosis; however, women with the disorder conceive at a lower rate and have a higher incidence of miscarriage and ectopic pregnancy. Often after childbirth, the symptoms of the disorder return.

MEDICAL ALERT:

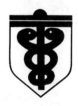

In the case of any abdominal pain, see your doctor before you attempt to treat yourself for endometriosis. The symptoms of this disorder can be very close to those of a tubal pregnancy, a urinary tract infection, and colitis.

STANDARD MEDICAL TREATMENT:

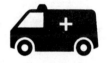

Endometriosis is difficult to diagnose. In order to do so a laparoscopy may be recommended. A small abdominal incision is made which allows the doctor to insert a lighted viewing device to examine the pelvic cavity. Your physician may choose to prescribe hormones which are contained in birth control pills, or a drug called Danazol. When taken over a period of months, these hormones reduce the flow of blood in menstruation. This reduction of blood allows for the destruction of existing abnormal tissue. Progesterone therapy or synthetic male hormones may also be used in more severe cases, which stop the menstrual cycle completely. In difficult cases, radiation therapy or surgery may be indicated. If drug therapy fails, a hysterectomy may be recommended.

Laser surgery through a laparoscopy can often find and destroy adhesions and cysts. Some new options include a procedure called a "near-contact" laparoscopy which has had some dramatic success. In this procedure all suspected growths or adhesions are removed from the entire pelvic cavity.

SIDE-EFFECTS: Oral contraceptives: Nausea, abdominal cramps, vaginal bleeding, changes in menstrual flow, breast tenderness, period of infertility after stopping the treatment, weight changes, headaches, rash, vaginal itching, vaginal infection, dizziness, nervousness, changes in appetite, changes in sex drive, and loss of hair.

Warning: Do not take any hormonal therapy if you are pregnant or nursing unless specified by your physician. Birth control pills should not be taken by anyone who suffers from high blood pressure, blood clots or strokes.

Success rating of standard medical treatment: fair. Surgical techniques can help control the symptoms of this disorder; however, it has a tendency to recur. The use of analgesics for pain and hormonal therapy are limited in their usefulness and can have significant side-effects. There is no known accepted cure for endometriosis in the medical community.

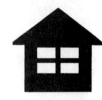

HOME SELF-CARE:

◆ Get in touch with the endometriosis association for additional support. Through this organization solutions and additional information can be shared through a large network.

◆ Exercise has been found to reduce estrogen levels, which can aggravate the progression of endometriosis. Regular walking is recommended as the best type of exercise. Thirty minute vigorous workouts are also good. Studies show that women who exercise regularly have less pain with endometriosis.

◆ Use a warm, moist heat on your abdomen and lower back.

◆ For some women, soft ice packs work better than heat to decrease pain. Ice wrapped in a towel and placed on the lower abdomen can provide some relief.

◆ Try using a lubricant if sexual intercourse is painful. A change of position may also eliminate pain.

◆ Use over-the-counter drugs that also act as antiprostaglandins. Prostaglandin, the hormone which causes uterine contractions, also causes menstrual cramping. Such drugs contain ibuprofen and are found in Advil, Medipren, or Nuprin

◆ Acupuncture and acupressure are routinely used by the Chinese for endometriosis and should be investigated as a viable option.

NUTRITIONAL APPROACH:

Eat a diet low in animal fats and high in linoleic acids found in vegetable sources. Avoid meats and dairy products. Increase your intake of fish. Fish is a natural antiprostaglandin and can help control cramping. Some theories maintain that hormones routinely given to fatten poultry, cattle and other livestock collect within the human system and may cause hormonal disorders.

Some studies have linked endometriosis with autoimmune diseases. Keep your immune system healthy by eating plenty of fresh fruits and vegetables and foods that are high in vitamin C. Avoid junk foods and refined sugars and flours which can stress the immune system.

◆ Avoid caffeine: Some women claim that caffeine increases the pain associated with endometriosis.
◆ Don't smoke: Nicotine can aggravate the symptoms of endometriosis.
◆ *Vitamin E:* Contributes to maintaining hormone balance and may help to control menstrual bleeding.
◆ *Vitamin A:* Some studies have found that vitamin A helped to normalize heavy periods, with blood loss significantly reduced.
◆ *Iron:* If periods are heavy, a deficiency of iron may occur with endometriosis.
◆ *Vitamin B complex:* Boosts blood cell production and hormone balance.
◆ *Vitamin C:* Assists in the healing process and strengthens capillary walls. Vitamin C also increases the absorption of iron and boosts the immune system.
◆ *Vitamin K and chlorophyll:* Have traditionally been associated with the control of excessive bleeding.
◆ *Calcium:* Some theories propose that endometriosis is related to the body's inability to absorb calcium.

HERBAL REMEDIES:

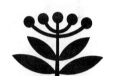

◆ *Black cohosh:* Works to balance hormones and strengthen uterine muscles.
◆ *Cramp bark:* A natural uterine relaxant.
◆ *Raspberry leaves:* A traditional herb used in treating disorders of the female reproductive system.
◆ *Dong quai:* Strengthens the uterus.
◆ *Siberian ginseng:* Helps to control abnormal bleeding.
◆ *False unicorn:* Stimulates ovarian hormones.
◆ *Gentian:* An herb which is high in iron and can help avoid the development of anemia with endometriosis.
◆ *Shepherd's purse:* An antihemorrhagic herb used traditionally for obstetric and gynecological purposes.

The following herbs in combination may be useful: Red raspberry leaves, blessed thistle, uva ursi, pien lien, false unicorn, squaw vine

Endometriosis Association, International Headquarters
Box Rd 8585 N. 76th Place
Milwaukee, WI 53223
800-992-3636

Epilepsy

DEFINITION:

Epilepsy has mystified and frightened people for generations. It has been associated with both the demonic and the divine and even today, is still misunderstood. Dispelling the myths that have become linked to epilepsy is necessary to fully appreciate the disorder and its effects. It may surprise some people to learn that epilepsy affects a vast portion of the world's population and that in most cases, epileptics live perfectly normal and productive lives.

Epilepsy does not refer to a specific disease but rather, to a group of symptoms caused by several conditions. It occurs when brain cells that normally communicate with one another send out signals that are abnormally strong. As a result, this sudden excess electrical discharge brings on an epileptic seizure. During a seizure, the electrical impulses of the brain become chaotic and unregulated.

This disorder usually begins in childhood or adolescence and is outgrown by one-third of its victims. There are several forms of epilepsy: generalized, partial and absence seizures. The type of seizure that occurs in epilepsy is dependent on its place of origin in the brain and how extensively it affects surrounding areas.

Generalized seizures, which cause a loss of consciousness, affect the entire brain and body. Grand mal seizures fall into this classification. Partial seizures include simple seizures, in which consciousness is maintained, and complex seizures where it becomes lost. Partial seizures may lead to a generalized seizure. Absence seizures refer to a condition where a momentary loss of consciousness occurs with no other sign of abnormal movement. Petit mal seizures fall into this category. This type of epilepsy is more common in children. This absence of consciousness can last from a just a few seconds to a minute. The child may appear to be daydreaming. This type of seizure can occur several times a day and hinder school work and activity. Approximately, one person in 200 suffers from epilepsy. There are close to 1 million epileptics in the United States.

CAUSES:

The exact cause of an epileptic seizure remains somewhat of a mystery. While certain injuries to the head can cause the onset of epilepsy, in two out of three individuals suffering from the disorder, no structural abnormalities or scar tissue is present. In one-third of epileptics, epilepsy is a secondary complication resulting from physical damage to the brain caused by traumatic birth, bacterial meningitis, malaria, rickets, rabies, tetanus, malnutrition, poisoning, cerebral palsy, mental retardation, brain tumors, hydrocephalus, stroke, lack of oxygen or injury to the head. Epilepsy runs in families.

SYMPTOMS:

Grand mal seizure (tonic-clonic): Sudden and complete loss of consciousness characterized by falling down, which can be accompanied by a high-pitched cry, a stiffening of the arms and legs, rhythmic muscle jerking, incontinence, and a cessation of breathing, which causes bluish skin. Following the seizure, which usually lasts two minutes, a relaxed state occurs in which the victim will feel sleepy, confused, and uncooperative for a period from 15 minutes to several hours. During this time, if you try to physically move or restrain the person, they may become combative.

Petit mal or absence seizures: This type of epilepsy is characterized by brief lapses of consciousness characterized by staring, rhythmic twitching of face muscles or eyelids, and a complete cessation of whatever activity the person was engaged in prior to the episode. After the seizure is over, normal activity is resumed. The person usually has no recollection of the seizure, which can occur up to several hundred times a day.

Complex partial seizures (psychomotor): This type of epilepsy can vary in its symptoms. An aura or warning can sometimes precede an attack which may include a feeling of apprehension, an unusual smell, a distortion in visual perception, or an abdominal sensation. After the aura, consciousness and speech are impaired. Repetitive movements, such as swallowing, hand movements, gestures etc. are also common. Confusion is typical and memory of the episode is lost.

Psychological: Epileptics have a tendency to feel that their condition is something to be ashamed of. While in the past, the disease may have been viewed as a social stigma, present knowledge and treatment of the disease provide a much more positive outlook for epileptics. With medication, the vast majority of epileptics lead a perfectly normal life.

Being overprotective of epileptics can create more psychological stress than anything else. Children with only minimal restrictions should be able to participate in sports and other activities, although increased supervision is encouraged. Adults with active seizures should avoid high-risk jobs such as construction, driving, or operating dangerous machinery. Anyone suffering from epilepsy should inform his or her co-workers and friends of the condition with instructions on what to do if a seizure occurs.

MEDICAL ALERT:

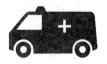

Seizures can be caused by a number of conditions such as fever, head trauma, infectious diseases or poisoning. Anyone who has suffered a seizure of any type should immediately see a physician.

WHAT TO DO IF SOMEONE HAS A SEIZURE:

- Move anything away from the victim that could cause injury. Gently place the person on a bed or the floor.
- Loosen tight clothing around the neck.
- If possible, turn the victim on his or her side.
- Call an ambulance.
- Stay calm. Witnessing a seizure can be very frightening. Frequently, the victim's face will turn blue due to a lack of oxygen. Seizures are usually brief and the incidence of death during a seizure is very low.
- Do not try to restrain the victim or put anything in the mouth.
- Do not attempt to move the victim unless there is danger of further injury.
- The most important things to consider when caring for someone who has a seizure is to let the convulsion run its course and to make sure the victim can breathe and will not be injured by furniture or other objects.

STANDARD MEDICAL TREATMENT:

An electroencephalogram (EEG) test will be ordered by your doctor. It is a painless procedure and involves tracking brain wave patterns through electrodes positioned on the head. A skull x-ray may also be required if a possibility exists that the seizures are being caused by infection or injury. In some cases, a CAT scan of the brain will prove helpful in making an accurate diagnosis. The possibility of a brain tumor must be ruled out.

Anticonvulsant drugs will be prescribed. A period of experimentation with several drugs may be necessary. Phenytoin (Dilantin) has been widely prescribed in the past for epilepsy. It targets the motor cortex of the brain and inhibits the electrical brain waves that cause seizure activity. Phenobarbital, cabamazepine (Tegretol), valproate (Depakote), and ethosuximide (Zarontin) are other drugs commonly prescribed for epilepsy. Epileptics need to see their doctor regularly for blood tests that can determine whether anticonvulsant drugs are at a therapeutic level.

Surgical options: Surgery is considered an option only in rare cases of epilepsy where a single area of brain damage exists, such as scar tissue in the temporal lobe.

Side-effects of anticonvulsant drugs: Dizziness, drowsiness, unsteadiness, nausea, blurred vision, confusion, hostility, loss of appetite, blood disorders, inability to concentrate, impaired memory, slowed mental and physical reflexes, insomnia, depression, and tremors.

WARNING: No anticonvulsant drug should be taken during pregnancy or if nursing unless your physician has specified that they be used. As strong correlation between the use of anticonvulsant drugs and birth defects exists.

Caution: Anyone taking anticonvulsant drugs should never stop taking them suddenly. The dose must be cut gradually to avoid bringing on seizures. This should be done only under a doctor's supervision. The negative side-effects of anticonvulsants can be decreased by careful attention to diet and exercise.

Success rating of standard medical treatment: good to excellent. With the proper use of medication, epilepsy can be well-controlled.

HOME SELF-CARE:

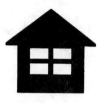

◆ One of the best things an epileptic can do is exercise on a regular basis. While water sports and high-risk activities might be discouraged, walking, jogging, playing tennis etc., can help keep the mind alert and help counteract the side-effects of drug therapy.

◆ Wear a tag or keep a card in your wallet which identifies you as a epileptic and carry it with you at all times.

◆ The possible value of hyperbaric therapy which involves high pressure oxygen should be investigated.

◆ Make sure you get adequate sleep every night. A lack of sleep can increase your risk for a seizure. Interrupted sleep patterns can also cause fatigue which, if severe enough, can result in seizure activity.

◆ Get involved with your local epileptic association. Chapters are located throughout the country.

NUTRITIONAL APPROACH:

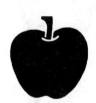

◆ Eat a diet high in the following foods: dark green leafy vegetables, carrots, raw fruits, fresh juices, whole grains, low-fat cheeses and low-fat meats.

◆ Avoid: Alcohol (which usually interacts with anticonvulsants), caffeine, coffee, tea, chocolates, artificial sweeteners, nicotine, refined sugars and flours.

◆ Eat regular, nutritious meals. Going without food for long periods of time can put significant stress on brain cells.

◆ *Vitamin D:* Danish medical studies done on a small scale indicate that when vitamin D supplements were given to epileptics being treated by anticonvulsants, the incidence of seizures was significantly reduced. Some epileptic medications interfere with the metabolism of vitamin D.

◆ *Vitamin B complex:* Especially folic acid and B12, which are destroyed if taking Dilantin or Phenobarbital

◆ *L-taurine and l-tyrosine:* These amino acids are important for the proper functioning of brain cells. Amino acids should be taken with your doctor's consent.

◆ *Calcium/magnesium:* Helps to facilitate normal nerve transmissions.

◆ *Manganese:* Some studies have indicated that a manganese deficiency is present in some epileptics.

◆ *Chromium picolinate:* Involved in the metabolism of sugar in brain cells.

- *Niacin and choline:* Needed to produce acetylcholine, which is a neuro-transmitter.
- *Acidophilus:* Important when taking any prolonged drug therapy. Helps to replace friendly bacteria essential for good health.

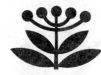

HERBAL REMEDIES:

NOTE: Herbs should never be used to take the place of anticonvulsant medication that is being taken for epilepsy. Herbal treatments can help to eventually decrease the dosage or to counteract drug-induced side-effects.
- *Black cohosh:* Considered a natural sedative and a tonic for the nervous system.
- *Lobelia:* A natural herbal relaxant.
- *Valerian tincture:* A natural tranquilizer and antispasmodic.
- *Ginkgo:* Helps to stimulate brain function and can boost memory capacity, which may be impaired by anticonvulsant drugs.
- *Skullcap:* A relaxant and restorative for the central nervous system.
- *Lady's slipper:* An herbal nervine which helps to relax the nervous system.

PREVENTION OF SEIZURES IF YOU HAVE EPILEPSY:

- Do not become overly fatigued or stressed. Use exercise, biofeedback and relaxation techniques, including meditation, to relax.
- Be more careful if you have an infectious illness, especially if a fever is present. This type of situation may increase your susceptibility to a seizure.
- Don't get up too quickly in the morning. Allow your body to slowly adjust to waking up. Perform stretching exercises while still in bed and take some deep breaths.
- Take your medication at the same time each day and in the exact prescribed dose.
- Some epileptics have effectively used biofeedback to avoid a seizure that they feel coming on. While this is not recommended alone, its possible value should be explored.
- Do not attempt to blow up balloons. For some epileptics this activity can precipitate a seizure.
- Do not engage in any abnormal visual activity such as prolonged staring at hidden 3D pictures.

The Epilepsy Foundation of America
4351 Garden City Drive, Suite 406
Landover, MD 20785
301-459-3700

Eye Infections (conjunctivitis)

DEFINITION:

You know it's going to be one of those days when you wake up and your eyelids are glued shut. Eye infections can appear suddenly and usually look a lot worse than they feel. Conjunctivitis is a common infection of the eye that is generally simple to treat.

Conjunctivitis, or pink eye, is medically described as an inflammation of the membrane that lines the eye and inner eyelids. The infection can be bacterial or viral, with viral infections being highly contagious and potentially serious. Most cases of conjunctivitis rarely affect vision. Every year, one person in 50 visits a physician with this particular eye complaint.

Newborn babies will occasionally come down with a type of conjunctivitis called neonatal ophthalmia, which is caused by an infection contracted from the mother's cervix. This type of infection needs immediate medical treatment. An inflammation of both the conjunctiva and the cornea can occur and is referred to as keratoconjunctivitis. Simple conjunctivitis is more commonly seen in children and will often clear up without medical treatment.

CAUSES:

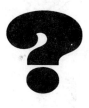

Irritants to the eye can cause conjunctivitis such as air pollutants, pool chlorine or other chemicals, fumes, smoke, blowing sand, extensive exposure to glare or a welder's arc, allergens (dust, pollen, etc.), some contact lens solutions, eye makeup, injury to the eye, the presence of a foreign body, and a viral or bacterial infection.

Most eye infections are caused by the staphylococci bacteria, which can be spread by hand-to-eye contact or by viruses associated with colds or sore throats. Minor conjunctivitis can accompany a cold and will usually resolve itself. When conjunctivitis is caused by the herpes virus, ulceration of the eye can result and vision may be impaired. Viral eye infections can occur in epidemics and spread rapidly in settings such as schools.

SYMPTOMS:

Physical: In bacterial infections, pus forms and causes a thick discharge from the eyes, which results in crusty eyelids that may be glued together upon waking up. Even in bacterial eye infections, a fever is not usually present. Eyes may become swollen and bloodshot, and in some cases may itch. Eye irritation that is not accompanied by a yellow or greenish discharge is probably not an infection.

Warning: People who wear contact lenses are more susceptible to eye infections.

If you wear contacts, remove them at the first sign of conjunctivitis. Continued use of contacts during an eye infection can cause serious corneal infections that could lead to blindness.

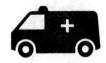

MEDICAL ALERT:

A herpes infection of the eye can be potentially serious. It can cause ulcers to form in the cornea and threaten vision. Certain symptoms may indicate the presence of serious eye conditions and need prompt medical attention. If you have any of the following symptoms, see your physician immediately:
◆ a decrease in vision or blurred vision
◆ irregular pupils
◆ eye pain upon light exposure
◆ seeing halos around lights
◆ a thick discharge from the eyes
◆ any injury to the eye needs immediate medical attention

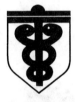

STANDARD MEDICAL TREATMENT:

Your physician will examine your vision, eye motion, eyelids and the reaction of your pupils to light. A slit-lamp examination may be done if you go to an ophthalmologist. Swabs may be taken to determine the cause of the infection, especially in the case of newborns. Antihistamines may be prescribed if the inflammation is caused by an allergy.

In addition, steroid eyedrops may be recommended to control allergic inflammation of the eye, but should not be used if an infection is present. Antibiotic eyedrops or ointments are frequently prescribed. If herpes is present, it will need special treatment. The use of antibiotic preparations in a herpes-based eye infection can actually intensify the infection.

Note: Antibiotic ointments are thought to be better than drops in that they cling to the eye more effectively. Request the ointment and squeeze about an inch of the cream into the space created by pulling your lower eyelid forward. Keep the tube there as the ointment is melting; then close your eyes and roll them around to promote good coverage. Your vision will be blurry for a few minutes. Polysporin is an over-the-counter antibiotic ointment which can be used if you cannot get prompt medical attention.

Success rating of standard medical treatment: very good to excellent. Antibiotic eye preparations can readily cure most cases of conjunctivitis.

HOME SELF-CARE:

◆ Over-the-counter eyedrops such as Murine or Visine may help take the redness out of the eye, but will not cure an eye infection. In addition, they contain tetrahydrozoline, a drug that can cause rebound eye vessel dilation in much the same way that nasal sprays do in the nose. Using these types of eyedrops for longer than three days can actually induce redness.

◆ If you have an eye infection, don't patch your eye. Covering the eye in this way can increase bacterial or viral proliferation by raising the temperature of the eye environment.

◆ Avoid exposure to any substance that is an eye irritant, such as smoke, certain chemicals, and dust.

◆ Wear dark glasses to avoid eye strain.

◆ Avoid swimming during an eye infection. Chlorine can aggravate eye irritations.

◆ Apply a warm compress to the eyes for 5 minutes at a time to reduce eye discomfort. Cold compresses are recommended if the eye inflammation is allergic in nature.

◆ Placing slices of raw potatoes on the eyes can help decrease swelling.

◆ Keep the eye area clean by swabbing away pus or crusty matter with cotton balls soaked in warm, sterile water. Sterile saline solution which can be purchased at any pharmacy is also good.

◆ Use antibiotic ointments right before going to sleep to decrease discharge during the night. This will help to lessen the crusting that can occur while you're sleeping.

NUTRITIONAL APPROACH:

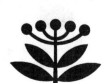

◆ Eliminate any foods which may be suspected of causing an allergic reaction such as dairy products, citrus fruits or wheat.

◆ A fruit juice or carrot juice fast is encouraged for one day to help clean the blood.

◆ *Vitamin A:* Good for promoting healthy eye function and immune response to bacterial or viral invasion.

◆ *Vitamin C:* Helps to promote healing and reduces inflammation.

◆ *Zinc:* Plays an important role in any disorder of the eye and boosts immune response to infection.

HERBAL REMEDIES:

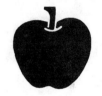

◆ Eyebright and golden seal tea (strained) can be used as an eyewash which is applied with an eye cup.

◆ *Agrimony:* An astringent for the mucous membranes of the eye which can be strained and diluted to create an eyewash.

◆ *Purple coneflower:* Take internally to fight infection.

◆ *Pot marigold:* Use a strained tea solution or tincture solution to create a compress for the eyes. This herb is a natural anti-inflammatory.

◆ Chamomile and fennel can be made into a tea and used as compresses on the eyes.

◆ *Ju hua*: An antibacterial, and anti-inflammatory herb. Follow directions for usage.

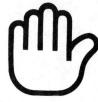

PREVENTION:

◆ Be sure to wash towels, pillowcases, washcloths or any other item which may come in contact with someone suffering from conjunctivitis to prevent further spread of the infection.

◆ If you are infected, wash your hands often with soap and water.

◆ Wear protective goggles if swimming in chlorinated water or exposed to toxic fumes, smoke, chemicals or other irritants.

◆ Don't rub your eyes if they feel itchy or irritated.

◆ Keep your hands and nails away from the mucosal tissue of the eye.

Fever

DEFINITION:

A fever is not a disease, but rather a symptom which indicates the presence of an illness. The presence of a fever usually indicates that the body is fighting some type of infection. Normal body temperature ranges from 98 to 99 degrees Fahrenheit. Temperature is generally at its lowest in the morning. Generally speaking, children have higher body temperatures than adults. Elevating the body's temperature is a natural reaction of the immune system to destroy bacteria and viruses.

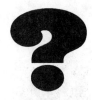

CAUSES:

Bacterial and viral infections are the most common cause of a fever and are present in colds, flu, sore throats, tonsillitis, typhoid, earaches, diarrhea, urinary tract infections, childhood diseases such as roseola, chicken pox, mumps, measles, pneumonia, appendicitis and meningitis.

When certain infections are present, proteins referred to as pyrogens are released which act on the temperature-controlling center of the brain. Other conditions that can cause a fever are dehydration, heat exhaustion, sunburn, heart attack, drug withdrawal and tumors of the lymphatic system.

Note: Overdressing a baby or small child or leaving a child in a hot car can cause life-threatening overheating.

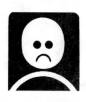

PHYSICAL SYMPTOMS:

Fever commonly causes hot, flushed skin, sweating, clammy skin, headache, shivering (a sensation of being cold can be experienced either by lowering the temperature of the surrounding environment or by raising the body temperature), goosebumps, increased hunger, thirst, rapid breathing, confusion, delirium, and in a very high fever, seizures and possible death.

Note: How high a fever climbs is not necessarily indicative of how serious the condition is that caused it.

MEDICAL ALERT:

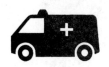

A doctor should be consulted immediately for any fever that goes above 102 in adults, 101 if over the age of 60, and 102 in a child. In addition, see a physician for any fever present in babies less than 3 months old, fevers that linger more than three days, fevers accompanied by rash, headache, stiff neck, back pain or painful urination, or any fever that accompanies diabetes, heart or lung disease. Chronic recurring fevers should also be checked out. A prolonged high fever can cause brain damage or dehydration. A fever may indicate the presence of a serious condition.

WARNING: Never administer aspirin to anyone under 21 who is feverish. If a viral infection is present, using aspirin increases the risk of Reye's syndrome, a potentially fatal condition.

STANDARD MEDICAL TREATMENT:

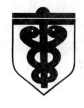

A physician will first want to determine if an infection is present. The eyes, throat, skin, lungs, glands and abdomen will be examined. Blood and urine tests may be ordered. In certain cases, a chest x-ray or spinal tap may be necessary to rule out pneumonia or spinal meningitis. If a bacterial infection is present, antibiotics will be prescribed. Antipyretic drugs to lower temperature are routinely recommended and are usually over-the-counter preparations.

HOME SELF-CARE:

Many physicians and health practitioners believe that a mild fever (under 100) can actually speed recovery from infection and should not be suppressed. By taking aspirin, ibuprofen or acetaminophen fevers can be reduced; however, the immune system can become suppressed to a certain extent by these medicines.
- ◆ Do not use a cold bath or an alcohol rub to bring down a fever. Tepid or warm baths are recommended so that body temperature is not brought down too quickly which can result in chills. Sponging the limbs with tepid or warm water is also effective
- ◆ Drink plenty of fluids. Fever can cause excessive sweating and loss of water. Keeping your fluids up can make it easier to bring a temperature down.

- Change clothing and bedding often if sweating is increased.
- Keep your activity down. Although increasing exercise is accepted by some as a way to promote sweating and eliminate toxins, exercising while you have a fever can stress the heart.
- Do not overdress infants or small children.

NUTRITIONAL APPROACH:

The value of "starving a fever" has been questioned. Fever actually increases the body's need for calories. Foods that are recommended are those high in liquid content such as fresh fruits and vegetables. In addition, mild foods are encouraged such as whole grains and yogurt. If a child with a fever refuses to eat, encourage drinking instead. Fluid intake is extremely important when a fever is present. Fruit and vegetable juices that are low in sodium are excellent.

- Fresh lemon juice in water.
- *Vitamin A:* Fights infection and boosts the functions of the immune system.
- *Protein supplement:* necessary for tissue repair. During periods of fever, tissue damage can occur.
- *Vitamin C:* Helps to reduce fevers and facilitates the elimination of toxins. Vitamin C powder can be mixed in water and taken as a fluid supplement also.
- *Barley water:* Helps keep fever down.

HERBAL REMEDIES:

- *Garlic:* A natural antibiotic and immunostimulant.
- *Lobelia extract or tincture:* Helps to lower fever.
- *Linden tea:* Can induce sweating and help to break a fever.
- *Black elder:* A traditional herbal treatment for fevers.
- *Elderflower and peppermint leaves:* Taken together as a tea help to induce sweating and lower body temperature.
- *Willow bark:* A natural analgesic rich in saliclylates, which are aspirin-related compounds. Use for adults only.
- *Echinacea:* Fights both bacterial and viral infections.
- *The following herbs in combination may be useful:* Echinacea, golden seal root, burdock, dandelion and capsicum.

PREVENTION:

- A fever is a normal reaction of the body's immune system and is an important part of combating infection. A fever should not be prevented; however, it should be watched and not allowed to climb too high. Fortifying the immune system so that resistance to infection is high and avoiding environments where exposure to infection is great can help avoid the illnesses commonly associated with fevers.

Gallstones

DEFINITION:

Gallbladder removal is one of the most common operations in the United States. The gallbladder collects bile, a cholesterol-rich fluid which comes from the liver and secretes bile when fatty substances are digested.

Gallstones occur when cholesterol crystallizes when combining with bile due to a chemical impairment. There can be between one and 10 stones present in the gallbladder. Gallstones are composed principally of cholesterol, but may also contain bile pigment and chalk.

Approximately 20 million people suffer from gallstones, with at least 1 million new cases diagnosed each year. Gallstones can vary in size from smaller than a pea to as large as an egg. Frequently, the presence of gallstones can go unnoticed. If a gallstone becomes stuck within a bile duct, severe pain usually results. Women who are over 40, obese and have had children are more likely to suffer from gallbladder disorders. Gallstones are rarely found in primitive cultures, another testament to the perils of our life-style and diet.

CAUSES:

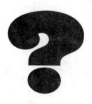

The high incidence of gallstones in the United States is thought to be directly related to Western dietary habits. Elevated levels of cholesterol in the blood increase the risk of developing gallstones. There is some speculation that food allergies may predispose one to gallstones by causing a swelling of the bile ducts, resulting in impaired bile flow from the gallbladder.

Interestingly and for unknown reasons, 70 percent of American Indian women over 30 years of age suffer from gallstones. The older one gets, the chances for developing gallstones increases. Hormonal factors play a role, in that each pregnancy increases the risk of gallstones.

Prolonged periods of fasting can also increase the risk of gallstones by causing bile to stagnate in the gallbladder. The use of birth control pills may cause gallstones to form earlier than normal.

SYMPTOMS:

Physical: Between one-third and one-half of people with gallstone have no symptoms; however, when the stones get stuck in the bile duct the following symptom can occur: severe pain in the upper right section of the abdomen or between the shoulder blades. This pain can build to a peak and then fade over a period of hours, and has been described as an intense, gnawing ache that may be accompanied by bloating, nausea, and vomiting.

A gallstone attack may occur after a meal high in fatty or fried foods. Drinking alcohol has also been related to gallstone attacks. If the symptoms subside, the stone may have fallen back into the gallbladder or been forced into the intestines.

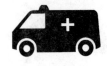

MEDICAL ALERT:

Any type of severe or prolonged abdominal pain should receive immediate medical attention.

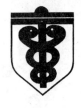

STANDARD MEDICAL TREATMENT:

If your physician suspects gallstones, he will take a blood sample, and may order a cholecytogram, which is a type of x-ray taken after ingesting a certain pill which enhances the visibility of the gallbladder. An ultrasound scan, which detects up to 95 percent of gallstones, or a CAT scan may also be recommended to detect gallstones which have not shown up in previous tests.

Standard treatment for gallstones usually involves surgically removing the gallbladder. New laser surgery techniques may be an option. This process of removing the gallbladder involves only a small incision and recovery is rapid.

A new treatment called lithotripsy is also available in which stones are fractured by an external machine. Another technique uses a tube inserted in the gallbladder, through which a strong solution which dissolves cholesterol is administered. The value and safety of both of these methods is still being evaluated. Drug therapy such as ursodiol (Actigall) may be suggested to dissolve small gallstones. This treatment is slow and is only effective with certain types of gallstones.

SIDE-EFFECTS: Ursodiol (Actigall): Nausea, vomiting, upset stomach, abdominal pain, bile pain, gallstone pain, metallic taste, constipation, gas, diarrhea, itching, rash, dry skin, sweating and hair loss. Headache, fatigue, sleep disturbances and joint pain have also been associated with the drug.

Success rating of standard medical treatment: gallbladder removal surgery: very good. Removing the gallbladder surgically is 100 percent effective in resolving the problem of gallstones, but is not without its risk.

Other forms of medical treatment vary in their effectiveness. Drug therapy is considered long and not very effectual. The treatment is expensive and does not prevent the formation of new stones. For some cases, the lithotripsy technique based on sound waves may prove of value, but is also not without its risks. As in a variety of other diseases, prevention, which is usually not stressed, should receive more emphasis.

HOME SELF-CARE:

◆ Drinking at least 6 to 8 glasses of water per day is very important in helping maintain the proper water content of bile from which gallstones are formed.
◆ Don't try any drastic home remedies such as taking large quantities of olive oil and fruit juice. Drastic measures like this one can actually increase the risk of a serious gallbladder attack.

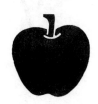

NUTRITIONAL APPROACH:

◆ Emphasize a low-fat diet high in raw foods such as yogurt, broiled fish, beets, carrots, apples, lemons, oranges, grapes, celery, garlic, onions, tomatoes, dates, melons, and fiber-rich foods. Make sure you get at least 20 percent of your calories from good fat sources such as olive or canola oil.
◆ Fiber is thought to help prevent the formation of gallstones by stimulating bile flow from the liver and by preventing bile reabsorption.
◆ Avoid fried foods, fatty foods, animal fat, saturated fat, margarine, commercial oils, chocolate and coffee. Minimize consumption of sugar and refined carbohydrates.
◆ Lose weight and learn to push away from the table before feeling uncomfortably full.
◆ Drink beet juice, which acts as a liver cleanser.
◆ *Vitamin C and vitamin E:* Some studies indicate that deficiencies of both vitamin C and E have been shown to cause gallstones in animals. Vitamin E also helps keep fats from becoming rancid.
◆ Vitamin D: Vitamin D may not be properly absorbed if the gallbladder is impaired.
◆ *Lecithin:* Some research suggests that low levels of lecithin in the bile may cause gallstones. Lecithin also helps to emulsify fats, which is important to proper cholesterol digestion.
◆ *Choline:* Important for cholesterol metabolism and in the proper functioning of the gallbladder and liver.
◆ *Fiber supplements:* Psyllium, pectin, and guar gum can decrease cholesterol levels.

HERBAL REMEDIES:

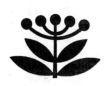

◆ *Dandelion root* and *artichoke leaves* have a favorable effect on the solubility of bile.
◆ *Alfalfa:* acts as a liver cleanser.
◆ *Barberry root bark:* Stimulates bile flow and helps to relieve liver congestion.
◆ *Fringe tree:* Stimulates liver function and the movement of bile.
◆ *Queen of the meadow:* Has a long history of use for gallbladder disorders.

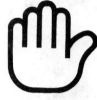

- *Buckthorn:* A natural bile stimulant.
- *Peppermint oil:* Used in some countries to help cleanse the gallbladder.
- *The following herbs in combination may be useful:* Red beet root, dandelion, Oregon grape, pan pien lien, yellow dock, bayberry and golden seal.

PREVENTION:

- Gallstones are thought to be much easier to prevent than to treat. Reducing your risk factors for the formation of gallstones is of primary importance.
- Eat a diet low in fats and especially low in cholesterol. Avoid animal and saturated fats, sugar, and fried foods. Minimize your consumption of animal protein. Vegetable proteins such as soy are believed to prevent the formation of gallstones.
- Emphasize the following foods: fresh fruits and vegetables, fiber (oat bran, flax seed, guar gum, pectin). Eating fiber regularly is believed to help prevent gallstones from forming.
- Do not become obese, which increases your risk for gallstones. Even slightly overweight people have twice the risk of developing gallstones. Lose weight safely and slowly. Losing weight too quickly can increase the risk of developing gallstones.
- Do not go on quick weight loss diets where no fat is allowed. An extremely low-fat diet can cause bile to sit in the gallbladder, increasing your chances of stone formation.

Glaucoma

DEFINITION:

Glaucoma is an insidious disease that silently robs eyesight with no obvious warning symptoms. Glaucoma is one of the most prevalent eye disorders in people over the age of 60. It is responsible for 15 percent of all blindness in the United States, afflicting approximately 2 million people, and is the second leading cause of blindness.

Glaucoma is a condition in which fluid pressure in the eye becomes high enough to cause damage to delicate optic nerves. Small internal blood vessels can become compressed or obstructed in the optic nerve, resulting in nerve fiber destruction, which can lead to partial or total blindness.

Chronic open-angle glaucoma is the most common form of the disease and usually begins after the age of 40. A blockage of fluid in the eye gradually increases the pressure over a period of years. Acute closed angle glaucoma refers to the sudden obstruction of fluid with a sudden rise in pressure. Congenital glaucoma results from structural abnormalities within the eye.

CAUSES:

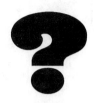

Acute closed angle glaucoma runs in families. Other possible causes of glaucoma are injury to the eye, a dislocation of the lens, adhesions that grow between the iris and the cornea, and diseases such as uveitis. Malnutrition and stress have also been linked to the disease. Impairment in collagen metabolism due to several syndromes is also associated with glaucoma.

There is some speculation that exposure to allergens both airborne or environmental can cause a rise in intraocular pressure, which could cause glaucoma-like symptoms. Certain drugs can hasten the onset of glaucoma. The following people are also at a higher risk for developing glaucoma: anyone who has a family history of the disease, the severely nearsighted, those with cataracts, diabetics, anyone over 65, and anyone taking certain blood pressure medication or cortisone. Black people have a higher incidence of glaucoma.

SYMPTOMS:

Chronic glaucoma can often progress without any symptoms, due to the very slow loss of peripheral vision. Unfortunately, it is usually only after the disease is in its later stages, after irreversible damage has occurred, that vision loss becomes obvious.

Possible symptoms of glaucoma include: A severe, dull ache or throbbing pain in the eye and sometimes above the eye, eye discomfort, which is usually worse in the morning, blurred or foggy vision, tunnel vision, inability to adjust to darkness, loss of peripheral vision, the perception of rainbow rings around lights, nausea, vomiting, a red, bloodshot appearance to the eyes, dilated pupils, and a hazy cornea.

MEDICAL ALERT:

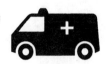

Acute closed-angle glaucoma is considered a medical emergency and requires immediate medical attention. Go to an emergency facility if you feel sudden eye pain, blurred vision, see halos around lights, and experience nausea or vomiting.

Note: The only way glaucoma can be detected in its early stages is with regular eye examinations. Applanation tonometry, which measures eye pressure, is used to detect the presence of the disease, along with visual field testing and gonioscopy,

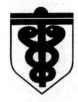

which measures the drainage angle in the eye. See an ophthalmologist, not an optician or an optometrist

STANDARD MEDICAL TREATMENT:

Chronic glaucoma is commonly controlled with eyedrops which reduce eye pressure. Timoptic (Timolol Maleate) reduces fluid formation and Pilocarpine decreases the size of the pupil, which increases fluid drainage. Propine (Dipivefrin) is considered a cornerstone drug in the treatment of glaucoma. Careful monitoring of the eyes must be done during treatment to ensure its effectiveness.

If pressure is still too high, other types of eyedrops may be used. In persistent cases, tablets or capsules such as Diamox (acetazolamide) may be prescribed, which are generally taken as lifelong medications. If drug therapy fails, laser surgery or regular surgery may be necessary to enlarge the drainage area or to create an artificial channel in which the fluid can drain. Laser surgery involves aiming a beam at the iris and making a tiny hole to relieve pressure.

Acute glaucoma is considered a medical emergency and requires immediate treatment. In this case, osmotic eye drops, oral medication and intravenous fluids may be administered to reduce eye pressure. Surgery will probably be recommended to prevent a reoccurrence of the problem. This procedure is called an iridectomy, and involves making a small incision in the area around the iris so the fluid can drain. Medications may be recommended following the surgery.

SIDE-EFFECTS: Timolol (Timoptic): used in eyedrop form. decreased heart rate, aggravation of congestive heart failure, decrease in blood pressure, tingling in arms and legs, lightheadedness, depression, inability to sleep, weakness, nausea, constipation, fatigue and mental disturbances.

Warning: Do not take this drug if you are pregnant or nursing without your doctor's approval.

SIDE-EFFECTS: Dipivefrin (Propine): Burning or stinging in the eye, conjunctivitis, allergic reaction, rapid heartbeat, irregular heartbeat, sleeplessness, and high blood pressure.

Warning: If you are pregnant or nursing, take this only with your doctor's consent.

SIDE-EFFECTS: Acetazolamide (Diamox): Tingling in the arms, legs, lips or anus, loss of appetite, increased frequency of urination, drowsiness, convulsions.

Note: Acetazolamide is considered a sulfa drug and can cause an allergic reaction in some individuals.

Warning: This drug should not be taken by pregnant or nursing women. It has been linked to birth defects and abnormal development.

Success rating of standard medical treatment: good. If caught early enough, glaucoma can be controlled through medication and surgery and blindness can be avoided. Normal vision can be restored if glaucoma has not progressed too far.

HOME SELF-CARE:

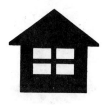

◆ Glaucoma self-tests can be administered with a self-tonometer, and should be done with the consent of your doctor.

◆ Avoid excessive or prolonged stress to the eye such as watching too much television, reading, or doing close-up work that puts extra strain on the eyes.

◆ Corticosteroids should not be used by anyone suffering from glaucoma due to their adverse affect on collagen structures within the eye. Cortisone also interferes with the fluid flow of the eye and can actually increase pressure

◆ Avoid taking decongestants or antihistamines, which can narrow eye drainage canals and increase intraocular pressure.

◆ If taking eyedrops for glaucoma take them regularly and don't miss any doses. The best way to apply eye drops is to lay down, pull down your lower eyelid, place a drop of fluid in, and then press against the tear duct in the corner of your eye with your finger.

◆ Regular exercise, especially cycling, appears to also help reduce pressure within the eye.

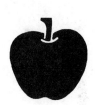

NUTRITIONAL APPROACH:

◆ Avoid: coffee, alcohol, nicotine, and all caffeine.

◆ Eat a diet high in whole grains and fresh fruits and vegetables and low in animal and saturated fats.

◆ Avoid salt and sugar.

◆ Try not to drink large amounts of fluid at once.

◆ *Vitamin B complex:* This vitamin, especially in injection form, may be helpful if glaucoma is stress-related.

◆ *Vitamin B6:* Helps to control intraocular pressure.

◆ *Inositol:* Important for the synthesis of healthy eye membranes.

◆ *Calcium/magnesium:* Functions in the production of healthy connective tissue in the eye.

◆ *Rutin:* Found in vitamin C complex. Helps to reduce pressure behind the eye.

◆ *Vitamin C and bioflavonoids:* Help to reduce intraocular pressure and is vital for proper collagen metabolism. Collagen gives strength to tissues within the eye. Studies have indicated that therapeutic levels of vitamin C can significantly reduce eye pressure, decrease eye fluid production and facilitate fluid movement. Check with your doctor before setting a dosage.

◆ *Vitamin A:* Excellent vitamin for the eyes. Vitamin A helps to prevent night blindness and works to protect the eye from irritants.

◆ *Niacin:* Helps to clear out fatty deposits that can accumulate in the blood vessels of the eye.

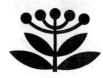

HERBAL REMEDIES:

◆ *Forskolin:* A derivative of the coleus plant which has had some positive effects in treating glaucoma in some university studies and should be investigated.

◆ *Bilberry:* Strengthens eye tissue.

◆ *Agrimony:* Helps to heal mucous membranes of the eye.

◆ *Eyebright:* Provides elasticity to nerves and eye tissue.

◆ Make an eye wash with fennel and chamomile teas. Steep these herbs and then strain the water well.

◆ Diuretic herbs that help to remove excess fluid from the tissues include parsely, uva ursi, marshmallow, cornsilk, shavegrass, watermelon seeds, pan pien lien, black cohosh, juniper berries and gravel root.

PREVENTION:

◆ See your eye doctor for a routine eye exam once a year, especially after age 40, for early detection of glaucoma.

◆ Avoid eye injury or eye strain.

◆ Wear protective goggles when involved in carpentry, metalwork, playing sports, chopping wood, etc.

◆ Make sure reading and work areas are well-lighted.

◆ Use glasses if needed and update your prescription periodically.

◆ Take breaks from tedious eye work such as computer entry, typing, and lab work. Toning down the brightness of computer screen images is also less stressful on the eyes. Try not to work in direct sunlight, and wear sunglasses if sun is bright or glare severe. However, try not to become dependent on tinted glasses by overusing them.

◆ Eat a diet that is low in salt, sugar and saturated fats and high in fresh fruits, vegetables and whole grains.

◆ Avoid prolonged allergic irritation of the eyes.

◆ Placing herbal tea bags on each eye that have been steeped in an herb tea such as eyebright and then cooled can help relieve stress and relax the eye.

Gout

DEFINITION:

Gout has traditionally been thought of as a disease of the aristocratic class. This particular association comes from the fact that royal figures, rather than regular "peons," often suffered from gout. This suggests that diets rich in meat, wine and fats have been associated with the development of "gouty" joints for generations. Ironically, the peasants, who ate plenty of grains and vegetables, enjoyed a diet that we know now was far superior to their king's table.

Gout is an arthritis-like metabolic disorder which results from an increased concentration of uric acid in the body. This uric acid becomes crystallized and is deposited in joints, tendons, the kidneys and other tissues, causing inflammation, swelling and damage. Uric acid forms as a byproduct of certain foods.

Today gout is a disease that primarily affects adult men over the age of 30. In women, gout occurs only after menopause. Approximately three adults in 1000 suffer from gout. Once an initial attack of gout is experienced, subsequent episodes are common; however, a small percentage never experience a second attack. Individuals that suffer from gout are typically obese, prone to high blood pressure and diabetes, and may have a history of cardiovascular disease.

CAUSES:

Gout is a diet-related condition. Obesity and stress have also been linked to gout. Enzyme defects are involved in gout and gout can result from chemotherapy used to treat cancer, due to the cellular destruction which releases large amounts of uric acid. Other disorders that can cause gout are cancer, chronic anemia, kidney dysfunction, and psoriasis. Cytotoxic drugs are also linked to the disease.

Diuretics used to treat high blood pressure and heart failure may impair the ability of the kidney to excrete uric acid. It is possible to live with elevated levels of uric acid and never have an attack of gout.

SYMPTOMS:

Physical: An attack of gout can be characterized by intense joint pain that resembles a dislocation. The first joint of the big toe is affected in 90 percent of people who suffer from gout. Gouty joints are swollen and red. Other symptoms of the disorder are fever and chills. Attacks of gout commonly occur at night. They can be aggravated by overeating, drinking alcohol, trauma to the body and certain drugs and surgical procedures.

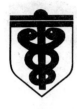

An untreated attack of gout will not usually last longer than a week. Common sites of gout are the ankle, heel, knee and wrist. The shoulder, back or the hip are rarely affected by gout. Victims of chronic gout may also increase their risk for the development or uric acid kidney stones.

STANDARD MEDICAL TREATMENT:

A diagnosis for gout may involve the drawing out of fluid from a painful joint and testing it for the presence of uric acid. This is not considered a completely conclusive test. An old, traditional approach for the treatment of gout is the administration of colchicine, an anti-inflammatory drug, which can have unpleasant side-effects. This drug dates back to the time of Hippocrates. This medicine is aimed at reducing inflammation rather than decreasing uric acid levels. Allupurinol (Zyloprim, Lopurin) is also a common drug used to treat gout and works by inhibiting the enzyme that produces uric acid. Other drugs used to treat gout are probenicid (Benemid) and sulfinpyrazone (Anturane).

Anti-inflammatory drugs such as Naprosyn, Motrin, Advil, Nuprin, Feldene, Clinoril and Indocin are also routinely prescribed for pain. A corticosteroid injection is sometimes administered into the joint to relieve severe inflammation and pain.

Side-effects: Colchicine. Vomiting, diarrhea, stomach pain, nausea, hair loss, skin rash, loss of appetite.

Warning: Do not take this drug if pregnant or nursing. Colchicine can cause birth defects and does pass through breast milk. Do not take this drug if you suffer from serious kidney, liver, stomach or cardiac disorder.

Side-effects: Allopurinol (Zyloprim): Rash, nausea, vomiting, diarrhea, stomach pains, drowsiness, inability to concentrate.

Warning: Do not take Allopurinol if pregnant or nursing. This drug has been linked to birth defects and does pass through breast milk. This drug should not be taken with iron supplements.

Side effects: Indocin: Severe stomach upset or gastrointestinal distress including ulcers, vomiting, nausea, gas, and loss of appetite. Other possible symptoms are blurred vision, headache, reduced mental alertness, reduced coordination.

Warning: If pregnant or nursing do not use Indocin. The possibility of birth defects exists.

Note: If blurred vision or headache occurs while on this drug, contact your physician immediately.

Success rating of standard medical treatment: very good. Gout can be effectively controlled by the use of drug therapy and should be used to avoid the risk of kidney disease. Traditionally, the medical profession places more emphasis on drug treatment than on dietary modifications. Some physicians believe that changes in the diet are not effective and the gout can only be controlled through drug preparations. Other individuals strongly support the idea that gout, like gallstones, is a diet-related disorder.

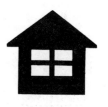

HOME SELF-CARE:

◆ Try to achieve an optimal weight through a nutritious diet with a regular exercise program.
◆ Do not lose weight too rapidly as uric acid levels may rise dramatically and result in an attack of gout.
◆ Keep the painful joint elevated. If pain is severe use an ice pack. Soft iced gel pack used for physical therapy are recommended.
◆ To keep the weight of bed sheets off of the affected joint use a box or make a frame to keep the joint uncovered when sheets or blankets are pulled up.
◆ A charcoal poultice made from activated powdered charcoal and water may provide some pain relief.

NUTRITIONAL APPROACH:

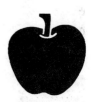

Although some physicians believe that dietary changes are an ineffective way of treating gout and prefer drug therapy, many health care providers support the idea that gout can be controlled by changes in dietary intake. This is a much more preferable approach to treating gout, rather than assuming that drug therapy will remedy poor eating habits. Nutritional changes and herbs should be tried by those who suffer with the disorder.

◆ A low purine diet is essential in treating and preventing gout. Purine foods to avoid are anchovies, meat gravies and broths, all organ meats, mincemeat, luncheon meats, asparagus, herring, sardines, mussels, and mushrooms, white flour and sugar. Additional foods to limit are dried beans, cauliflower, fish, lentils, oatmeal, peas, poultry, spinach, yeast products, saturated fats.
◆ Do not consume alcohol as it can increase the production of uric acid and significantly inhibit its elimination from the kidneys.
◆ Drink large amounts of fluid (water) to keep the urine diluted and promote the excretion of uric acid through the kidneys. Becoming dehydrated can increase your chances of an attack of gout.
◆ Foods to emphasize are raw fruits and vegetables, fresh juices (carrot, celery, parsley), grains, vegetable broths, seeds and nuts and high-fiber foods including complex carbohydrates.
◆ *Cherry juice:* Helps to neutralize uric acid.
◆ Cherries, hawthorne berries, blueberries and strawberries have shown through studies to be effective agents in lowering levels of uric acid and in preventing collagen destruction. Eating large amounts of cherries regularly is highly recommended if you are prone to gout.

- *Folic acid:* Important in facilitating nucleoprotein breakdown and inhibits the production of the enzyme responsible for the production of uric acid.
- *Vitamin C:* Helps to lower levels of uric acid but should not be taken in megadoses, as an increase in uric acid may result.
- *Vitamin E and selenium:* Help to keep the production of leukotrienes down, which inflame the joints in gout.
- *Zinc:* Involved in the breakdown of protein and in tissue repair.
- *Eicosapentaenoic acid:* A supplement that inhibits the production of the inflammatory agents released in gout.
- *Germanium:* Works to help control swelling and pain.
- *Kelp:* Has components which are good for reducing uric acid levels.
- *Bromelain:* An enzyme of the pineapple plant which functions as an effective anti-inflammatory.
- *Alanine, aspartic acid, and glycine:* These are amino acids which have been shown to reduce levels of uric acid. Before taking any amino acids, you should consult your doctor.

Note: Individuals who suffer from gout should not take high doses of niacin, as niacin may decrease the rate in which uric acid is excreted.

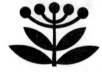

HERBAL REMEDIES:

- *Devil's claw:* An old folk medicine favorite for treating gout and arthritis. Helps to relieve joint pain and also reduces the cholesterol and uric acid content of the blood.
- *Celery:* Helps to clear uric acid from the joint. Can be used in seed or capsule form.
- *Wall germander:* Can be combined with yarrow and celery seed to help facilitate uric acid secretion. Do not exceed recommended doses.
- *Chaparral:* Helps to clear uric acid from the blood.
- *Hydrangea:* Helps the kidneys eliminate uric acid.
- *Saffron:* Helps to neutralize uric acid buildup in the system.
- Tea tree oil can be used externally by massaging it into the affected joints
- *The following herbs in combination may be useful:* Yucca, comfrey root, burdock, willow, redmond clay and pan pien lien.

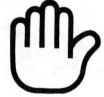

PREVENTION:

- Avoid a diet high in meat, alcohol and rich foods.
- If you are taking high blood pressure medication, you are at higher risk for developing gout. Watch your diet carefully, reduce salt, exercise and stay away from culprit foods and alcohols related to gout
- Eat cherries and other dark red or blue berries on a regular basis.

- Drink at least 5 to 8 glasses of water per day to make sure waste products such as uric acid can be excreted easier by the kidneys.
- Protect your joints from injury. Joints that have been traumatized seem more susceptible to gout.
- Don't overuse diuretics. The abuse of these agents can impair the kidney's ability to excrete uric acid.
- Do not consume large quantities of protein or take an excess of protein supplements.

Hantavirus

DEFINITION:

Hantavirus is a relatively new term referring to a life-threatening disease which first surfaced on Navajo reservations in New Mexico and has resulted in dozens of fatalities to date. This virally caused infection may have been around for years and would have gone unnoticed until the recent unexplained deaths of six people in 1993 resulted in a careful investigation of the virus.

The disease can strike suddenly and can become fatal within a short period of time. Hantavirus can be mistaken for an unexplained respiratory infection and is also referred to as hantaviral pulmonary syndrome. It is considered one of several recently discovered virally caused respiratory diseases that can in its initial stages mimic the flu, but progresses rapidly to a life threatening level.

Particular attention to the disease has been given in the southwest's four corner area where New Mexico, Arizona, Utah and Colorado meet. A 971-mile Navajo reservation located in New Mexico and Arizona was recently investigated by epidemiologists from the Federal Center for Disease Control and Prevention to try to find the cause of this mysterious disease. Seventy-three cases of hantavirus have been reported in 18 states, with 42 fatalities. Currently, there is no cure for the disease. As a result, prevention has been stressed.

The hantavirus family name originates from the Hantaan River in Korea, where the first strain of the virus was discovered several years ago.

CAUSES:

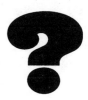

Hantavirus is transmitted by inhaling the virus or virus-containing material carried by rodent urine, droppings or saliva. Deer mice droppings and urine can emit airborne particles which can be inhaled by humans. Three strains of hantavirus have been discovered to date. Factors which may increase the risk of hantavirus are heavy winter precipitation, which can result in an abundance of pinon nuts which feed rodents, and unclean living conditions which attract rodents.

SYMPTOMS:

Physical: Hantavirus symptoms mirror those of influenza. Possible symptoms include fever, muscle aches, coughing, red eyes, headache and in later stages, fluid-filled lungs which inhibit breathing. These symptoms usually develop two weeks after exposure and rapidly progress as the lungs fill with fluid. This viral infection invades the lung capillaries and causes them to leak. Hantavirus circulates in the bloodstream while initial symptoms appear and then seems to intensify when the immune system is activated against the virus.

STANDARD MEDICAL TREATMENT:

An experimental antiviral drug called Ribavirin is considered the most promising treatment for hantavirus. This drug prevents the virus from reproducing in laboratory studies and may be effective in humans. Using artificial oxygenation can help to keep the victim of hantavirus from drowning in lung fluid.

Bradykinin antagonists are another family of experimental drugs which can interfere with the viral attack on the lungs. This drug has only been used on patients who are not expected to survive. Supportive measures such as intravenous feedings are also used to facilitate recovery.

Success rating of standard medical treatment: poor. Hantavirus has a 60 percent fatality rate.

Note: This disease requires immediate hospitalization. Home self-care, nutritional guidelines and herbal treatments can help support rehabilitation in some individuals after they are on the way to recovery. The volatile nature of the disease makes the utilization of many of the following suggestions difficult. Often the disease is not thought to be serious until it has progressed to its final stage.

NUTRITIONAL APPROACH:

◆ *Vitamin C with bioflavonoids in therapeutic doses:* Vitamin C is an antiviral agent that also helps to strengthen capillary walls, which are directly attacked by the hantavirus. Megadoses of vitamin C are recommended. Appropriate amounts should be discussed with a doctor.
◆ *Zinc:* Helps to boost the immune system to fight viral infection.
◆ *Vitamin A emulsion:* A powerful antioxidant which can enter the system quickly and fortify the immune system when under the stress of viral infection.
◆ *Germanium:* Helps to intensify immune responses.

◆ *L-cysteine:* An amino acid that helps to protect against viral infection.
◆ *Chlorophyll:* Helps to remove toxins from the bloodstream.

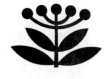

HERBAL REMEDIES:

◆ *Echinacea tea:* Drink a strong brew several times a day. Echinacea has significant antiviral properties.
◆ *Pau d'arco tea:* Drink this tea daily. It also is considered an herbal antiviral.
◆ *Catnip:* good to help bring down fevers which accompany viruses.
◆ *Comfrey and fenugreek:* Help to rebuild damaged lung tissue and promote drainage of lung fluids.
◆ *Garlic capsules:* Considered a natural antiviral substance.
◆ *Siberian ginseng:* Helps to heal respiratory passageways and promotes energy and recovery from debilitating conditions.
◆ *Buckwheat:* Rich in rutin, which helps to repair damaged capillary walls.
◆ *Heartsease:* Promotes healing of capillary walls.
◆ *Burdock root:* Helps to purify the blood and detoxify poisons.

PREVENTION:

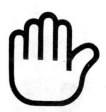

◆ Keep living areas clean.
◆ Decontaminate rodent nests and use spring-loaded traps baited with food to catch mice. Place the trap in newspaper that has been sprinkled with flea powder. Nests can be sprayed or dusted with insecticide for fleas. Wait one day and then disinfect with the procedures listed below.
◆ Don't leave old cars or junk piles in yards, where rodents might nest.
◆ Store all food in sealed containers.
◆ Place garbage in rodent-proof containers.
◆ Don't sleep on the ground or floor.
◆ Plug holes and crevices where rodents can enter. Even cracks as small as a quarter of an inch can allow a mouse to enter.
◆ If a live rodent is found is the home, use a trap and then spray the trap and the caught mouse with a disinfectant. Pick it up with a shovel or disposable rubber gloves and put rodent and trap in a double plastic bag. Place it in the garbage, or if in rural areas, bury it.
◆ If you have touched a rodent, wash your hands well and use a disinfectant rinse.
◆ If you have rodent infestation, do not sweep or vacuum until the area has been disinfected.
◆ Lysol or a mixture of 1 1/2 cups of chlorine bleach to a gallon of water can be used to mop and clean the area. Disinfect every item you used to clean with and throw everything away that was used for cleaning in sealed plastic bags.
◆ If you are in an area that is heavily infested by rodents, use a hepa filter mask to set traps and disinfect.

Heart Attack/Angina (myocardial infarction)

DEFINITION:

There are few things as frightening as either experiencing or witnessing a heart attack. Being able to recognize the signs of a heart attack can be extremely important, in that getting to a hospital as fast as possible can dramatically increase the chances for survival.

A heart attack refers to the sudden death of part of the heart muscle due to a lack of oxygen. An estimated 1 million heart attacks occur in the United States each year, and one-third of these are fatal. Heart attacks are considered the single most common cause of death in developed countries of the world.

Men are more susceptible to heart attacks than women. If you have had a heart attack, you have an increased risk of having another unless significant life-style changes are adopted. Many heart attack victims have a history of angina, which usually indicates the presence of coronary artery disease (see chapter on angina).

Because heart disease occurs far less frequently in primitive societies, Western life-style and diet must be viewed as the first and foremost contributing factor to heart related disorders and deaths.

CAUSES:

A heart attack results when blood supply to heart muscle is interrupted by a blockage of some kind, which causes the death of heart tissue. Atherosclerosis of the coronary arteries, in which cholesterol deposits (plaque) build up, is the most common cause of a heart attack. This buildup of fatty deposits develops on the inner lining of the arteries restricting blood flow and encouraging the formation of clots, which can result in the sudden blockage of blood flow to the heart.

Risk factors which increase your chances of having a heart attack are a familial history of heart disease, cigarette smoking, high blood pressure, obesity, high blood cholesterol, physical inactivity and coronary artery disease, which can develop from all of the risk factors listed here. Factors which are thought to trigger a heart attack include an emotional crisis, a heavy meal, physical overexertion or heavy lifting.

SYMPTOMS:

Physical: The pain of a heart attack usually comes on suddenly and ranges from a tight ache to an intense, crushing pain. It is persistent and does not decrease with rest. Heart attack pain can be characterized by the following:

◆   A feeling of central chest pressure, squeezing or tightness.

◆ Chest pain which radiates down the left arm, which may cause weakness in the arm muscles.

◆ Chest pain which radiates into the jaw area and through the back.

◆ Pain in the upper abdomen which may be mistaken for indigestion or heartburn.

Other symptoms of a heart attack include: shortness of breath, cold clammy skin, nausea, vomiting, diarrhea, anxiety, or loss of consciousness. If the attack is severe enough, heart failure can result after the heart has gone into an arrhythmia referred to as ventricular fibrillation.

Note: Twenty percent of heart attacks are painless, and usually occur in elderly people or diabetics.

Long-term complications of a heart attack include: mitral valve damage and a weakened heart which may require surgical repair.

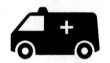

MEDICAL ALERT:

If you or someone else is experiencing any of the above symptoms, call an ambulance immediately. Any type of chest pain requires immediate medical evaluation. The use of electrical defibrillation and clot-dissolving drugs can save lives if administered quickly enough. Most heart-attack deaths occur before the victim ever reaches the hospital.

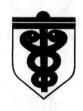

STANDARD MEDICAL TREATMENT:

An ECG will be taken immediately to assess the severity of the heart blockage. A blood sample will be tested for the presence of a certain enzyme which is released into the bloodstream from damaged heart muscle. Emergency coronary artery angiography may be indicated if surgery is being considered. Standard medical procedures to treat a heart attack include administering pain-killers and oxygen therapy. Diuretic drugs may be given to treat heart failure, which can lead to fluid accumulation in the lungs. IV fluids will be given to prevent shock, and antiarrhythmic drugs may be administered to control heart arrhythmias. Beta-blocker drugs are given in some cases to prevent further damage to heart muscle.

In cases where the victim of a heart attack arrives at a hospital within three to six hours of the attack, thrombolytic drugs to dissolve blood clots can be given and significantly increase the chances of survival. TPA (tissue plasminogen activator) is used to dissolve clots and is considered the best treatment for a heart attack. Streptokinase is another clot dissolver which is not considered as effective as TPA. Blood thinners will be given to prevent the formation of another clot until an angiogram can be done.

Following this test, an angioplasty, which widens the narrowed coronary arteries, or bypass surgery may be indicated. An angioplasty involves inserting a thin flexible tube into an artery located in the arm or leg and guiding it into the affected coronary artery. A small balloon is inflated in the artery, which usually eliminates the clot obstruction.

Surgical options: Coronary bypass surgery may be required to remove the blocked section of the artery and reconnect or reroute arterial blood flow by grafting in healthy vessels.

Success rating of standard medical treatment: very good. While doctors cannot cure the damage which results from a heart attack, cardiac care and drug therapy can save lives. Medical science is better at treating cardiac arrests and arrhythmias than heart failure, which results from a weak or damaged heart.

MEDICAL UPDATE:

◆ Recent studies done in Barcelona, Spain suggest that high fibrinogen levels in the blood may be a better predictor of heart attack than high cholesterol levels. As a result, fibrinogen testing will become a routine part of identifying patients at risk for having a heart attack. Ask your doctor about this new testing.

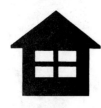

HOME SELF-CARE:

After you have sufficiently recovered, incorporate a sensible daily exercise regimen such as walking for 15 minutes a day. (Begin this only after you have received your doctor's approval.) Watch out for overprotective family members, who may have a tendency to inhibit your participation in exercise. Discouraging much-needed exercise in heart disease patients can do more harm than good. Make sure your spouse or family member is well educated on the benefits of exercise for the recovering heart patient.

◆ Avoid sexual intercourse for four to five weeks following a heart attack.
◆ Do not smoke. It not only impairs circulation, but also keeps substances that help to clear cholesterol out of artery walls from working properly. The bottom line is that regardless of what cigarette companies might claim, smoking can increase your risk of having a heart attack as well as a host of other diseases.

NUTRITIONAL APPROACH:

◆ Follow a diet which is high in fiber and low in animal fats and refined sugars. Add the following foods to your diet: whole grains, almonds, plenty of fresh fruits and vegetables, all kinds of legumes, white skinless turkey or chicken and fish.
◆ Avoid: Caffeine, red meats, and refined carbohydrates such as white sugar and white flour. These can cause wide fluctuations in blood sugar, which can strain the heart.

◆ Minimize your intake of dairy products. Use low-fat varieties. Homogenized dairy products contain an enzyme called xanthine oxidase which is believed to cause artery damage which could lead to arteriosclerosis.

◆ Avoid palm oil, coconut oil, peanut oil, cottonseed oil, shortening and butter. Only use margarine which is made from safflower or sunflower oils. Olive oil and canola oil are also good unsaturated oils that contain essential fatty acids.

◆ Use the following oils: Safflower, sunflower and corn oil, which are high in linoleic acid. Olive oil is monounsaturated and should be added to the diet along with polyunsaturated oils

◆ Decrease or eliminate salt and salty foods from your diet.

◆ Add plenty of raw onion and garlic to your diet. Both of these decrease the risk of blood clots.

◆ Pectin, which is found in fresh fruits and vegetables and can also be purchased as a supplement, can help to inhibit cholesterol build up and provide fiber.

◆ Drinking barley water is a traditional old-fashioned tonic which is considered high in its overall health benefits.

◆ Do not use alcohol.

◆ *Choline, inositol and lecithin:* These compounds are vital for the proper emulsification of fats in the bloodstream, which is directly linked with coronary artery disease. Polyunsaturated lecithin is recommended.

◆ *Coenzyme Q10:* Helps to facilitate oxygenation of heart muscle.

◆ *Vitamin C with bioflavonoids:* Helps prevent blood clots and strengthens capillary and blood vessel walls. Some studies indicate that vitamin C can protect arteries from becoming clogged and may contribute to reversing heart disease.

◆ *Vitamin C complex:* A thiamine deficiency (vitamin B1) can lead to heart disease.

◆ *Vitamin E:* While scientific confirmation is slow to surface, the benefits of vitamin E for heart-related disorders is supported by overwhelming individual case studies. Vitamin E is an antioxidant and is also considered a natural blood thinner.

◆ *Selenium and copper:* A lack of selenium and copper has been associated with the development of heart disease.

◆ *Calcium and magnesium chelate:* Vital for the proper function of heart muscle in maintaining normal heart rhythm and blood pressure. Both of these minerals contribute to the normal contraction and relaxation of heart muscle.

◆ *L-carnatine, l-cysteine and l-methionine:* These amino acids can help prevent heart disease by reducing fat levels in the blood.

◆ *Glucomannan:* Can help to control wide fluctuations in blood sugar.

◆ Unsaturated fatty acid supplements such as primrose or salmon oil can protect heart muscle.

◆ *Omega-3 EPA:* Helps prevent blood cells from clumping together, which decreases the risk of blood clot formation. Taking this supplement can keep the

blood thinned without the side-effects of aspirin therapy.
- ◆ Taking 2 teaspoons of wheat germ oil daily is also recommended for any heart-related disorder.

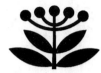

HERBAL REMEDIES:

- ◆ *Hawthorne berries:* Can be taken in capsule or syrup form. This is an excellent herbal tonic for the heart which helps to compensate for valvular insufficiency. Hawthorne helps to reduce high blood pressure and prevent hardening of the arteries. It is also good for controlling low blood sugar levels.
- ◆ *Mistletoe:* Can lower blood pressure and reduce stress on the heart by strengthening capillary walls.
- ◆ *Garlic capsules:* Garlic promotes blood circulation and is considered beneficial to the heart. In several studies, garlic has been shown to decrease blood cholesterol levels even after a fatty meal was consumed. Garlic also helps to lower blood pressure and inhibit clot formation.
- ◆ *Ginkgo:* Relaxes blood vessels and improves blood flow, even in constricted arteries.
- ◆ *Heartsease:* Contains flavonoids which strengthen blood vessel walls.
- ◆ *Oolong tea:* Contains phenols which can inhibit cholesterol absorption and help prevent coronary artery disease.
- ◆ *Capsicum:* Helps to clean and nourish blood vessels.
- ◆ *Rosemary tea:* Considered a traditional heart tonic, this herb helps to promote circulation and lower blood pressure.
- ◆ Chinese mushroom (*auricularia polytricha*) is a natural blood thinner. A tablespoon of soaked mushrooms eaten four times a week may be as valuable as aspirin therapy without the risk of hemorrhage or stomach irritation.
- ◆ Saffron: Reduces cholesterol levels and strengthens heart muscle.
- ◆ *The following herbs in combination may be useful:* hawthorn berries, capsicum and garlic.
- ◆ *The following herbs in combination may be useful:* capsicum, pan pien lien, and hawthorne.

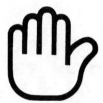

PREVENTION:

- ◆ The best way to prevent a heart attack or heart disease is to build good habits of eating, exercise and relaxation, which protect coronary arteries from damage.
- ◆ Keep serum cholesterol levels low: High serum cholesterol is the most important predictor of a heart attack. Cholesterol-reducing drugs should be used only as a last resort. Atherosclerosis can be stopped and even reversed without the use of drugs if dietary changes are implemented.
- ◆ Don't smoke: Nicotine constricts arteries, impairs circulation and raises blood pressure. It also reduces the capacity of the blood to carry oxygen and increases

the risk of blood clot formation. Smoking is a great contributor to coronary heart disease and the incidence of heart attacks.

◆ Exercise daily, incorporating a routine of 30 minutes of aerobic exercise five days per week. Exercise has a multitude of physical as well as emotional benefits. It improves the efficiency of the heart, reduces cholesterol levels and the chance of blood clot formation and improves circulation in the heart muscle itself. Brisk walking is considered an excellent aerobic exercise.

◆ Make relaxation techniques an integral part of your life. Reduce and manage stress, which can actually elevate blood cholesterol and clotting. Stress releases adrenalin, which causes the heart to work harder. Excessive adrenal stimulation which can occur in periods of prolonged stress not only increase the chance of arterial spasms and heart attacks but can decrease your chance of surviving a heart attack as well. Use methods such as biofeedback, music therapy, yoga, and self-hypnosis to control stress.

◆ Evaluate your emotional status. If you are resentful, fearful or angry, get rid of these toxic reactions to the events of life. Make the pursuit of joy and serenity a daily goal. The power of prayer and meditation should not be minimized.

◆ Maintain an optimal weight: Obesity increases the risk of heart disease, high blood pressure, diabetes and a number of other diseases.

◆ Keep your blood pressure normal: High blood pressure can significantly increase demands on the heart and may accelerate the development of coronary artery disease (see chapter on coronary artery disease).

Heartburn/Indigestion

DEFINITION:

Heartburn is a not-so-subtle reminder that sometimes you have to pay the piper for overeating or for choosing the wrong things to eat. The fiery, burning sensation that characterizes heartburn can quickly spoil after-dinner conversation and demands attention. Unfortunately, the fast-paced nature of our society and the disappearance of leisurely meals have also made heartburn a routine occurrence.

Heartburn is also called gastroesophageal reflux, and refers to a burning sensation which originates from the stomach, but is usually experienced in the chest region. This feeling may travel from the breastbone to the throat and can come and go. It is caused when hydrochloric acid, which promotes digestion, backs up from the stomach into the esophagus. Occasional heartburn is no cause for alarm.

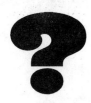

CAUSES:

Heartburn occurs when there is too much pressure on the stomach or when the sphincter muscle, which separates the esophagus from the stomach, does not completely close. Excessive consumption of certain foods such as fried, fatty, spicy, rich or acidic foods can increase the risk for heartburn. In addition, alcohol and smoking increase the risk for heartburn. Overusing aspirin and caffeine have also been linked to an increased incidence of heartburn.

Heartburn may also be caused by an enzyme deficiency, a hiatal hernia, stomach ulcers, gallbladder disorders, allergies, stress or heart problems. Chronic constipation can also contribute to heartburn by causing straining during bowel movements, which can put added pressure on the abdomen.

Recurring heartburn may indicate the presence of esophagitis, which indicates the inability of the lower segment of the esophagus to completely close off from the stomach. Lying down in a certain position or bending over after a meal can also result in heartburn. Pregnancy can cause heartburn due to the added pressure placed on the stomach by the growing fetus.

Certain drugs including some antidepressants, birth control pills, antihistamines and certain sedatives like valium can also increase your risk for heartburn.

SYMPTOMS:

Physical: Heartburn is characterized by a burning pain or sensation that can feel like it's moving from the upper stomach area to the throat. Heartburn is sometimes accompanied by bloating, belching and an uncomfortable feeling of fullness. Headache and nausea can also be present. Sometimes the sensation of pain that surrounds the chest area is mistaken for a symptoms of a heart attack.

Psychological: Heartburn, like a number of other physical conditions, can be brought on by anxiety and stress. It is important that during meal or right after eating, the mind is relaxed and tension alleviated. "Nerves" can result in adrenalin surges which can cause poor digestion and excess stomach acid. If you have trouble with heartburn, do not eat on the run, and try to make mealtime a pleasant experience. Avoid topics of conversation which may cause intense emotional reactions. Make the eating environment tranquil and relaxing, and slow down.

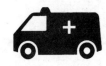

MEDICAL ALERT:

If heartburn is accompanied by the vomiting of black or bloody material, passing a tar-like stool, chest pain that radiates to the back or shoulder, difficulty swallowing, shortness of breath, or dizziness, see your doctor immediately. These symptoms may indicate the presence of ulcers, an obstruction of the esophagus or a heart attack.

Note: If you experience heartburn on a regular basis, see your doctor. Repeated episodes of heartburn can damage the esophagus or cause ulcers.

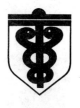

STANDARD MEDICAL TREATMENT:

Your doctor will have to determine whether or not your symptoms are the result of stomach acid. Medications that decrease the secretion of acid may be prescribed. An upper GI x-ray may be indicated if the presence of an ulcer or hiatal hernia is suspected. Antacids will be recommended.

Side-effects: Antacid (magnesium and aluminum products): Diarrhea and constipation. Calcium and sodium products may produce a rebound effect where more acid is produced. Aluminum compounds have been associated with Alzheimer's disease, although the link is not widely accepted among medical professionals.

Warning: Do not take antacids over a long period of time if you have high blood pressure, heart trouble or kidney disease. Check with your doctor for the best kind of antacid to use.

Note: Pregnant or nursing mothers can take antacids in moderation; however, always check with your doctor before doing so.

HOME SELF-CARE:

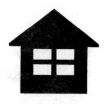

- ◆ Don't smoke: Nicotine adversely affects the tone of the esophageal sphincter muscle and can directly contribute to heartburn.
- ◆ Over-the-counter antacids can be effective but can contain undesirable ingredients. Try to avoid products that contain sodium or aluminum. Antacids such as Maalox, Mylanta or Gelusil may provide relief but should be used with caution by people who suffer from heart disease or high blood pressure. Tums is recommended because it contains calcium carbonate. Milk of Magnesia is also free of aluminum and sodium. There is some speculation that using antacids on a regular basis can actually encourage further stomach acid secretion. The continued use of antacids may also result in a depletion of calcium.
- ◆ Calcium carbonate can function as an antacid and can be purchased as a powder. It is also contained in Tums.
- ◆ Do not use sodium bicarbonate (baking soda) as a home remedy. It contains sodium and if misused, it can upset the acid/alkaline balance of the body and cause a potentially dangerous condition.
- ◆ While drinking milk can sometimes help to relieve the symptoms of heartburn initially, dairy products increase the stomach's production of hydrochloric acid.
- ◆ Review other medications that you are taking to see if they are the cause of your heartburn. Certain high blood pressure drugs (calcium channel blockers) can cause stomach acid to back up into the esophagus. Birth control pills, antihistamines, and certain tranquilizers like Valium can also promote heartburn.

◆ Loosen constrictive clothing or tight belts.
◆ Learn to eat slowly, chew thoroughly and relax during mealtime.
◆ Do not eat on the run or get involved in unpleasant discussions during a meal.

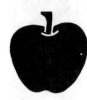

NUTRITIONAL APPROACH:

◆ Avoid culprit foods: fried foods, fatty foods, citrus fruits, coffee, alcohol, spicy foods, chocolate, tomato-based foods, onions (although if cooked thoroughly they are considerably less likely to cause trouble; certain varieties of onions such as the walla and maui are considerably milder) rich dairy products and carbonated beverages. These substances can irritate the lining of the esophagus or cause the sphincter muscle to relax, which allows acid to escape. Soda pop can cause a sensation of bloating which puts pressure on the abdominal sphincter.
◆ Eat smaller, more frequent meals and avoid overeating.
◆ Apple cider vinegar (1 teaspoon to half a glass of water) sipped slowly seems to counteract heartburn.
◆ *Pancreatin:* A proteolytic enzyme which can facilitate digestion.

HERBAL REMEDIES:

◆ *Ginger:* An excellent herb for heartburn due to is ability to absorb excess stomach acid. Can be taken in capsule form.
◆ *Comfrey and pepsin:* Soothes the digestive tract.
◆ Papaya tablets are good to help with any problem related to indigestion. They quickly help relieve stomach distress.
◆ *Papaya and peppermint:* Natural acid neutralizers.
◆ *Peppermint tea:* Acts as a sedative for the stomach. Helps to calm a nervous stomach.
◆ *Angelica root:* Helps to relieve gas and other stomach ailments.
◆ *Fennel:* Works as an anti-inflammatory for the stomach.
◆ *Algin:* A gel derived from algae that can help to quiet heartburn and protect the lining of the esophagus.
◆ *Lemon balm:* Relaxes a nervous stomach, which can help decrease the level of acid output.
◆ *The following herbs in combination may be useful:* Papaya, ginger, peppermint, wild yam, fennel, dong quai, spearmint and catnip.

PREVENTION:

◆ Don't smoke. Smoking may actually weaken the sphincter muscle of the stomach.

- Eat slowly, take small bites, and chew your food thoroughly. Gulping food down can place stress on the stomach and impair digestion.
- Avoid rich, fatty, fried foods, carbonated drinks, or highly spiced foods. Most fast food is high in fat. Fat slows the emptying of the stomach.
- Do not use caffeine or alcohol.
- Do not eat while on the run or in situations of high stress. Make mealtime a time to relax your body and mind.
- Do not lay down after a meal, especially on your right side. Laying on the right side after eating can produce uncomfortable bloating.
- Take a leisurely walk after dinner. This movement helps to facilitate digestion, but don't run after eating or engage in strenuous exercise.
- Do not consume large quantities of liquid with your meals, as digestion may become impaired. Some professionals believe that drinking small amounts of water throughout your meal can help wash away and neutralize stomach acids that may migrate into the esophagus.
- At the first sign of heartburn, drink a glass of water.
- Do not over-use aspirin and ibuprofen, which can promote the production of excess stomach acid.
- Elevating the head of the bed may help to prevent the backflow of acid from the stomach into the esophagus.
- Don't wear clothing that is too constricting while eating.
- Don't eat too close to bedtime.
- Don't become constipated. Eat plenty of fiber and drink lots of water every day. Frequent straining during difficult bowel movements can place pressure on the stomach and increase your risk for heartburn.

Hemorrhoids

DEFINITION:

While varicose veins in the legs are routinely discussed, many people are not aware that a hemorrhoid is nothing more than a varicose vein located in the rectum. Hemorrhoids can be particularly bothersome and create a great deal of discomfort, especially if you have to sit for extended periods of time. Technically, hemorrhoids refers to a condition characterized by distended veins that form in the lining of the anus. Internal hemorrhoids may be located near the beginning of the anal canal or close to the anal opening (ecteranl hemorrhoids). When hemorrhoids protrude outside the anal opening, they are referred to as prolapsed hemorrhoids.

Hemorrhoids are very common and may begin in the early twenties, but usually do not become obvious until the thirties. Approximately 50 percent of people over 50 have hemorrhoidal symptoms. Up to one-third of the total population of the United States have hemorrhoids to some extent. While hemorrhoids are painful, they are rarely dangerous.

CAUSES:

Gravity causes continual stress on the delicate vessels which supply blood to the anus. In addition, abdominal pressure of any kind can aggravate the pressure placed on these veins. Hemorrhoids can be the result of pregnancy, which puts added weight and pressure on the rectum, a complication of childbirth, a congenital weakness in the veins of the anus, or from repeated straining during attempts to move hard feces.

In addition, the repeated use of laxatives, prolonged hard coughing, violent sneezing, physical exertion, lifting the wrong way, and standing or sitting for long periods of time can also initiate the formation of hemorrhoids. Hemorrhoids can sometimes develop as a complication of liver disease.

SYMPTOMS:

Physical: Hemorrhoids commonly cause rectal bleeding, pain and discomfort, inflammation, throbbing, especially during a bowel movement, mucus discharge, and itching. If a clot forms in the vein of a prolapsed hemorrhoid, intense pain can result. If hemorrhoidal bleeding is prolonged, iron deficiency anemia can occur.

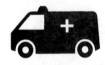

MEDICAL ALERT:

If you find blood in the stool, or experience a change in bowel habits, see your doctor immediately. Other causes of rectal bleeding are anal fissures, intestinal disorders and colon cancer.

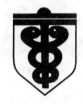

STANDARD MEDICAL TREATMENT:

A proctoscopy will be done by your doctor, where the rectum is viewed and examined for the possible presence of cancer. A barium enema and a sigmoidoscopy may be recommended, if cancer is suspected. In mild cases, hemorrhoids are traditionally treated with high-fiber diets, increased liquids, rectal suppositories, anorectal pads and creams which contain corticosteroid drugs to reduce swelling and inflammation.

Internal hemorrhoids must be treated on an outpatient basis using the proctoscope. Some types of hemorrhoids can be treated by constricting them with tight rubber bands which causes them to wither within a few days.

Using liquid nitrogen (cryosurgery) is another method of removing hemorrhoidal distensions. A procedure referred to as monopolar direct current therapy is another outpatient technique where Procaine solution is injected into the hemorrhoid. This approach has had some success and for some physicians is the treatment of choice; however, for large hemorrhoids it is sometimes ineffective. If these measures prove unsuccessful, a hemorrhoidectomy may be recommended.

Surgical options: A hemorrhoidectomy refers to a procedure which is done under general or epidural anesthesia, whereby the hemorrhoid is clamped, secured with a suture and then surgically cut off.

Medical update:

♦ A new laser technique developed in Europe is now available in the United States. This procedure does not require hospitalization or general anesthesia and should be investigated as an option.

Success rating of standard medical treatment: good. Most hemorrhoids can be taken care of medically; however, the methods that have been employed are viewed by the victim of hemorrhoids as unpleasant. Laser surgery and monopolar therapy seem to be generally regarded as better therapies. Hemorrhoids typically recur.

Home self-care:

♦ When applying any ointment, cream or preparation to the anal area, make sure the surface has been cleaned and dried. Bacteria can become trapped under creams and ointments, which can cause additional inflammation.
♦ Using witch hazel on hemorrhoids is an old traditional treatment. Witch hazel is an astringent which constricts blood vessels. It is an ingredient found in Tucks, Preparation H and other hemorrhoidal treatments. It can be purchased in a bottle and applied with cotton. Soaking a piece of cotton in witch hazel and leaving it on the anal opening overnight may provide additional relief.
♦ Using petroleum jelly on the anal area can help to reduce pain. A cotton ball works nicely for application.
♦ *Zinc oxide cream:* This inexpensive over-the-counter ointment is also good for pain and swelling. Zinc oxide powder is also available. These preparations also help to toughen the skin over the hemorrhoid, which lessens the risk for additional irritation.
♦ A and D ointments or vitamin E ointments are also good for pain and lubrication.
♦ *Aloe vera gel:* Soothes and cools the area and promotes healing.
♦ Avoid topical anesthetic preparations which contain benzocaine. These may numb the area temporarily but can also cause more irritation. Preparation H is considered an effective ointment, which is made from a combination of yeast

culture and shark liver extract.

◆ An ice pack applied to the anal area may also decrease swelling and pain. A product called Anurex is specifically designed to reduce the swelling and pain of hemorrhoids.

◆ Controlled exhaling and inhaling while lifting a heavy object or during a bowel movement helps to minimize abdominal pressure. Singing while on the toilet has also been suggested as a way to minimize straining. If you suffer from hemorrhoids, don't lift heavy objects.

◆ Sit in a tub of warm water. All you need is 4 to 5 inches of warm water. Stay in the tub for at least 10 minutes. A good temperature is between 100 and 105 degrees Fahrenheit.

◆ Sitting on a doughnut pillow which can be purchased at a pharmacy can greatly help relieve pressure on anal tissue and provide some relief from pain.

◆ Try not to postpone bowel movements when you feel the urge. Constipation can result from this practice, which may initiate difficult bowel movements. Sitting on the toilet for long periods of time may also aggravate hemorrhoids.

◆ Keep the anal area clean but do not use abrasive toilet paper. Use a pre-moistened wipe, then pat dry with toilet paper. Scented or colored toilet paper may cause additional irritation. If using toilet paper, moisten it first with witch hazel.

◆ Exercise regularly to keep your bowels active. Brisk walks, low-impact aerobics, yoga or dance classes are all excellent ways to exercise.

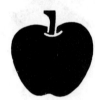

NUTRITIONAL APPROACH:

◆ Hemorrhoids are rarely seen in cultures where high-fiber diets are consumed. Like so many other disorders, hemorrhoids could be controlled with a diet low in refined, processed foods and high in whole grains, raw fruits and vegetables.

◆ Eat a high-fiber diet (oat bran, whole grains, dried prunes, dates, raw fruits and vegetables and beans). Individuals who do not get enough bulk fiber in their diets tend to strain during bowel movements due to the formation of small and hard feces.

◆ Avoid refined white flour, white sugar, and the empty calories found in high-fat junk foods. In addition, coffee, and alcohol are discouraged. There is some speculation that hot peppers can make hemorrhoids more painful. Those that disagree point out that the peppers would be broken down before reaching the lower intestine.

◆ Avoid salt: Salt can cause hemorrhoidal tissue to swell more due to the retention of fluid.

◆ Guar gum and psyllium seed are natural bulking agents that can significantly reduce constipation and straining during bowel movements. These compounds are less irritating to the bowel than whole wheat or cellulose products.

◆ Drink 6 to 8 glasses of water per day to avoid constipation and hard stool.

◆ *Bioflavonoids:* Beneficial in the treatment of any varicose veins. Help to strengthen the integrity of vein walls and increase the muscular tone of the veins. Bioflavanoids are contained in certain berries such as hawthorne, cherries, blueberries, and blackberries.

◆ *Rutin:* A component of vitamin C: rutin combats fragility of the capillaries. It is contained in buckwheat, rose hips, grapes, plums, apricots, and all citrus fruits.

◆ *Vitamin E:* Promotes tissue healing and helps control bleeding.

◆ *Calcium and magnesium:* Helps to prevent colon disorders and promote the clotting of blood.

◆ *Vitamin A and beta carotene:* Help promote healing of mucous membranes and damaged tissue.

◆ *Zinc:* Helps to decrease inflammation.

◆ *Vitamin K:* Good if hemorrhoidal bleeding is present. Can be found in alfalfa, kale and other dark green leafy vegetables.

◆ *Onion and garlic:* Help to break down fibrin, which can be deposited in tissues near to varicose veins.

◆ *Bromelain:* An enzyme from the pineapple plant which helps to prevent the formation of hard and lumpy skin which surrounds varicose veins in the rectum or anus.

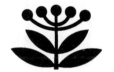

Herbal remedies:

◆ *Butcher's broom:* Has a long history in the treatment of hemorrhoids. It contains compounds which act as vasoconstrictors to help shrink hemorrhoidal tissue. Can be used both externally and internally.

◆ *Linseed oil:* Can help to soften hard stools.

◆ *Buckthorn bark:* Promotes vein integrity and helps to strengthen vein walls.

◆ *Pilewort:* An astringent herb that can help to stop bleeding. Use as a topical ointment.

◆ *Huaijiao:* A cooling anti-inflammatory that also helps to prevent constipation.

◆ *Capsicum and ginger:* Increase the breakdown of fibrin, which can contribute to the formation of distended veins. Take internally in capsule form.

◆ *Tormentil:* Can be used externally on the surface of the hemorrhoid.

◆ *Yarrow extract and white oat bark:* Applied externally can help heal and decrease inflammation.

◆ Stoneroot can be swabbed on the hemorrhoids as a tincture or taken as capsules. This herb has been particularly effective in treating hemorrhoids. It promotes vein strength and structure.

◆ *Elderberry poultice:* Can be applied directly on inflamed area. Helps to relieve hemorrhoidal pain.

Prevention:

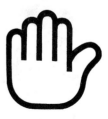

◆ A diet high in fiber is the best way to prevent the formation of hemorrhoids. Eat plenty of vegetables, fruits, legumes, and grains.

◆ Do not stand or sit for long periods of time. If you have a choice between driving or walking, walk. Exercise regularly to promote good muscle tone and to prevent constipation.
◆ Keep weight in a desireable range.
◆ When lifting heavy objects, do so in such a way as to minimize abdominal pressure.

Hepatitis (infectious)

DEFINITION:

The heart and the brain are usually the most praised organs of the human body. However, the liver is truly a marvel and without its incredible functions, human life could not be sustained. Because of its vital importance to maintaining health, any disease that affects the liver is considered serious.

Hepatitis is characterized by an inflammation of the liver that can be caused by a virus, exposure to toxins or by a bacterial infection. Viral hepatitis is the most common kind and is most prevalent among adolescent girls. Viral hepatitis ranks among the top four infectious diseases in the United States and is typically divided into three types: A, B, and Non-A/Non-B. Type A, or infectious hepatitis, is highly contagious.

The incubation period for infectious hepatitis is between 14 and 40 days and the onset of the disease is typically sudden. Autumn and winter are peak seasons for this type of hepatitis. Travelers run a high risk of exposure to the disease if they are going to areas where hygiene is poor such as parts of Asia, South America and Africa.

CAUSES:

Infectious hepatitis can be spread by contaminated milk or water, certain foods such as shellfish, through animal contact or by swimming in infected water. Fecal contamination of food commonly occurs in restaurants, which can cause an epidemic outbreak of the disease.

SYMPTOMS:

Physical: Hepatitis can be a symptomless disease or a flulike illness. It is sometimes followed by jaundice, but not always. Jaundice (yellowing of the whites of the eyes), fever, malaise, chills, itching, headache, lack of appetite, vomiting, diarrhea, constipation, dark urine, upper abdominal pain and cramping and joint pain can also accompany hepatitis. Any fever present will usually disappear when the jaundice becomes apparent. Stools appear chalky and cream-colored during the infection and a skin rash may develop.

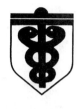

STANDARD MEDICAL TREATMENT:

Diagnosis is made by identifying the virus through the detection of certain antibodies to the virus in the blood. A blood alanine aminotransferase test will be administered to determine the presence of hepatitis. In some cases, corticosteroid drugs may be employed to reduce liver inflammation.

Antiviral agents have not been very successful in the treatment of virally caused hepatitis. Plenty of rest and a specific diet will be suggested to the victim of hepatitis. Subsequent lab tests will monitor recovery and watch for symptoms of chronic hepatitis, which rarely occur with infectious hepatitis.

Success rating of standard medical treatment: good. Hepatitis is a serous disease that requires the care of a physician. While there is little that can be done to treat virally caused hepatitis, medical care to monitor the presence of the infection is vital. Drugs stress the liver and are discouraged unless absolutely necessary. In cases of viral infection, natural therapies can have a very beneficial effect.

MEDICAL UPDATE:

◆ A new test that can detect the Non-A and Non-B form of hepatitis that can be spread through blood transfusions will be available shortly. This type of hepatitis affects more than 150,000 Americans each year. A new vaccine for travelers is also currently available.

HOME SELF-CARE:

◆ Rest and proper nutrition are the best home-care strategies for effecting a full and rapid recovery.
◆ Avoid using any drugs or antibiotics (assuming the infection is viral), as these tax the liver. Acetaminophen and iron supplements are particularly irritating to the liver during a hepatitis infection.
◆ A hot castor oil pack can be used over the liver area for 15 minutes a day to stimulate circulation. A hot water bottle can also be used.

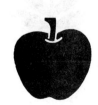

NUTRITIONAL APPROACH:

◆ The liver has a wonderful ability to restore and regenerate itself if given the proper tools. The right nutritional choices can work wonders in treating hepatitis.
◆ Do not eat excessive protein. One way to help the liver heal is to lighten its

workload by not taxing it with too much protein.

- Restrict your intake of fats while the liver is healing. Avoid high protein foods and concentrate on complex carbohydrates and fresh fruits and vegetables. A vegetarian diet is preferable as the disease runs its course.
- Don't use any protein or amino acid supplements. When the liver is stressed these are not recommended. Methionine is one exception which is seen as beneficial in its ability to detoxify the liver.
- Avoid fried foods and animal fats and stay away from very hot or very cold foods. Do not consume white sugar or highly processed and refined foods. Avoid shellfish and eat no raw fish or animal flesh while the liver is healing. Reduce your salt intake also.
- Make breakfast the most nutritious meal of the day. Appetites are generally very poor with hepatitis, and morning is the best time to get a child or adult to eat.
- Drink plenty of water and get a great deal of rest. Fresh lemon juice in warm water is recommended. Other juices that are particularly good for liver ailments are beet, celery, carrot, apple, and spinach.
- Eat plenty of strawberries, grapes and cherries, which are rich in bioflavonoids. Other foods to emphasize include artichokes, cauliflower, collards, endive, spinach and green peppers.
- *Coenzyme Q10:* Helps to boost the immune system in fighting viral infections.
- *Germanium:* Facilitates cell oxygenation and helps to control pain.
- *Lecithin:* Works as a cell protectant and helps to prevent fat buildup in an inflamed liver.
- *Vitamin A:* Promotes digestion and proper food assimilation.
- *Vitamin B complex:* Helps normalize the liver and its function.
- *Vitamin C with bioflavonoids:* Helps to counteract inflammation, fights infections and promotes tissue regeneration. Large doses of vitamin C have had dramatic results in speeding the rate of recovery from hepatitis.
- *Vitamin E:* Helps to reduce uric acid and also contributes to the control of scarring in living tissue.
- *Liver extracts:* Help to promote liver cell regeneration.
- Do not under any circumstance drink alcoholic beverages.
- Do not take iron or zinc.

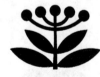

HERBAL REMEDIES:

- *Milk thistle:* Facilitates liver cell regeneration. European research has shown that this herb can also protect the liver from toxic damage. Take in capsule form.
- An herbal tonic can be made by placing 1/2 teaspoon of nutmeg and a pinch of cardamon in 1 cup of hot water. This combination works to stimulate pancreatic juices, which help to strengthen and rebuild the liver.
- *Burdock:* Helps to restore liver functions.
- *Gentian:* A bitter tonic that is considered a liver stimulant.

- *Dandelion:* A restorative herb for the liver which promotes bile flow. Dandelion root tea is excellent and should be taken throughout your recovery period. Herbalists all over the world recognize dandelion as an excellent liver ailment remedy.
- *Chai hu and ho shou wu:* Encourage liver health and proper liver function.
- Oregon grape root tincture taken in water two to three times a day can help to remove toxins from the blood, especially if liver function is compromised.
- *Artichoke:* This herb has a long folk history of use in the treatment of several liver diseases. It also contributes to liver tissue growth and expedites the movement of bile from the liver.
- *Schizandra berries:* A Chinese medicinal herb which can help promote liver tissue healing, especially when liver inflammation is present in conditions like hepatitis.
- *Pau d'arco:* Protects liver tissue from damage.
- *Saffron:* Helps to digest fats, which puts less stress on the liver while it heals.
- *Golden seal:* Use in tea form as an antiviral agent.
- *Blue vervain, devil's claw:* Both considered traditional liver tonics.
- *The following herbs in combination may be useful:* Golden seal root, yellow dock, Oregon grape, pan pien lien, dandelion, and red beet root.
- *Licorice:* An effective antiviral herb in the treatment of liver infection.

PREVENTION:

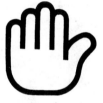

- Wash your hands frequently with soap and water or an antiseptic solution if you handle raw food.
- Keep a family member who has hepatitis as isolated as possible from the bathroom other people use. Use disposable eating utensils, cups and plates and do not let the infected person participate in meal preparation.
- Launder the linens, clothing, towels etc. in a separate wash load and use chlorine bleach in the water.
- For non-immune travelers at risk, passive immunization with immunoglobulin combined with good hygiene and careful selection of food and drink can help prevent becoming infected with the hepatitis virus.
- Vaccines are available for Type B hepatitis and are usually only recommended for those who are at a high risk for this type of hepatitis, which include health care workers, male homosexuals drug addicts and children born to mothers who carry the virus.
- Observe good hygiene by washing hands and utensils often when preparing food, and always washing hands after using the bathroom.
- Never share a needle, even for ear piercing or tattooing.
- Don't drink water from a questionable source even if it looks pure.
- Do not consume alcohol, drugs or a high-fat and high-animal protein diet. All of these factors can tax the liver and make it more susceptible to infection.

High Blood Pressure (hypertension)

DEFINITION:

Having high blood pressure should never be taken lightly. High blood pressure is considered one of the major medical problems of our age and is considered a liability of 20th century life-styles and diet. Of all the risk factors, high blood pressure is the most accurate predictor of future cardiovascular disease in people over the age of 65.

Hypertension, or high blood pressure, refers to a condition where too much pressure is exerted on the arteries when the blood is pumped by the heart. In high blood pressure, the heart has to pump the blood through the circulatory system with greater force, resulting in added strain on the entire cardiovascular system.

When measuring blood pressure, both the systolic and diastolic pressure is read. Systolic pressure refers to the highest pressure which occurs when the heart contracts. Diastolic pressure is the pressure at the moment when the heart relaxes, which permits the in flow of blood to be pumped out. A reading of 120 over 70 refers to a systolic pressure of 120 over a diastolic reading of 70.

There are two types of high blood pressure: essential hypertension, which results for no apparent reason, and secondary hypertension, which is a complication of another condition. Essential hypertension comprises 92 percent of all diagnosed cases of high blood pressure. High blood pressure is extremely common in North America. Approximately one in ten Americans suffers from hypertension (60 million).

The incidence of high blood pressure dramatically rises with age and is twice as high among black Americans. Men are more affected than women. A normal blood pressure reading is 120 over 80; however, acceptable blood pressure readings can vary from 110 over 70 to 140 over 90.

A condition referred as malignant hypertension is a rare form of high blood pressure which comes on suddenly and shoots up dramatically. It requires immediate medical attention. If left untreated it can result in serious kidney, eye or brain damage. It is a potentially fatal condition.

CAUSES:

The exact cause of most high blood pressure remains somewhat of a mystery. What is known is that high blood pressure runs in families, and is also linked to obesity, diet, cigarette smoking, alcohol consumption, stress, the excessive use of stimulants, drug abuse and high sodium intake.

The incidence of high blood pressure increases with age and is higher among blacks. High blood pressure can also result from arteriosclerosis, atherosclerosis, congestive heart failure, kidney disease, diabetes, hormonal disorders, taking birth control pills, pregnancy, and smoking.

Some studies have shown a connection between exposure to heavy metals such as lead and cadmium and elevated blood pressure. Genetic research suggests that two specific genes may identify children who will develop high blood pressure later in their lives.

SYMPTOMS:

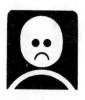

Physical: High blood pressure can be a symptomless disease. Symptoms of advanced hypertension include dizziness, headache, rapid pulse, sweating and visual disturbances. Frequent nosebleeds have also been linked to high blood pressure.

Psychological: While high blood pressure affects every cultural class to some extent, there is some speculation that certain types of personalities seem more prone to the disorder. The type A personality, which is usually typified by perfectionism, ambition, high levels of motivation and high standards of achievement is thought to be more susceptible to stress-related high blood pressure. Some studies indicate that people who are always in a rush, have a tendency to look at their watches often, have trouble sleeping and don't find time to relax need to monitor their blood pressure and take steps to counteract stress. Regular exercise, music therapy, breathing techniques, yoga, etc. can greatly help in reducing tension.

Several physicians believe that high blood pressure is a physiological condition which cannot result from anxiety or tension alone. Their approach to the value of relaxation and stress reduction therapy on the disease is skeptical at best.

MEDICAL ALERT:

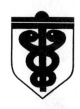

Anyone who is suffering from high blood pressure should be under a doctor's care. Because high blood pressure is often asymptomatic, it should be monitored every six months to a year. High blood pressure is a serious condition which should not be taken lightly. Prolonged high blood pressure can result in heart disease, kidney damage, stroke and atherosclerosis. Untreated high blood pressure can significantly reduce life expectancy.

STANDARD MEDICAL TREATMENT:

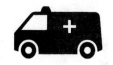

High blood pressure is generally treated with either diuretic drugs or beta-adrenergic drugs. Hypotensive drugs which include vaso-dilators and reserpine alkaloids are also used. Your doctor will have to choose from diuretics, beta-blockers, alpha-blockers, calcium blockers, vasodilators, or alpha-simulators. Angiotensin-converting enzymes are currently considered a good treatment with the lowest incidence of side-effects, and are known under the names Capoten, Prinivil, Zestril, or Vasotec.

SIDE-EFFECTS: Any diuretic drug will make urination more frequent. As a result, potassium stores may become depleted. Eating potassium-rich foods, such as bananas and oranges, and taking potassium supplements is recommended.

Warning: If pregnant or nursing do not take any type of diuretic without consulting your physician.

Side-effects: Vasodilators: Dizziness, fainting, weakness, headache, fatigue, palpitations, nausea, stuffy nose, sinus irritation, tingling in hands and feet, bloating, inability to sleep.

Warning: If pregnant or nursing do not take this drug without your doctor's consent.

Side-effects: Angiotensin-converting enzyme: Dizziness, headache, tiredness, mild rash, cough, itching, fever, chest pain, loss of taste perception, stomach pain, low blood pressure.

Warning: If pregnant or nursing do not take this drug unless advised to do so by your physician. The effects on the developing fetus are unknown. It is also unknown if angiotensin-converting enzymes pass through breast milk.

NOTE: If you take high blood pressure drugs purchase a blood pressure cuff and chart your readings. Don't stop drug therapy if you feel good. High blood pressure is a silent disease. Overusing diuretics and other high blood pressure medication can cause hypotension or very low blood pressure. This condition is seen in elderly people and medication levels should be checked if fainting, headaches or weakness results.

Success rating of standard medical treatment: good to very good. While blood pressure-reducing drugs are effective and may be necessary, many cases of high blood pressure can be controlled through changes in diet and life-style. The fact that blood pressure-reducing drugs are so widely prescribed implies that changes in lifestyle and diet are not considered as effective as a form of treatment as drug therapy.

MEDICAL UPDATE:

Auriculin, a synthetic heart hormone, is currently being tested as a new drug which is very effective in lowering blood pressure.

The first in a new class of antihypertensive agents has been recently tested and results have been promising. Losartan, a new angiotensin II antagonist, has been found to be as effective as current high blood pressure medications, but without some of their adverse side-effects. With this particular drug, the troublesome cough which is commonly experienced with some high blood pressure pills does not occur.

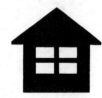

HOME SELF-CARE:

◆ Buy a blood pressure monitor so you can chart your daily readings and evaluate drug therapy.

◆ Stop smoking: A definite link exists between smoking and coronary artery disease which can also cause high blood pressure. Giving up smoking can decrease your risk for high blood pressure by half. In addition, smokers often have higher concentrations of lead and cadmium in their systems than non-smokers.

◆ If you are overweight, choose a gradual weight reduction and exercise plan. Stay away from weight lifting or isometric exercises, which can actually raise blood pressure. Try low-impact aerobics, such as walking. While reaching an optimal weight is no guarantee that hypertension will disappear, thin people are much less prone to high blood pressure and the diseases which cause it.

◆ Reduce or eliminate salt: Salt can cause fluid retention, which can raise the water content of the blood, thus contributing to high blood pressure.

◆ Don't take antihistamines without consulting your doctor.

◆ Learn to relax and fight stress. Use breathing techniques, yoga, exercise, or music to inhibit tension. When you feel tense, stop and use visualization techniques to achieve tranquility. Slow down if your pace of living has become too stressful.

◆ Get a pet or set up a fish aquarium. Stroking a pet and watching an aquarium are both activities which can help reduce stress and consequently lower blood pressure.

◆ Don't drink alcohol. Even moderate amounts of alcohol can produce an immediate rise in blood pressure due to increased adrenalin secretion. The continual consumption of alcohol is considered a significant predictor of hypertension.

NUTRITIONAL APPROACH:

◆ Reduce salt intake in the diet, which can promote the retention of fluids and increase blood pressure. Look for the symbol "NA" or the word "sodium" in products. Watch for hidden salts. Avoid ingesting monosodium glutamate (Accent), some canned vegetables and soups, ibuprofen medications, such as Advil and Nuprin, diet sodas, meat tenderizers, most sugar substitutes, soy sauce and softened water.

◆ Many salt substitutes contain up to 50 percent sodium chloride. Check your ingredient label.

◆ Avoid the following foods: Smoked or aged cheeses and meats, chocolate, animal fats, gravies, boullions, and processed foods.

◆ Avoid using NutraSweet, which contains phenylalanine.

◆ Do not consume caffeine: Caffeine can temporarily elevate blood pressure.

◆ Watch your intake of white sugar. Some studies have shown that ingesting white sugar can increase sodium retention and can also stimulate adrenaline production, which can cause blood vessel constriction.

◆ Emphasize a low-fat, high-fiber diet. Eat plenty of oat bran, pectin fruits, bananas, apples, melons, broccoli, cabbage, green leafy vegetables, peas, prunes, beets, carrots, spinach and essential fatty acids. The incidence of high blood pressure is considerably lower in vegetarians.

- ◆ *Calcium and magnesium:* Some studies have found a correlation between high blood pressure and a calcium deficiency. Several clinical studies have shown that calcium supplementation lowers blood pressure. Magnesium has been recommended as therapy for hypertension for several decades. A cellular deficiency of magnesium has been found in some people suffering from high blood pressure.
- ◆ *Potassium:* Studies suggest that the excessive consumption of salt in combination with low levels of potassium can cause an increase in the fluid volume of the blood. A high-potassium, low-sodium diet can help to reduce blood pressure.
- ◆ *L-carnatine:* An amino acid which helps to prevent heart disease. Amino acids should be taken only after your physician has been consulted.
- ◆ *Selenium:* A connection between heart disease and a lack of selenium exists.
- ◆ *Zinc:* some studies suggest that zinc can help counteract cadmium-induced high blood pressure.
- ◆ *Coenzyme Q10:* Helps to lower blood pressure through its involvement in metabolic processes.
- ◆ *Lecithin:* Helps with the emulsification of fats and can contribute to lower blood pressure.
- ◆ *Essential fatty acids* (linoleic) found in vegetable oils have been found to reduce of high blood pressure.
- ◆ *Vitamin C:* Some studies have shown that the lower the serum vitamin C level in men, the higher the blood pressure. Whether vitamin C directly affects hypertension has not been determined; however, the possible validity of its relationship to the disorder should be considered.
- ◆ *Vitamin E:* Improves function of the heart.
- ◆ *Primrose oil, black currant oil, flaxseed and olive oil:* Good sources of unsaturated fats, which can promote better circulation.
- ◆ Eating celery has a beneficial effect on high blood pressure. Studies have suggested that eating celery every day can help to bring blood pressure down. Celery oil and celery seed have been used for generations by folk healers and Chinese physicians in the treatment of high blood pressure.

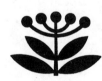

Herbal remedies:

- ◆ *Cayenne:* Helps to clean out the veins.
- ◆ *Hops:* Works to help relax veins and nerves.
- ◆ *Garlic:* Garlic has been shown to be effective in not only lowering high blood pressure, but also in decreasing cholesterol and triglyceride levels in the blood. Garlic may be eaten fresh, in cooked foods or taken in capsule form. Because most people do not receive therapeutic levels of garlic from their diets, odorless capsules are recommended. Onion has some of the same benefits as garlic.
- ◆ *Parsley:* A natural diuretic that does not have the negative side-effects of prescription drugs.

◆ *Mistletoe:* This is a potentially toxic herb and should be used with caution and under proper supervision. It has been used traditionally for lowering blood pressure.

◆ *Hawthorn berry:* This herb has been extensively used in Europe for its blood pressure reducing properties. It helps to reduce blood pressure as well as lower serum cholesterol levels. This herb also helps prevent the buildup of cholesterol on artery walls, which can in itself cause hypertension. This herb also functions to dilate larger blood vessels.

◆ *Suma tea:* Helps to improve circulation.

◆ *Ju hua:* Promotes the dilation of coronary arteries and increases blood flow.

◆ *Yarrow:* Works to relax peripheral blood vessels and improves circulation.

◆ *Wood betony:* A circulatory relaxant.

◆ Guelder rose: Relaxes smooth muscle and helps lower diastolic blood pressure.

◆ *The following herbs in combination may be useful:* Garlic, capsicum, parsley, ginger, Siberian ginseng and golden seal.

PREVENTION:

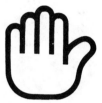

◆ Keep your diet low in fat and salt and high in fiber and fresh fruits and vegetables.

◆ Keep your weight down. Obesity directly contributes to the development of high blood pressure

◆ Do not smoke. Smoking is directly linked with the development of coronary artery disease

◆ Do not consume alcohol.

◆ Keep stress levels down or learn to manage stress through mediation, relaxation, exercise, etc.

◆ Talk quietly and slowly and learn to have a sense of humor. In other words, don't take life too seriously.

◆ Try to drink water that has not been softened. Softened water often has higher concentrations of lead due to the acidity of the water. Exposure to lead and cadmium can cause elevated blood pressure. In these cases, bottled drinking water is recommended.

Hyperactivity (Attention Deficit Disorder)

DEFINITION:

Having a child with attention deficit disorder can teach a parent the true meaning of patience and endurance. The exuberance and energy of normal children can be amazing and sometimes trying in and of itself. When these normal childhood traits are intensified to the point of becoming out of control, your child may be suffering from hyperactivity.

Hyperactivity is not the result of poor parenting and should not be viewed as a sign of parental failure. Hyperactivity is technically thought of as a behavioral disorder of the central nervous system caused by a chemical imbalance. It is also referred to as attention deficit disorder with hyperactivity (ADHD). It is usually limited to children but can affects adults as well.

Typical signs of hyperactivity are a short attention span, impulsive behavior, inappropriate responses, and poor concentration for the mental and chronological age of the child. Hyperactivity has been diagnosed in 4 to 20 percent of school-age children, or approximately 2 million children in the United States. Because an accurate diagnosis is difficult, the figures could be considerably less. Boys are four times more likely to be hyperactive than girls.

Hyperactivity will usually occur by the age of 3, although the disorder may not be suspected until the child is in school. In some cases, hyperactivity disappears at puberty. The hyperactive child can become moody, depressed and feel antisocial. Occasionally, the symptoms of hyperactivity persist into adulthood. In some cases, hyperactive children who gave their parents a great deal of grief in their childhood develop into energetic and creative adults.

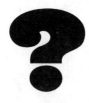

CAUSES:

The general consensus regarding the cause of hyperactivity is that it is the result of an insufficient amount of one or several chemicals found in the nervous system that regulate concentration and attention. Factors that have been linked to hyperactivity are heredity, food allergens, artificial food additives, heavy metal poisoning (lead), glucose intolerance, smoking during pregnancy, oxygen deprivation during birth, and phosphate additives.

SYMPTOMS:

Physical and psychological: NOTE: A child will usually manifest only some of the following symptoms of hyperactivity, depending on the severity of the disorder.

Hyperactivity typically causes emotional instability, short attention span, inability to get things finished, poor concentration, distractibility, impatience, impulsive behavior, abrupt changes of activity and thought, inappropriate jumping and running, head knocking, self-destructiveness, and temper tantrums.

In addition, memory and thought impairment, motor or speech defects, and poor performance in school or other structured environments can also occur. Lack of coordination, clumsiness, sleep disorders, and aggressive behavior toward other children or adults is commonly seen with hyperactivity. Hyperactive children will sometimes show neurological abnormalities including electroencephalogram irregularities.

Attention: It is possible for a teacher to mistakingly label a child hyperactive when in actuality the child is suffering from another type of learning disability, poor vision, impaired hearing or a language problem.

Standard medical treatment:

Before a child is assumed to be hyperactive and subsequently treated with drugs, a careful medical evaluation is necessary to eliminate other possible conditions. Accepted treatments for hyperactivity and attention deficit disorder are methylphenidate or dextroamphetamine (Dexedrine), which are used in extreme cases. Ironically, stimulant drugs (amphetamines or methylphenidate) are used to treat hyperactivity. It is thought that the midbrain may actually be understimulated in hyperactivity, causing a lack of control. Stimulating the midbrain actually causes a suppression of the extra activity.

The use of Ritalin (methylphenidate) has been the subject of widespread controversy. It is estimated that this drug is currently being taken by over 1 million children in the United States. The question is whether Ritalin is prescribed too quickly and before other alternatives have been explored. Unquestionably, in severe cases of hyperactivity, drug therapy may be required. Behavior therapy and counseling are also useful.

Side-effects: Methylphenidate (Ritalin): Nervousness, sleep disorders, loss of appetite, stomach pains, weight loss, abnormal heart rhythms.

Warning: If pregnant or nursing do not take this drug without your doctor's consent. It may cause birth defects. Ritalin does pass through breast milk.

NOTE: Chronic or abusive use of Ritalin can cause addiction or dependence. This drug can cause severe psychotic disorders.

Success rating of standard medical treatment: fair. The widespread use of Ritalin is cause for concern. Even the Journal of the American Medical Association questioned the extent of the current use of drugs prescribed for hyperactivity. Every four to seven years the number of children receiving medication for hyperactivity is thought to be doubling. It must be remembered, however, that in some severe cases of hyperactivity, Ritalin can be considered a life saver.

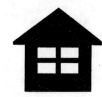

HOME SELF-CARE:

Locate a good counseling service for the entire family. Dealing with a hyperactive child can be extremely stressful and additional outside support is necessary. Often parents become so callous to the demands of a hyperactive child they have a tendency to ignore the child more, which usually aggravates aggressive behavior. Child abuse may become a factor when the hyperactive child is unusually difficult. Preventive measures should be taken to avoid this type of situation.

◆ A hyperactive child, just like any other child, needs a structured, disciplined environment. Consistency is vital and follow-through a must. A hyperactive child, more than a normal child, must be trained to remember and to complete tasks.

◆ It is essential that parents present a united front to the child and decide together on rules, expectations and discipline.

◆ Break up every task the child is asked to do in step-by-step requests. Don't give general instructions, but specific ones designed to bring the child to a conclusion. Use a brightly colored chart to help the child succeed. List tasks one by one such as get out of bed, brush your teeth, take off your pajamas, make your bed, etc. A reward system can be used, such as so many stars equals going to the movies.

◆ Choose the right kind of activities for your child. Working on puzzles or long-term visual activities requiring exact hand-eye coordination are not recommended, although some hyperactive children are very adept at putting together mechanical objects. Hyperactive children usually enjoy activities such as swimming or soccer rather than baseball or football.

◆ Some studies found that a regular jogging program was as effective as low-dose medication in controlling hyperactivity.

◆ The home environment should not be overstimulating. Avoid blaring TV's, video games, loud stereos, etc.

◆ Give the child simple responsibilities such as sweeping the floor, and use a great deal of praise to reinforce good behavior.

◆ Don't neglect other members of the family and involve them in regular family meetings where feelings can be openly expressed.

NUTRITIONAL APPROACH:

The role that food additives play in hyperactivity and attention deficit disorder has been widely debated and researched over the last few years. The Feingold hypothesis proposes that food additives such as BHT, BHA, artificial colors and flavorings, emulsifiers, nitrates and sulphites induces hyperactivity in children. Feingold came up with 3,000 food additives that should be investigated.

While the final verdict of the National Advisory Committee on hyperkinesis and food additives was that there was no significant connection between the two, ongoing studies suggest that a definite correlation exists. In controlled experiments, up to 50 percent of hyperactive children improved when their diets were modified. By controlling the ingestion of food additives, sugar and eliminating possible food allergens, some health care professionals believe hyperactivity and attention deficit disorder can be managed.

◆ Eliminate white sugar from the diet. Several studies suggest that hyperactive children have impaired glucose tolerance. A tendency toward hypoglycemia in hyperactive children also supports the negative emotional effects which sugar could induce. Diet, violent behavior, hypoglycemia and hyperactivity have all been linked together by certain studies.

◆ Eliminate not only food additives but also possible food allergens such as BHA, BHT, red dye, yellow dye, blue dye, preservatives, cow's milk, chocolate, grape flavoring, orange flavoring, cane sugar, eggs, peanuts, and tomatoes. It is widely accepted that food allergens like sugar, can cause mood shifts.

◆ Eliminate salt, soda pop, catsup, mustard, soy sauce, cider vinegar, colored cheeses, boxed dinners, lunchmeats, hot dogs, smoked meats, ham, wheat, corn, colored butter, margarine, ice cream, candy, and perfumes.

◆ Do not use foods with salicylates which include almonds, apples, apricots, cherries, currants, berries, peaches, plums, prunes, tomatoes, cucumbers and oranges.

◆ Emphasize fruits and vegetables that are not on the elimination list, cereals, breads, crackers that only contain rice or oats, or millet. Keep a chart for a week of foods consumed and any emotional reaction that may be linked with those foods.

◆ Some university studies have revealed that a carbohydrate-and sugar-rich breakfast can lead to an increase in hyperactive behavior. If protein was eaten at breakfast, hyperactivity was reduced. Some theories linked increases in serotonin levels with the ingesting of carbohydrates and sugars.

◆ Give the child a good multivitamin and mineral supplement.

◆ *Calcium and magnesium:* Work to help calm the nervous system.

◆ *Vitamin B complex with extra niacin, B5, B6, and B12:* Essential for proper functioning of the brain.

◆ *Vitamin C:* Considered an anti-stress vitamin.

◆ *Vitamin A:* Helps to boost the immune system and fight allergies.

◆ *Iron:* Any form of malnutrition can result in impaired learning and concentration. An iron deficiency is common among American children and can produce symptoms very similar to those of attention deficit disorder.

◆ Make sure your child has not been exposed or is currently being exposed to any heavy metal, lead in particular. Childhood learning disorders can be related to body stores of heavy metals, especially lead. If a hair analysis reveals a high level of metals, l-cysteine, an amino acid, may be helpful. Check with your doctor before using any amino acid.

◆ Some studies have shown that giving GABA (gamma-amino butyric acid) can help to decrease hyperactivity as well as benefit children with learning disorders.

HERBAL REMEDIES:

- *Valerian root:* Can be used as an extract. It has a sedating effect. Use only recommended dosages.
- *Gotu kola:* Considered a food for the brain.
- *Catnip:* A natural relaxant.
- *Hops and lady's slipper:* Have a natural calming effect on the nervous system.
- *Xia ku cao:* Has traditionally been used in Chinese medicine to calm overexcitability.
- *Chamomile and wood betony:* Considered calming nervine herbs.
- *The following herbs in combination may be useful:* Valerian root, wood betony, hops, skullcap, black cohosh, mistletoe, pan pien lien, capsicum, lady's slipper, juniper berries and periwinkle.

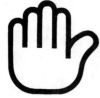

PREVENTION:

There is some speculation that breast feeding and slowly introducing cow's milk, wheat and citrus fruits into a baby's diet may make that child less prone to food allergies. The link between infant diet and future allergic sensitivities exists. How it relates to increasing or decreasing the risk of hyperactivity is not known.

- Keep your child on a nutritious diet that is low in refined sugars and high in natural foods.
- Establish codes of behavior, household chores, etc. early in the child's life.
- Keep noise and distraction to a minimum within the home environment.
- Keep your children involved in activities where they can expend energy such as swimming, jogging, gymnastics, and soccer.

Hyperthyroidism   (Graves Disease)

DEFINITION:

When former first lady Barbara Bush was diagnosed with Grave's disease, many of us became aware, for the first time, of thyroid disorders and how they affect the body. An overactive thyroid gland can make you feel nervous and overly anxious and can be difficult to treat.

Medically speaking, hyperthyroidism refers to a disorder which causes the thyroid gland to overproduce thyroxine, which subsequently creates an overactive metabolism. The digestive system is particularly affected, resulting in the poor absorption of nutrients.

Hyperthyroidism is an autoimmune disease and affects more women than men. It is a fairly uncommon disorder, and its most common form is called Grave's disease. Hyperthyroidism affects 1 percent of the adult population of the U.S. targeting mostly young to middle-aged women. The prognosis for this disease varies with each individual case, with total recovery possible.

CAUSES:

A malfunctioning thyroid gland can be the result of a number of illnesses. In addition, the development of nodules on the thyroid gland can create symptoms of an overactive gland. People who have an overactive thyroid gland generally contain an abnormal antibody in their blood which is referred to as a long-acting thyroid stimulator (LATS). This antibody causes the pituitary gland, which controls the thyroid gland to malfunction. As a result, an overstimulation of the thyroid gland can occur.

SYMPTOMS:

Physical: Hyperthyroidism can cause nervousness, irritability, insomnia, fatigue, weight loss, increased perspiration, hair loss, tremors, weakness, rapid heartbeat, heart palpitations, increased appetite, breathlessness, and the separation of the nails from the nail bed.

Patients with overactive thyroid glands also experience frequent bowel movements, muscle weakness and wasting, have a heat intolerance and sometimes have smooth skin and fine hair and a decrease in menstrual flow.

A swelling in the neck referred to as a goiter may also develop; however, this may also be present in hypothyroidism. In some cases, the eyes may protrude from the eye sockets. The thyroid gland plays an integral part in the proper functioning of the sex glands, the pituitary gland and the parathyroid glands. Consequently, a malfunction of the thyroid gland directly influences the entire endocrine system.

Psychological: Hyperthyroidism may be confused with psychological disturbances such as anxiety disorders or depression.

STANDARD MEDICAL TREATMENT:

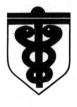

In the case of young people suffering from hyperthyroidism, drugs that block the production of thyroxine such as methimazole may be prescribed by your doctor. These must be taken every day for an extended period of time, after which treatment is stopped to check the function of the thyroid gland.

If this treatment is not effective, the thyroid gland may have to be destroyed. An injection or drink of radioactive iodine (RAI) is commonly used. The radiation is quickly picked up by the thyroid gland due to its iodine content. This treatment is rarely used for children and is used as a last resort in people who are under 30. The goal of this treatment is to destroy only enough of the gland so that overproduction of thyroxine will not continue. To determine how much thyroxine is released after this procedure, regular thyroid tests must be done on a regular basis.

Surgical options: Surgery to remove part of the gland is still routinely performed on children. Surgical treatment of hyperthyroidism successfully cures the disorder in approximately 90 percent of cases.

Side-effects: Methimazole: Itching, dizziness, numbness, stomach pain, loss of taste, joint pains, nausea and vomiting, tingling fingers and skin rash.

Success rating of standard medical treatment: good. Most people suffering from hyperthyroidism can be helped by conventional medical treatment, although those treatments are sometimes radical in nature. Administering radioactive iodine will usually destroy too much of the thyroid gland, which results in a thyroid deficiency (hypothyroidism). Both radiation and surgery should only be considered after diet changes have been attempted and fail. While side-effects to both procedures are considered negligible by medical professionals, both treatments carry a certain amount of risk.

HOME SELF-CARE:

♦ A thyroid self-test can be taken by shaking down a thermometer before going to bed and immediately upon rising, placing it in your armpit for 10 minutes. A reading below 97.8 may suggest a thyroid deficiency. An elevated temperature may indicate the presence of an infection or an overactive thyroid.
♦ Practice a yoga posture called a shoulder stand at least once a day for 10 to 20 minutes. This position can help to stimulate the thyroid gland and normalize its function.

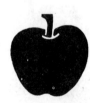

NUTRITIONAL APPROACH:

♦ Emphasize the following foods: broccoli, cabbage, kale, peaches, pears, soybeans, spinach and cauliflower. These foods help to suppress thyroxine production.
♦ Foods which nourish the thyroid glands include alfalfa sprouts, avocado, figs, olive oil, rice, bran, rye, yams and dark green vegetables.
♦ Avoid all dairy products and do not consume alcohol or caffeine.
♦ *Essential fatty acids:* Vital to correct glandular function. Evening primrose oil has been particularly effective in treating diseases of the thyroid.
♦ Take a good multivitamin that emphasizes the B-complex vitamins.
♦ *Vitamin A:* Assists with normal glandular function.
♦ *Vitamin C with bioflavonoids:* A vitamin C deficiency has been found in some people suffering from thyroid diseases. This vitamin is particularly beneficial if you have received radiation therapy for hyperthyroidism.

◆ *Iodine:* Promotes the proper metabolism of thyroxine and prevents goiters.
◆ *Lecithin:* Contributes to the proper digestion of fats and protects cell linings.
◆ *Calcium/magnesium:* Assists in all metabolic functions and helps to calm jittery nerves, which can accompany hyperthyroidism.
◆ Magnesium, phosphorus and potassium are all essential to the maintenance of healthy gland function and hormone production.

HERBAL REMEDIES:

◆ *Black walnut:* A traditional herbal treatment for goiter.
◆ *Kelp, dandelion and alfalfa:* Considered a tonic for the thyroid gland, this combination can help to normalize its function.
◆ *The following combination of herbs may be useful:* Irish moss, Norwegian kelp, black walnut, parsley, watercress, Iceland moss and capsicum.
◆ *Norwegian kelp:* A natural source of iodine.

PREVENTION:

◆ Take a daily supplement of Norwegian kelp to supply the thyroid gland with iodine.
◆ Keep the immune system healthy through proper diet and exercise and eliminate tobacco, alcohol and caffeine.

Hypoglycemia

DEFINITION:

Hypoglycemia is buzzword of the 80's and 90's and has come under substantial attack from the medical profession, who generally view it as a bogus disorder. Hypoglycemia, also known as "sugar shakes," has been blamed for everything from marital breakups to infertility.

Technically, hypoglycemia occurs when the pancreas produces an excess of insulin, which results in an abnormally low level of blood sugar. True hypoglycemia is considered an extremely rare disorder and usually occurs in people suffering from diabetes mellitus who have an excess of administered insulin in their bloodstream .

Functional hypoglycemia is a relatively new term which refers to hypoglycemia that is directly related to dietary habits rather than physiological abnormalities. This type of hypoglycemia has been the subject of ongoing debate. While some doctors accept it as a valid disorder, most deny its existence.

There is also some evidence to support the fact that if you routinely experience "sugar shakes" you may be a candidate for diabetes. This theory is based on the fact that the pancreas is not functioning properly by secreting too much insulin and that it will eventually fail altogether.

CAUSES:

True hypoglycemia can be a complication in people suffering from insulin-dependent diabetes, from ingesting large amounts of alcohol, or from an insulinoma, which is an insulin-producing tumor of the pancreas. Other glandular disorders such as thyroid abnormalities or glandular tumors may also cause hypoglycemia. Functional hypoglycemia can also result from inherited tendencies and dietary factors.

SYMPTOMS:

Physical: Hypoglycemia commonly causes dizziness, fatigue, irritability, mood swings, anxiety, sweating, cold sweats, weakness, fainting, tremors, strong sensation of hunger, food cravings, eye pain, visual disturbances, palpitations, insomnia, mental disturbances, and swollen feet. In severe cases of hypoglycemia, the person may lapse into a coma.

Psychological: It is a well-established fact that abrupt drops in blood glucose levels can cause dramatic mood swings, irritability, combativeness and depression. Low blood sugar can result in feelings of confusion, impatience and the inability to cope. The brain is highly dependent on sugar as an energy source. Several studies indicate that psychiatric patients have a higher incidence of low blood sugar.

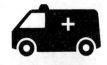

MEDICAL ALERT:

A large number of people who suffer from the symptoms of hypoglycemia have reduced thyroid function and should see a physician. Persistent symptoms of hypoglycemia may indicate the presence of a serious disorder.

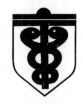

STANDARD MEDICAL TREATMENT:

A five hour glucose tolerance test (GTT) will be administered by your doctor, where a large amount of sugar water is consumed and subsequent blood tests are taken at intervals to determine glucose levels. Hypoglycemia that does not have a specific physical cause is considered by some physicians as a "fad" disease that does not truly exist. Some critics of the glucose tolerance test also point out that giving the body such high levels of glucose may result in false readings.

Success rating of standard medical treatment: poor for functional hypoglycemia. Insulin-dependent hypoglycemia can be quickly remedied with an injection of glucagon. Functional hypoglycemia, however is often not taken seriously. The five hour glucose test is generally considered unreliable.

If a physician determines that low blood sugar exists, diet changes where protein is stressed and carbohydrates are minimized will be recommended. There is some controversy surrounding this approach. Some health care professionals believe that complex carbohydrates should be stressed and protein kept to a minimum.

In addition, some doctors will suggest eating a piece of candy when symptoms of hypoglycemia begin. Critics of this approach point out that by quickly raising the blood glucose level with refined, quickly assimilated sugars, blood sugar may later drop down even lower to compensate. This is referred to as reactive hypoglycemia.

HOME SELF-CARE:

◆ If you are an insulin-dependent diabetic, always carry sugar cubes with you and take them at the first sign of a hypoglycemic reaction.

◆ Taking injections of B vitamins has produced some good results in keeping the pancreas from oversecreting insulin when certain foods are ingested.

◆ Lose weight if you need to. The relationship of fat stores to the metabolism of sugar has been firmly established.

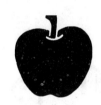

◆ Exercise is extremely beneficial in helping the body regulate sugar metabolism.

NUTRITIONAL APPROACH:

◆ Designing the right kind of diet is vital to controlling hypoglycemia. Eat the kind of sugars that come from complex carbohydrates, which are assimilated more slowly.

◆ Avoid the following foods: sugars, refined and processed foods, white flour, soda pop, salt, caffeine, alcohol, extremely sweet fruits, dried fruits and juices which can be diluted with water, noodles, gravy, white rice, and corn. Presweetened cold cereals are especially prone to cause a rapid rise in blood sugar and can precipitate the over-secretion of insulin.

◆ Alcohol can induce a drop in blood sugar. Eating sugar and consuming alcohol aggravates the cycle of hypoglycemia.

◆ Emphasize fresh fruits and vegetables, sprouts, brown rice, seeds, grains, nuts, cottage cheese, lean meats, fish, high fiber foods such as oat bran, popcorn, and other whole grains.

◆ Eat several small meals a day to prevent the onset of low blood sugar. Carry apples with you.

◆ *Chromium:* Important component in proper glucose metabolism. The picolinate form is recommended.

- *Vitamin B complex with extra niacin, B1, B3, B12 and B5:* This complex is vital in the utilization of carbohydrates.
- *Brewer's yeast:* Contains both B vitamins and chromium.
- *Vitamin C:* Helps the adrenal glands, which in some cases of hypoglycemia do not function normally.
- *Calcium/magnesium:* Participates in the normal assimilation of sugars.
- *L-carnatine:* An amino acid which helps to convert fat stores into energy. Before taking amino acids, check with your doctor.
- *L-cysteine:* An amino acid which can help to block the action of insulin, therefore keeping blood sugar level normal. Before taking amino acids, check with your doctor.
- *Manganese:* Some hypoglycemics have shown a deficiency of this mineral.
- *Zinc:* Some studies indicate that hypoglycemics are low in zinc.
- *Spirulina:* Can help to balance blood glucose levels in between meals by stabilizing blood sugar.

Herbal remedies:

- *Glucomannan:* Helps to normalize blood sugar.
- *Licorice:* Stimulates the adrenal glands and helps counteract stress.
- *Lady's slipper:* Helps the adrenal glands to function normally.
- *Lobelia and mullein:* Considered herbal glandular foods.
- *The following herbs in combination may be useful:* Dandelion root, licorice root, wild yam, juniper berries, and horseradish.

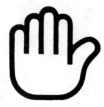

Prevention:

If you are an insulin-dependent diabetic there are several ways to help prevent hypoglycemia. Refer to the diabetes chapter.

Good dietary habits combined with regular exercise are the formula to help prevent not only low blood sugar, but also several other common diseases of our age. A low-fat diet, high in fiber, fresh fruits and vegetables and complex carbohydrates is invaluable in helping to prevent functional hypoglycemia.

- Keep yourself at an ideal weight.
- Do not consume alcohol.
- Do not consume an excess of white sugar products, candy, cakes, sugared cereals, or desserts. Reach for fruit instead.
- Eating small meals several times of day may be preferable to two or three large meals, which can shoot blood sugar level up.

American Diabetes Association
Two Park Avenue
New York, NY 10016
212-683-7444

Impotence

DEFINITION:

Impotence has traditionally caused feelings of humiliation and shame in males who suffer from it. Men who experience impotence usually assume the worst, and may believe that their sex life is over. Impotence refers to the inability to achieve or to maintain a penile erection. It happens to most men at one time or another and is usually reversible and temporary. Impotence can also refer to premature ejaculation or the inability to ejaculate.

Impotence is the most common sexual disorder among males. It is estimated that more than 10 million American men are chronically impotent. By the age of 75, 55 percent of men report suffering from impotence. Aging increases the chances of impotence due to lowered levels of testosterone and decreased circulation.

At one time, impotence was considered an emotional disorder. Recently, physicians have to come to accept that at least half of all cases of impotence have a physiological component as well.

CAUSES:

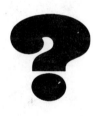

Impotence can be the result of psychological factors such as stress, performance anxiety, fatigue, boredom, anxiety, guilt, depression, marital discord, and age. Physiological conditions that can result in impotence are diabetes mellitus, peripheral vascular disease, Parkinson's disease, liver or kidney disease, stroke, epilepsy, Alzheimer's disease, lower back problems, hormonal diseases, neurological disorders, alcoholism, and spinal cord damage.

Various drugs are associated with impotence including antipsychotics, antidepressants, some tranquilizers such as Valium, antihypertensives and diuretics. Some over-the-counter antihistamines and decongestants have also been linked to bouts of temporary impotence.

SYMPTOMS:

Psychological: If the causes of impotence are psychological in nature, sex counseling or psychotherapy may be helpful, although it is vital that you choose a therapist that has good credentials and is respected in his or her field. Traditional methods of psychotherapy have not enjoyed a great deal of success in treating impotence. A sex therapist may be more qualified in this area. If alcoholism is a factor, it will have to be treated appropriately.

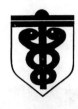

STANDARD MEDICAL TREATMENT:

Tests will be ordered to rule out the possibility of a physical cause. A test to determine if blood flow to the penis is adequate may be performed by your doctor. The health of the spinal cord will also be determined. A history will be taken and a blood glucose test may be ordered to eliminate the possibility of diabetes. In addition, a testosterone level test should be performed. Certain medications may be stopped or dosages adjusted.

If depression is a factor, it is usually treated with antidepressants and counseling. Testosterone shots may be recommended. Thyroxine is another name for a testosterone medication that can be effective in some cases. Determining and administering the best levels of testosterone is difficult. A testosterone patch is currently being developed and will be used by men who experience sexual dysfunction as the result of a physical disorder.

Note: An old drug which is considered a sexual enhancer is yohimbine, which is synthesized from the bark of an African tree and has been traditionally thought of as an aphrodisiac. It is available as a prescription drug under the brand names Yocon, Yohimex or Aphrodyne.

Attention: A urologist may need to be consulted if the problem is severe. A urologist can discuss surgical options available.

Surgical options: If blood insufficiency to the penis is the cause of the impotence, a surgical procedure to unblock the arteries involved may be necessary.
◆ Special vacuum devices can be surgically implanted which draw blood into the penis.
◆ Penile implants: These are surgically implanted prosthetic devices which facilitate an erection.

Side-effects: Testosterone (Android, Metandren, Oreton Methyl, Testred, Virilon): Chronic erection of the penis, breast enlargement, impotence, changes in libido, flushing of the skin, acne, excitation, chills, sleeplessness, water retention, nausea, vomiting, diarrhea, and possible change in blood cholesterol level.

Warning: Older men using this drug run an increased risk of developing prostate enlargement or prostate cancer.

NOTE: testosterone and other androgens are potent drugs and should be taken exactly as prescribed and strictly under a doctor's supervision.

Side-effects: Pumps and vacuums: these devices can cause prolonged erections that can last for hours and become quite painful. If the erection lasts too long it can cause damage and medical treatment is required immediately. Taking Dudafed or other sinus or hay fever medications can sometimes help resolve the problem. Apparently the adrenalinlike substances in these over-the-counter medications decease the blood flow to the penis.

Success rating of standard medical treatment: good. With new scientific advances, impotence treatment is seeing more success than it did 20 years ago. Medical doctors take the disorder more seriously today and will want to address both psychological and physical factors involved.

MEDICAL UPDATE:

◆ For men over 40, taking the following high blood pressure drugs may cause impotence: Inderal, Aldomet and Catapres. In addition, taking Tagamet for ulcers may also cause impotence.
◆ Home impotence tests exist which are used to determine whether impotence is psychologically caused or has an organic source. These are set up prior to sleeping and determine if any erections occurred during sleep. If there are no erections while sleeping, there may be a mechanical malfunction causing the impotence. Contact a urologist if this is the case. If you discover that erections do occur during sleep, but you still experience impotence when awake, then the problem has a psychological basis and an appropriate counselor may be consulted.

HOME SELF-CARE:

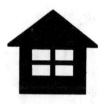

◆ Discuss your problem openly with your partner. Express your feelings, especially if you have negative feelings toward your partner. Anger, frustration or tension can cause impotence and need to be addressed.
◆ There is some speculation that exercising right before sex directs blood away from the penis and may hinder achieving an erection.
◆ Use relaxation techniques such as yoga, and biofeedback to counteract the negative effects of stress and tension.
◆ Don't drink alcohol to relax. Consuming alcohol can cause impotence by depressing the nervous system.
◆ Do not become preoccupied with the physical aspects of an erection. Relax and do not set your expectations unrealistically high.
◆ Don't smoke: Nicotene impairs blood flow to the penis and contributes to hardening of the arteries, which in itself can cause impotence.

NUTRITIONAL APPROACH:

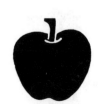

◆ Losing weight, exercising and eating a low-fat, high-fiber diet can help to improve circulation and counteract impotence that is caused by reduced blood flow. A diet high in fats can contribute to clogging the arteries that supply blood to the penis. If your cholesterol count is too high, lower it through the elimination of saturated fats, animal meats and rich dairy products and exercise regularly.
◆ *Vitamin E:* Is referred to as the "fertility vitamin" and helps strengthen both male and female reproductive organs.
◆ *Vitamin C:* Helps to maintain proper circulation and works to keep arteries

clean. It is also known as the antistress vitamin.

◆ *Zinc:* Important in maintaining healthy reproductive organs and contributes to normal prostate gland function.

◆ *Astrelin:* This compound is used in Europe and is considered an effective treatment for impotence.

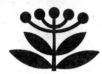

HERBAL REMEDIES:

◆ *Ginseng:* Contains male hormone precursors and can help in correcting impotence.

◆ *Gotu kola:* Functions as a normalizer of hormones.

◆ *Damiana:* Considered a tonic to the glands.

◆ *Sarsaparilla:* Contains a natural form of testosterone.

◆ Yohimbe bark is sometimes available in health food stores and is the basis for yohimbine, which is sometimes prescribed by doctors for impotence.

◆ *The following herbs in combination may be useful:* Siberian ginseng, damiana, suma, gotu kola, fo-ti, saw palmetto, ho-shou-wu, nettle, and licorice.

PREVENTION:

◆ The Boston University School of Medicine has recently found that a man's overall health is the key predictor of impotence. Men who suffered from high blood pressure, heart disease or diabetes were one to four times more likely to become completely impotent later in their lives. Having a low level of HDL cholesterol was also linked to eventually becoming impotent.

◆ Do not drink alcohol: Impotence among men in their late 40s and early 50s is associated with the excessive consumption of alcohol.

◆ Don't smoke: Smoking impairs circulation and contributes to hardening of the arteries, which can affect erections.

◆ Try to maintain an active, healthy and regular sex life. It is thought that testosterone levels stay higher when sex is more frequent.

◆ Try not to become obsessed with sexual performance. Performance anxiety can lead to psychological impotence.

◆ Learn to relax and to counteract stress and fatigue with exercise and relaxation techniques such as yoga, and music therapy.

◆ Eat a diet that is low in fat and high in fiber. Cholesterol deposits can affect the arteries that supply blood to the penis also.

Infertility

DEFINITION:

The inability to get pregnant is one of the most heartbreaking situations a couple can face. Most everyone who gets married naturally assumes that conception will be easily achieved. When pregnancy doesn't occur, a great deal of frustration and disappointment can result. Consequently, "trying" to get pregnant can become a long and difficult process.

Infertility refers to the inability to conceive after a year or more of normal sexual intercourse. It may also refer to the inability to carry a pregnancy to full term. Infertility is an increasingly common problem among American couples. As many as one in six couples will have to seek the aid of an infertility specialist.

Roughly 30 percent of infertility cases are due to factors that affect the male. Another 30 percent are due to female problems, and the remaining 40 percent are caused by a combination of the two. The good news is that there are several medical options to help encourage the stork's arrival, and many of these methods are eventually successful.

CAUSES:

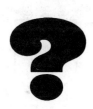

A hormonal imbalance is the most common cause of infertility. Other possible causes are chlamydia, pelvic inflammatory disease, an allergic reaction to sperm, endometriosis, obstruction of the fallopian tubes due to cysts or scar tissue, and physical injury to reproductive organs. Cervical mucus which provides a hostile environment to sperm, allergy to sperm, chromosomal abnormalities, and congenital defects or deformities can also cause infertility.

A low sperm count in male semen due to varicocele (a varicose vein in the scrotum), prostate infections, mumps, alcohol use, nicotine, illness or fatigue, and impotence can be contributing factors as well.

Diets that are deficient in certain vitamins have also been linked with infertility. There has been some speculation that the increased rate of infertility is due to the consumption of refined sugars and flours which do not provide natural sources of vitamin E found in whole grains. Adolescent eating disorders may also contribute to subsequent infertility if severe enough.

SYMPTOMS:

Psychological: While it is not completely understood, unquestionably the ability to relax seems connected to increasing your chances of conception. Often it is best to concentrate on passion and forget about mechanics or temperature charts. Going on a cruise or other restful type of vacation is recommended. A prescribed sexual regimen to achieve fertility can also result in a lack of interest in sex, which can become more of a chore than anything else. Women are sometimes impatient with men, who are perceived as uncooperative or resistant. Some men can mistakingly view infertility as a sign that they lack virility.

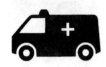

MEDICAL ALERT:

Consult an OB/GYN if the following applies:

You or your partner has had a venereal disease (especially chlamydia) which can cause fallopian tube damage and ductal scarring in men.

Your menstrual periods are irregular or abnormally scant.

You have a history of endometriosis, pelvic infections, abdominal or urinary tract surgery, mumps, measles, excessively high fevers, polycystic ovary disease, exposure to toxic chemicals such as lead, or significant exposure to radiation.

You can find no evidence that ovulation is occurring (taking temperature, using standard ovulation kits).

You have symptoms of too much male hormone in that you have hair growth on your chest, upper lip, or chin.

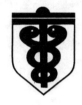

STANDARD MEDICAL TREATMENT:

Usually your physician will take a complete history and evaluation of both physical and psychological factors which may be related to infertility. Separate interviews of both partners are sometimes conducted where sexual habits are discussed. If the problem is physical, you will be referred to a fertility clinic where the first lab test is usually a sperm count. If sperm production is normal (at least 60 million sperm per milliliter of ejaculate), the female reproductive system will be examined. A sample of the cervical mucus and a biopsy of the uterine lining will be taken and tested to see if ovulation is occurring.

You may be asked to keep a chart of morning temperatures with a basal thermometer to confirm ovulation, which is usually marked by a rise in temperature of 1 to 2 degrees. A post-coital semen test may also be ordered.

If ovulation is absent, a fertility drug may be advised. In addition, the fallopian tubes may be tested with a hysterosalpingography to check for any obstruction. A laparoscopy, which involves inserting a scope through the abdominal wall, may be suggested if the presence of adhesions, scar tissue, fibroid tumors, endometriosis, a tipped uterus, cysts or tumors is suspected, and in some cases, surgical correction can take place at the same time.

In cases involving low sperm count, artificial insemination with the male semen may be successful. If sperm count is low because of an endocrine imbalance, drugs such as domiphene or gonadotropin may be prescribed. Artificial insemination with donor sperm is also a possibility and should be done only if both partners agree.

Surrogate pregnancy is another option that should be explored only if attitudes permit and all legalities are discussed.

In vitro fertilization (test tube baby), where an egg and sperm meet inside of test tube with subsequent implantation into the woman's uterus, is another possibility. In vitro fertilization is expensive, at $6000 or more for each attempt. Sometimes adopting a baby seems to increase chances for conception for reasons that are not totally understood.

Success rating of standard medical treatment: fair to good. Approximately half of all couples who seek professional infertility treatment will achieve conception.

MEDICAL UPDATE:

◆ Research in Great Britain confirms that in vitro fertilization success rates decline with age. The study found that conception and live birth rates fell 20.2 percent and 14.4 percent respectively in women over the age of 40 who had attempted five in vitro cycles. In contrast, more than 50% of women between the ages of 20 and 34 conceived after five cycles.

HOME SELF CARE:

◆ Home ovulation kits such as Ovu-stick can be purchased to determine the most optimal time for conception to take place. The test is simple and is done by using a chemically treated stick which is placed in a urine sample. A positive result indicates that ovulation will occur within 12 to 36 hours.

◆ Usually couples under 30 are advised to try to achieve conception for a year before consulting a fertility specialist. Fertility does decrease with age. Often women in their 30s and 40s do not regularly ovulate, which significantly reduces the probability of conception.

◆ Avoid extreme exercise and the repeated use of hot saunas, which can induce changes in normal ovulation. Exercising for more than an hour per day is not recommended.

◆ Men should not take hot showers, baths, or saunas which may reduce sperm count. In addition, stay away from electric blankets and occupational exposure to high temperatures.

◆ Take a cold bath 30 minutes before intercourse. There is some speculation that the cold water not only increases the sperm count but also makes them more active.

◆ Do not use commercial vaginal douches. Douching can disturb the natural pH balance of the vagina, which may impair or actually kill sperm.

◆ Use a vaginal lubricant that won't disturb the natural acid/alkaline balance of the vagina. Egg white has been suggested as being the least disruptive to normal sperm motility. Use the egg white after it has reached room temperature just prior to intercourse on fertile days. Using Vaseline or K-Y jelly may decrease your chances of conception.

◆ If you are thin, gain enough weight to put you close to or at your ideal weight. Stored body fat can produce estrogen.

◆ Women should remain lying down and try proping their feet up for at least 20 minutes after intercourse.

◆ Men should not take any kind of steroids, which can adversely affect the pituitary gland also damage the testicles.

◆ Men should avoid tight underwear or athletic supporters, which may also decrease sperm count. Boxer shorts are preferred over the tight-fitting jockey shorts.

◆ Abstain for at least two days prior to ovulation or fertile days to increase sperm count.

◆ Don't smoke.

◆ Some medications can decrease sperm count or impair motility. Tagamet, certain antibiotics and antiseizure preparations are among these drugs. Get off any over-the-counter or prescription drugs that aren't necessary

◆ Some doctors have suggested that women take cough syrup containing guaifenesin four times a day during ovulation. This substance has a tendency to thin the cervical mucous which makes it easier for sperm to travel.

NUTRITIONAL FACTORS:

◆ Avoid caffeine: Some recent studies have linked caffeine consumption with infertility. Give up coffee, cola beverages and chocolate.

◆ *Vitamin E:* Called "the fertility vitamin" it plays an essential role hormonal balance and can help increase sperm count.

◆ *Vitamin C with bioflavonoids:* Some European studies suggest that bioflavonoids may help women prone to miscarriages to sustain the pregnancy. Bioflavonoids in conjunction with vitamin C can help to strengthen blood vessels.

◆ *Zinc:* An important mineral for the prostate gland and the normal function of the reproductive organs.

HERBAL REMEDIES:

◆ *Dong quai:* Strengthens female reproductive organs.

◆ *Damiana:* Considered a tonic for male reproductive organs and can help in stimulating testosterone.

◆ *Gotu kola:* Helps to achieve hormone balance and works as a nerve relaxant.

◆ *Scullcap:* An herb traditionally used to treat infertility which also acts as a relaxant.

◆ *False unicorn:* A uterine stimulant which is also used for impotence. It is useful in

the treatment of irregular periods.
◆ *Ginseng:* Helps increase sperm count.
◆ *Sarsaparilla:* Plays a role in the stimulation of progesterone.

PREVENTION:

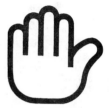

While there is no real way of knowing if you might be infertile when you are young, eating right and taking care of your body cannot be overemphasized. Drinking, smoking, using illicit drugs and not getting the right nutrients as a teenager can eventually take its toll. Eating disorders like anorexia and bulimia can lead to sterility and can be devastating to the body. The bottom line is to take care of yourself long before you try to get pregnant. Bad habits have a way of catching up with us.

Insect Bites

If you love to camp or go on sunny afternoon picnics, then you know firsthand how annoying insect bites can be. For some reason, biting flies, gnats, mosquitos and some spiders find human flesh irresistible. Most insect bites are aggravating but rarely need medical attention; however, in some cases, special attention is required.

Insect bites can vary in their seriousness from mild to potentially fatal. Some insect bites carry diseases such as deer ticks, responsible for Lyme disease (see chapter on Lyme disease). Bites from mosquitoes, lice, midges, gnats, horseflies, sand flies, fleas, bedbugs, bees, spiders, ticks and mites are common during summer months.

SYMPTOMS:

Physical symptoms of minor insect bites: Pain, redness, swelling, itching and burning. If multiple stings have occurred, muscle cramps, headaches, fever, drowsiness, weakness or unconsciousness can occur.

MEDICAL ALERT:

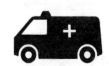

Any insect bite that causes weakness, difficulty breathing, wheezing, abdominal pain, fainting, hives or a skin rash should receive immediate medical attention.

STANDARD FIRST AID:

◆ Remove the stinger without using tweezers
◆ Wash the area with soap and water
◆ Apply an ice pack or cold compress to the area.

SPIDER BITES:

Spider bites can be dangerous for children or elderly people. There are three varieties of poisonous spiders found in the United States. They are the black widow, the brown recluse, and the tarantula.

PHYSICAL SYMPTOMS FROM A BLACK WIDOW BITE:

◆ Abdominal cramps, hard abdomen, difficult breathing, grunting, nausea, vomiting, headache, sweating, twitching, shaking and tingling sensations in the hand.
 Note: Bites from a brown recluse spider, which have a violin pattern on their backs, cause significant pain and local reactions and are generally considered more dangerous than the black widow spider. The toxin from a brown recluse spider can cause a sore to form that is slow to heal.
◆ First aid: Put an ice pack or cold compress on the bite and seek medical attention as soon as possible.

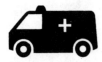

MEDICAL ALERT:

The bite of a black widow or brown recluse spider requires immediate medical attention.

ANT, MOSQUITO OR CHIGGER BITES:

◆ First aid: wash the area with soap and water. Apply a paste made of baking soda and water. In the case of chigger bites, use a brush and scrub the area. Use ice packs if swelling or pain is present

BEE STINGS:

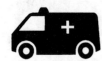

MEDICAL ALERT:

The sting of bumblebees, wasps, hornets, fire ants and yellow jackets can cause an allergic reaction in 5 out of 1,000 people. This reaction can be life-threatening and requires immediate medical treatment. (See the bee sting section in allergy chapter).

◆ First aid for simple bee stings: Remove the stinger with a clean, sharp blade scraped against the skin. Using a pair of tweezers may squeeze a venom sac located at the end of the stinger and cause more pain and inflammation. Wash the area with soap and water.

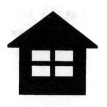

HOME SELF-CARE:

◆ A charcoal paste can be applied to bites to help draw out poisons and reduce inflammation.
◆ Taking antihistamines or Benedryl can help to lessen allergic-type symptoms that sometimes accompany insect bites.
◆ Calamine lotion helps with itching.
◆ Insect repellents such as "deet," which contain M-diethyltoluamide, can repel mosquitos and ticks. Some allergic reactions to this substance have been reported and it should be used with caution on children. Insect repellents containing R-11 have been banned by the EPA as being potentially hazardous to humans. Don't use any insect repellent on broken skin.
◆ Apply distilled witch hazel to inflamed area for a soothing effect.
◆ Apply a slice of fresh onion on insect stings for pain relief.
◆ Rubbing meat tenderizer on an insect bite can reduce pain. A paste can be made with meat tenderizer and water.
◆ Lotions such as Alpha Keri and Skin-So-Soft which is an Avon product, have been reported to repel bugs. Vick's Vaporub seems to have the same effect.
◆ Lindane and Crotamiton, both prescription drugs, can kill mites and alleviate itching.
◆ Topical steroid creams like Cortaid can be used for itching if not used for prolonged periods of time. Use an antibiotic cream if it looks as though the bite has become infected.
◆ Applying wet clay or making a mudpack and applying it to the bite can also help with pain and swelling.
◆ After removing the stinger, apply honey to the bite area.

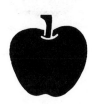

NUTRITIONAL APPROACH:

◆ Some studies have suggested that people whose diets are high in thiamine or vitamin B1 are not as attractive to insects, possibly due to a body odor given off in perspiration which cannot be detected by humans, but is repellent to insects. Taking a thiamine supplement three times a day when camping is recommended, or one 100 mg. tablet before going on a picnic.
◆ Eating a lot of onions and garlic can also make you repugnant to flying bugs. Use a good mouthwash or chew on fresh lemon and parsley or you might repel people as well!

◆ Large doses of vitamin C have been used to treat bites by venomous insects such as the brown recluse spider.
◆ Applying a mixture of PABA with alcohol has had good results with large and persistent mosquito bites.

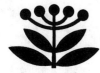

HERBAL REMEDIES:

◆ Rub a paste of vitamin C, aloe vera gel, myrrh oil and wintergreen on the bite area to control inflammation and pain.
◆ Chickweed cream can draw out insect stings.
◆ Plaintain or lemon balm applied to insect bites can reduce swelling and pain. Lemon balm oil also acts as an insect repellant.
◆ *Comfrey:* Mix dry comfrey powder with aloe vera juice to promote healing and reduce swelling.
◆ *Papaya:* Contains papain, an enzyme which is also found in some meat tenderizers. Applying papaya to an insect bite promotes healing and reduces inflammation.
◆ Elecampane is considered a natural insect repellent when used externally.
◆ Hanging dried tomato leaves in each room of the house is a traditional way to repel insects of all kinds.
◆ Oil of lavender and oil of collinsonia (citronella) are also good herbal insect repellents.
◆ Pennyroyal applied to the skin can repel mosquitoes and gnats.
◆ Take the following herbs in combination if you have suffered a systemic reaction to an insect bite: licorice, red clover, sarsaparilla, chaparral and burdock.
◆ Herbal ointments containing myrrh, aloe vera, Irish moss, and wintergreen are also recommended.

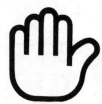

PREVENTION:

◆ Where light colored clothing that does not have brightly colored patterns.
◆ Avoid wearing perfumes, sweet smelling soaps, lotions, hair sprays, suntan oil or metallic jewelry.
◆ Don't eat sweet, drippy foods outside, such as watermelon or ice cream.
◆ If attacked by a swarm of insects, lie down and cover your head.
◆ Don't wear sandals or loose-fitting, short-sleeved clothing. Tuck your pants inside of your shoes.
◆ Avoid alcoholic drinks, which cause the skin to flush and blood vessels to dilate, which can attract mosquitos and flies.
◆ Black widows like to nest in dark woodpiles. Exercise caution when going into these kinds of areas. Spray woodpiles regularly for spiders.
◆ Use Skin-So-Soft by Avon or Vicks Vaporub to repel flying insects.

◆ Eating a lot of onions and garlic can help to repel some bugs.
◆ Use a bug repellant that contains deet on exposed areas; however, don't use it near your eyes or on small children. Follow instructions closely.

Insomnia

DEFINITION:

Your head hits the pillow and you close your eyes, eagerly looking forward to a good and restful night's sleep. Hours later, you're pacing the floor, or watching an old-time horror movie. Sleep has once again escaped you and you feel irritable and frustrated. There are some 120 million Americans who just can't seem to get to sleep at night, all victims of a malady called insomnia.

Insomnia simply refers to having trouble falling asleep or staying asleep. It is a very common problem with an incidence of one in three adults in the United States. Sleep needs greatly vary in each individual and can range from 4 hours to 10 hours per night. Generally speaking, the older one gets, the less sleep is required. Frequently, an individual who assumes he is suffering from insomnia is getting more sleep than he thinks. Sleeping pills or hypnotics are among the most widely prescribed drugs in the United States. The vast numbers of people suffering from insomnia reveals that most Americans have not properly learned to relax.

CAUSES:

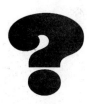

The most common cause of insomnia is anxiety, which results from worrying about a problem. Other possible causes include caffeine consumption, malnutrition, sleep apnea, indigestion, low blood glucose and some over-the-counter and prescription drugs. In addition, lack of exercise, pain, a feeling of restlessness in the legs, overwork, and the misuse of sedative drugs can contribute to insomnia.

The withdrawal from certain drugs such as sleeping pills, antidepressants, tranquilizers, illicit drugs or alcohol can also result in the inability to sleep. Poor sleeping routines such as sleeping late or excess napping are also contributory factors.

SYMPTOMS:

Physical: People who suffer from insomnia generally also complain of daytime fatigue, irritability, impatience and the inability to concentrate. Nightly routines can involve tossing and turning, short intervals of sleep, the inability to get comfortable, getting up several times at night and a generally frustrated feeling.

Psychological: Insomnia can also be symptomatic of a psychiatric illness. People who suffer from anxiety disorders and depression often have difficulty sleeping. The typical pattern in these instances is to awaken very early in the morning and not be able to resume sleeping. Manic-depressives usually sleep much less than normal and schizophrenics often pace at night. Victims of dementia may become afraid of the dark and act confused and restless at night.

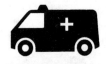

MEDICAL ALERT:

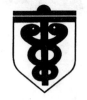

If a physical problem is keeping you awake, such as chest pain, shortness of breath, or heart palpitations, consult your doctor as soon as possible.

STANDARD MEDICAL TREATMENT:

If a physical or psychological cause for insomnia is discovered, it is treated accordingly. In cases of persistent insomnia which has no apparent cause, an EEG may be recommended to evaluate brain wave patterns during periods of rest.

If your physician determines that you have a sleeping disorder, such as sleep apnea, you may be referred to a specialist. Most cases of insomnia are treated with sedative-hypnotic drugs such as the barbiturates: Seconal, Nembutal, Tuinal and the Benzodiazepines Valium, Librium.

SIDE-EFFECTS: Barbiturates: This class of drugs depress the central nervous system and can cause death if taken in too large a dose.

Warning: Combining any barbiturate with alcohol can be fatal.

NOTE: Prescription sleeping pills induce an unnatural sleep which is not necessarily restful. Consequently, they may leave you feeling more tired than before, which may prompt an increased dosage of the drug. This cycle of disturbed sleep with continual drug treatment is referred to as drug-dependent insomnia and is thought to plague a significant number of Americans.

Caution: Any type of sedative-hypnotic can create a psychological and physical dependency in its users.

Success rating of standard medical treatment: very poor. Hypnotics are among the most widely prescribed drugs in the United States. Sleeping pills are not a cure for insomnia. On the contrary, they can actually worsen the condition and create an aggravated sense of fatigue upon arising. Insomnia is often treated as a disease by physicians, when, in fact, it may be more a result of poor sleeping habits. Relaxation techniques such as biofeedback and self-hypnosis and herbal medicines are preferable to drug therapy.

HOME SELF-CARE:

◆ Eliminate any over-the-counter or prescription drugs you do not need to take. Barbiturates and benzodiazepines can actively interfere with the sleep cycle.

◆ Go to bed at the same time every night to establish a sleeping and waking routine for the body.

◆ Exercise regularly. The value of exercise in enabling the body to relax at night cannot be overestimated. Exercise earlier in the day and not too close to bedtime. Twenty to thirty minutes of aerobic exercise at least three days a week is recommended.

◆ A leisurely outside stroll prior to bed is recommended.

◆ Avoid drinking alcohol, especially in the evening. Alcohol can temporarily induce sleep; however, waking up in the middle of the night after a nightcap is common.

◆ Don't use nicotine. Smokers have more difficulty going to sleep.

◆ Don't eat a large meal prior to bedtime. Not only can this result in insomnia, it can cause nightmares as well.

◆ Try to keep the bedroom as tranquil as possible, making it a place exclusively for sleep. Keep noise low, and if necessary, purchase curtains that effectively block out light.

◆ A white noise machine, which can be purchased, emits a sound that masks other sounds and can help lull a person to sleep. A fish aquarium filter can produce the same effect.

◆ Make sure your bedroom is not too hot and is well-ventilated.

◆ Some people sleep better with an electric blanket or hot water bottle. Electric blankets with timers are recommended so that the heat shuts off after you fall asleep.

◆ Try switching to pure cotton or linen sheets. Often the fabric that comes in contact with our skin can cause a subconscious annoyance.

◆ Make sure your pillow is not too high or puffy. Feather pillows that compress down or special pillows designed to support your neck may be much more comfortable.

◆ Never sleep in what you wore during the day. Use a light pajama or nightgown that is not too constricting or heavy.

◆ Get in bed and do breathing exercises while gently stretching your limbs. Listening to a stress-reducing tape which plays the sound of rain falling or ocean waves may also be helpful.

◆ Relax and unwind before you go to bed by reading, watching TV, listening to music, or taking a bath.

◆ Try some aromatherapy. The smell of lavender is recommended for its ability to relax the body.

◆ A bedtime snack is often helpful. The traditional home remedy of drinking a warm glass of milk has a scientific basis. Milk contain l-tryptophan, which does

help to induce sleep.
- If you can't sleep, get up and read until you feel sleepy.
- Yoga is an effective meditative technique for combating insomnia.

NUTRITIONAL APPROACH:

- An old remedy for insomnia is to take 2 teaspoons of cider vinegar, and 1 teaspoon of honey to a cup of warm water.
- A traditional nightcap for insomnia used in Spain is made by mixing 2 tablespoons of honey and the juice of one lemon in a glass of buttermilk.
- Recently some controversy has surrounded the use of the amino acid l-tryptophan to induce sleep. Do not take this amino acid without specific instructions from a physician.
- Foods that are naturally high in tryptophan are bananas, turkey, figs, tuna, dates, yogurt, and milk.
- Avoid eating highly spiced foods, chocolate, smoked meats, sauerkraut and tomatoes too close to bedtime. There is some speculation that these foods stimulate a release of norepinephrine, a brain chemical stimulant.
- Low blood glucose levels at night have been associated with insomnia and may require a small prebedtime snack to be stabilized. A plain baked potato or piece of bread eaten 30 minutes prior to retiring may be helpful.
- *B-vitamins and inositol:* A lack of the B vitamins can contribute to feelings of anxiety, depression and insomnia.
- Niacin is thought to have a sedating effect due to the role it plays in tryptophan metabolism.
- *Vitamin C with bioflavonoids:* Helps to keep nerve cells healthy.
- *Calcium and magnesium:* Work to calm the nerves and help relax the system. A lack of these two minerals can result in impaired sleep. Take calcium lactate or calcium chelate after meals and before retiring.
- *Folic acid:* There is some indication that people who can't sleep because they are compelled to keep moving their legs may suffer from a folate deficiency.
- *Vitamin E:* In some studies vitamin E helped to control repeated muscle jerks that some people experience while going to sleep or during sleep.

HERBAL REMEDIES:

- Herbal remedies for insomnia are much safer than sleeping pills and provide a non-addicting alternative to the use of drugs.
- Herb teas taken before bed can be especially calming.
- Hops and chamomile tea taken before retiring can be quite relaxing. Both help to calm excess excitability. If you do not like teas, these herbs can be taken in capsule form.

◆ *Wood betony*: An effective herbal nervine and sedative.
◆ *Valerian root*: A traditional folk medicine remedy which can significantly improve sleep and reduce insomnia without morning sleepiness.
◆ *Lavender*: An herbal sedative and analgesic. Can be used as an oil which can be massaged into the temples, and as aromatherapy. The fragrance of lavender helps to promote relaxation.
◆ *California poppy*: A non-addictive natural hypnotic.
◆ *Wild lettuce*: Considered a natural sedative and can be used in combination with passion flower and valerian.
◆ *Hops*: An herbal sleep inducer.
◆ *Lobelia*: A powerful nerve relaxant.
◆ *Passion flower*: This herb has traditionally been used by the Aztecs as a natural sedative.
◆ *The following herbs in combination may be useful*: Valerian root, kava kava, catnip, scullcap, hops, chamomile and passion flower.
◆ Herbal baths can be quite relaxing and can be made by filling a muslin bag with lavender or other herbs and attaching it to the faucet so that hot water runs through it as the tub fills.

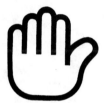

PREVENTION:

◆ Exercise regularly. People who exercise sleep better at night. Do not exercise vigorously too close to bedtime.
◆ Avoid ingesting caffeine, nicotine or alcohol. All three of these substances can alter natural sleep patterns.
◆ Learn to relax and "destress" before bedtime by listening to music, taking a hot bath or by some form of meditation. Relaxation tapes that contain the sound of rain falling or birds singing may also help achieve a "destressed" state of mind before going to bed.
◆ Establish a routine with set sleeping and waking hours.
◆ Make your bedtime environment as soothing and comfortable as possible.
◆ Avoid the use of over-the-counter and prescription drugs to induce sleep. These can end up promoting insomnia and are often counterproductive.
◆ Don't sleep in too late. Taking daytime naps may actually help you sleep better at night, although it is generally recommended that sleeping during the day be avoided. When Ben Franklin said "Early to bed, early to rise, makes a man healthy, wealthy and wise" he knew what he was talking about.

Kidney Stones

DEFINITION:

Trying to pass a kidney stone is one of the most painful experiences one might have the misfortune of enduring. Kidney stones have plagued humans for thousands of years. Michelangelo's letters record his own miserable encounter with them.

Today, over 10 percent of all males and 5 percent of females will suffer from a kidney stone sometime during their lifetime. Approximately 6 percent of the entire United States population develops kidney stones, which accounts for a great number of hospital admissions yearly.

Kidney stones occur when either calcium oxalate, uric acid or phosphates crystallize into stones. Seventy percent of all stones are calcium-oxalate based. Normally, these compounds stay in liquid form; however, when a chemical disruption occurs, stones can form and lodge anywhere within the urinary tract, causing a great deal of pain.

The incidence of kidney stones seems to be increasing and like other western diseases, such as gallstones and gout, may be directly linked with western diet and life-style. Once you have had a kidney stone, you are at somewhat of a higher risk of getting another, although it is not uncommon to pass one stone and never have one again. Approximately 60 percent of patients treated for a stone, will develop another within seven years.

Interestingly, more kidney stones are reported during the summer months, which may suggest that due to excess sweating, the urine can become more concentrated, increasing the chances of stone formation. Small stones that are present in the kidney will often cause no symptoms until they start to pass down into the ureter.

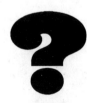

CAUSES:

Several conditions can cause the formation of kidney stones. Among them are an excess of vitamin D, Cushing's syndrome, degenerative bone disease, hyperparathyroidism, cystinuria, sarcoidosis, gout, and kidney disease. Other possible factors include deformities of the kidney, ingesting aluminum salts, excessive intake of milk and alkali (antacids), prolonged immobility, and an excess of vitamin C.

Anticancer drugs, high-protein diets, high alcohol consumption and exposure to certain heavy metals such as cadmium are also seen as contributing factors. A hereditary susceptibility exists with kidney stones as well. If your mother or father had trouble with kidney stones, your chances of getting them are increased.

SYMPTOMS:

Physical: Kidney stones typically cause upper back pain (acute and sharp) which can radiate to the lower abdomen and groin area and usually comes and goes. Kidney stone pain almost always occurs on one side of the body at a time and is so painful that it usually causes "doubling up." The following symptoms may also occur with kidney stones: chills, vomiting, fever, frequent urination, which can contain pus or blood, or impaired urination with poor flow rate or dribbling.

MEDICAL ALERT:

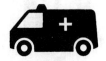

Contact a physician immediately if you are experiencing any type of unexplained intense pain or the presence of blood in the urine. If you have passed a stone, save it for laboratory analysis. The most serious complication of an obstructive kidney stone that is not treated is infection, which can lead to kidney damage.

STANDARD MEDICAL TREATMENT:

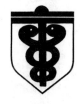

It is vital that the type of kidney stone you have be diagnosed, in order to design an effective treatment base on the stone's composition. Your doctor will use chemical analysis to classify the stone. The urine will be examined, which may contain the presence of stone crystals. Approximately 90 percent of urinary tract kidney stones will show up on an x-ray.

The use of intravenous or retrograde pyelography (IVP) can confirm the site of the stone. This test can also indicate any obstruction of the tract above the stone which can be monitored by ultrasound scanning. A chemical analysis of the blood and urine may be required, if another physical condition is thought to have caused the stone.

The usual treatment for a small kidney stone is bed rest accompanied by the use of narcotic analgesics. Increased fluid intake is encouraged. The majority of stones that are less than 0.2 inches in diameter can be passed without too much difficulty.

In the case of a larger stone, surgical treatment may be indicated to prevent kidney damage. Stones that are located in the bladder and the lower ureter can be crushed and removed using cystoscopy which is threaded up through the urethra into the bladder. Ultrasound lithotripsy uses an ultrasonic probe to break up larger stones. The shock-wave lithotritor can actually disintegrate stones using a focused shock wave. This method is continually being improved and is preferable to surgery.

Surgical options: The surgery described above should only be done as a last resort. Surgery to remove kidney stones is invasive and causes considerable trauma to the area affected.

Success rating of standard medical treatment: fair. There is really no satisfactory medical treatment for kidney stones that do not flush out on their own. If stones are being caused by other medical conditions, certain drugs can be prescribed to help inhibit the formation of future stones. Surgery should be considered only as a last resort. Recent advances in ultrasonic and shock-wave therapy offer better treatment options.

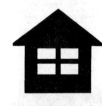
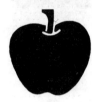

HOME SELF-CARE:

◆ At the first sign of a kidney stone, drink large quantities of water to help flush out the stone.
◆ Over-the-counter analgesics can help if the pain is not too severe.

NUTRITIONAL APPROACH:

◆ Drink plenty of fluids every day—at least 6 to 8 glasses of water (preferably more).
◆ Drink the juice from a freshly squeezed lemon in water first thing in the morning and at night.
◆ Drinking large amounts of cranberry or cherry juice has long been considered a folk remedy for kidney stones. Most physicians believe that in order to make the urine acid enough, unrealistic quantities of these juices would have to be consumed. The majority of the scientific community sees cranberry and cherry juice as just other ways to increase fluid intake, which is seen as desirable. Cherry juice contains bioflavonoids which can help reduce inflammation and heal damaged tissue.
◆ Calcium-based kidney stones, which make up the majority of kidney stones, can be the result of dietary patterns characterized by low fiber, high alcohol consumption, high fat, high animal protein, high sugar and high salt diets. Several studies indicate that vegetarians, as a whole, have a decreased risk of developing kidney stones. Because calcium-rich foods can also create stones, reduce the amount of milk, butter, cheese and other dairy products that you consume.
◆ Supplement the diet with fiber by changing to whole grains exclusively. Research has indicated that increasing fiber intake can lower the calcium content of urine.
◆ Avoid white sugar and refined carbohydrates. After ingesting sugar, a rise in urinary calcium can occur.
◆ Limit dairy products and try to avoid those fortified with vitamin D, which is thought to contribute to the formation of stones.
◆ Avoid foods that are high in oxalate such as cocoa, black tea, beet leaves, spinach, parsley, celery, grapes, blueberries, strawberries, summer squash and

nuts.

◆ Watch your protein intake (meats, cheeses, poultry and fish). Eating too much protein can increase the presence of urinary calcium, phosphate and uric acid.

◆ Cut your daily salt intake. Cutting down on salt helps to decrease the concentration of urinary calcium. Watch hidden sources of salt or sodium found in ketchup, mustard, pickled foods, smoked meats, chips, pops and pretzels.

◆ *Magnesium and vitamin B6:* Lab tests with animals have shown that a magnesium-deficient diet produces kidney stones. Magnesium increases that solubility of calcium. Magnesium supplemented with vitamin B6 has been shown to be effective in preventing the recurrence of kidney stones. Magnesium oxide or magnesium chloride are both good. The combination of magnesium and B6 has had dramatic results in curtailing the incidence of kidney stone recurrence, with a success rate in some studies as high as 90 percent.

◆ *Vitamin K:* Vitamin K plays a significant role in the synthesis of urinary proteins necessary to keep calcium oxalate from crystallizing. Vitamin K is found in green leafy vegetables and fat-soluble chlorophyll.

◆ *Citrate:* Found in potassium citrate or sodium citrate. A low level of citrate is often found in people who suffer from kidney stones. A decreased level of citrate can be the result of chronic diarrhea, urinary tract infections or acidosis. Citrate supplementation is thought to be of significant value in preventing kidney stones.

◆ *Vitamin A:* Helps to promote healing if the urinary tract has been damaged from the stone. Vitamin A can also help to discourage the formation of future stones.

◆ *Vitamin C:* Do not take megadoses. Too much vitamin C can cause the formation of kidney stones. Check with your doctor on an appropriate dietary dosage.

◆ Avoid ingesting vitamin D fortified milk and the prolonged use of antacids. This combination can increase the level of urinary calcium concentrations.

◆ Avoid ingesting large amounts of vitamin D supplements. Do not exceed 400 international units per day.

HERBAL REMEDIES:

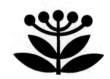

◆ *Aloe vera:* Reduces the growth rate of urinary calcium. It can be used in prevention as well as to reduce the size of an existing stone. Take in juice form.

◆ *Ginkgo biloba extract:* Used in China for its tonifying effect on the urinary system.

◆ *Goldenrod:* A traditional treatment for kidney stones due to its cleansing and eliminative action.

◆ *Agrimony:* Helps to allow fluids to pass more readily through the kidneys.

◆ *Queen of the meadow:* A traditional herb used for an ailment of the kidney or urinary tract.

- *Hydrangea:* Helps with the pain caused by the presence of stones in the ureters.
- *Khella:* Used by the ancient Egyptians for the treatment of kidney stones. It works by relaxing the ureter and allowing the stone to pass.
- *The following herbs in combination may be useful:* Golden seal root, marshmallow, juniper berries, watermelon seeds, uva ursi, pan pien lien and ginger.

PREVENTION:

- There is a sizable consensus that the majority of kidney stones can be prevented through dietary changes.
- Make sure you supplement your diet with adequate doses of magnesium and vitamin B6.
- Increase your daily fluid intake. Drink 6 to 8 glasses of pure water per day. If you have a hard water supply, drink bottled water that is lower in mineral content. Magnesium should be ingested and calcium avoided.
- Increase dietary fiber, complex carbohydrates and green leafy vegetables.
- Avoid excess sugar, salt, simple carbohydrates, animal fats and meats.
- Limit your intake of dairy products, especially those that have been fortified with vitamin D.
- Limit your intake of animal protein, which can lead to losing calcium which ends up in the urine. Uric acid kidney stones can also form from a diet that is too high in purines.
- Keep yourself at an ideal weight. Excess weight may lead to an insensitivity to insulin, which can cause hypercalciuria, a condition which increases your risk for stone formation.
- Do not use calcium-based stomach medications or antacids such as Tums, and avoid aluminum compounds.
- Keep yourself active. Exercise regularly. Prolonged inactivity can cause calcium levels in the blood to rise. Exercising helps to pull calcium out of the bloodstream and back into the bones.

Lyme Disease

DEFINITION:

Lyme disease was first described in Old Lyme, Connecticut in 1975. Approximately, 14,000 cases of Lyme disease have been reported in the United States and more cases occur every year. The disease has received a great deal of media attention and has resulted in some apprehension about going outdoors. Some simple precautions can go a long way to protect individuals against becoming infected with Lyme disease.

The disorder, which is transmitted through the bite of a tick, is characterized by changes in the skin, flulike symptoms and joint inflammation and swelling. The majority of cases of Lyme disease have occurred in the northeastern United States, which is inhabited by the white-tail deer, although the disease has been reported in other parts of the country. Ninety percent of all cases of Lyme disease have occurred in New Jersey, Minnesota, Connecticut, California, Massachusetts, New York, Rhode Island and Wisconsin. Migratory birds have transported the disease to southern areas of the United States.

Because tick bites are often painless and undetected, this disease may escape diagnosis for months or years. It usually takes three to twenty days following the bite of an infected tick for symptoms to appear. Ninety percent of all cases occurr between the months of June and September.

CAUSES:

Lyme disease is caused by the bacterium borrelia burgdorferi, which is transmitted through a tick bite. These ticks, called ixodes dammini, typically infest deer, but can also be found on some dogs and house cats. The white-footed field mouse found in the Eastern states can also carry the tick. Lizards and jackrabbits can also be carriers.

SYMPTOMS:

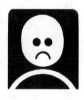

Physical: The symptoms of Lyme disease vary greatly with each individual. Frequently, no single symptoms appear in all cited cases and the sequence of symptoms can remain unpredictable. There are usually three phases to the disease. The following symptoms are typical of each phase:

Phase one: A distinctive oval rash is one of the earliest symptoms of Lyme disease. This rash may appear on several areas of the body. Along with this rash, other possible symptoms are flulike, including fever, headache, lethargy, muscle pain, stiff neck, backache, nausea, and vomiting.

Phase two: Approximately 20 percent of untreated victims will experience heart rhythm abnormalities, impaired motor coordination and partial facial paralysis during phase two.

Phase three: Approximately 50 percent of untreated cases will develop intermittent or chronic arthritis, which may not appear for up to two years from the time of infection. Joint inflammation with redness and swelling which typically affects the knees and other large joints is common.

Other possible symptoms of Lyme disease include: enlarged spleen and lymph nodes.

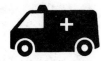

MEDICAL ALERT:

The symptoms of this disease have been misdiagnosed as rheumatoid arthritis and subsequently, mistreated. Any generalized, unexplained rash should be seen by a physician, especially in areas where Lyme disease is a problem. It is important that if you are suffering from the above symptoms, and have been exposed to tick infested environments, that you tell your physician. Family pets, especially cats, have been found to harbor the deer-tick and have been responsible for several cases of Lyme disease.

Unless the disease is diagnosed and properly treated, symptoms can persist for years, although their severity usually decreases. Complications such as an inflammation of the heart muscle or meningitis can occur in some cases. The symptoms of Lyme disease are also similar to chronic fatigue syndrome, multiple sclerosis, and gout.

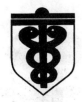

STANDARD MEDICAL TREATMENT:

If Lyme disease is diagnosed before joint inflammation occurs, it is easily treated with antibiotics. Doxycycline is the drug of choice. Your doctor will give you a blood test that has been devised to help identify Lyme disease, in which the presence of certain antibodies are found. Unfortunately, the tests are not particularly reliable.

In the future, a urine test which can detect the presence of the bacteria responsible for the disease will be available. In more advanced cases of Lyme disease, non-steroidal anti-inflammatory drugs or corticosteroid drugs may be needed. In these cases, a cure usually takes longer.

A three-week course of several antibiotics can work in the first stage and even in the second; however, only half the cases which have gone on to the third stage are cured with antibiotics.

Side-effects: Doxycycline (Doryx, Dory-caps, Doxychel, Vibramycin, Vibra-tabs): Stomach upset, cramps, nausea, vomiting, diarrhea, rash, hairy tongue, and itching.

Warning: Children under the age of 9 should avoid doxycylcine, which can produce serious discoloration of the teeth and impair the development of long bones. Pregnant women and nursing mothers should not use this drug.

Success rate of standard medical treatment: very good to excellent if diagnosed correctly. If Lyme disease is allowed to progress to the third stage, it is much more difficult to treat and may result in serious complications.

MEDICAL UPDATE:

◆ Connaught Laboratories are currently testing a vaccine for Lyme disease in over 10,000 volunteers. In the fall, results of the studies will be submitted to the FDA for evaluation and the vaccine may be available as early as 1996.

HOME SELF-CARE:

◆ Take hot baths or whirlpool treatments for joint pain.
◆ If experiencing joint pain, use the therapies suggested in the section on arthritis.

NUTRITIONAL APPROACH:

◆ Emphasize fresh fruit and fruit juices, which can help the body get rid of toxins. Apple and pineapple juice are recommended.
◆ *Germanium:* Helps strengthen immune functions.
◆ *Vitamin C:* Considered an anti-inflammatory which helps fight infection.
◆ *Vitamin A:* acts as an antioxidant, promotes tissue healing and boosts the immune system.
◆ *Acidophilus:* If under antibiotic therapy, use a supplement every day to replenish friendly intestinal bacteria.
◆ *Kelp:* Helps to detoxify the system.

HERBAL REMEDIES:

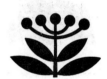

◆ *Echinacea:* Fights any type of infection both viral and bacterial.
◆ *Garlic:* An excellent anti-bacterial agent that boosts the immune system.
◆ *Golden seal:* Considered a natural antibiotic.
◆ *Red clover:* Considered a good blood cleanser and tonic.
◆ *Black walnut:* Can help to kill parasites and bacteria.

PREVENTION:

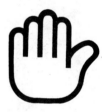

Use precautions when going into wooded areas, especially areas inhabited by white-tail deer. Leave as little skin exposed as possible. Cover your arms and legs, wear a hat and always wear long socks. High-necked shirts, scarves and gloves are also recommended. Wearing light colored clothing makes ticks easier to spot.

Use N-diethyl metatoluamide (Deet), a repellant, on any exposed area except the face. This can also be used on clothing. Use this minimally on children. Note: This chemical can be fatal if ingested so keep out of the reach of children.

◆ Stay near the center of trails in overgrown areas.
◆ Always check yourself after an outing for any raised bumps. Have someone else check your head and back.
◆ Taking your clothes off outside is also recommended.
◆ Checking children for ticks before they go to bed is also advisable.
◆ If your pets have any possibility of picking up the tick, delouse them frequently.
◆ Ticks on clothing can be killed by putting the clothing in the dryer on high for at least 30 minutes. Laundering clothing does not always kill ticks.

HOW TO REMOVE A TICK:

◆ Use a pair of tweezers and grab the head-not the swollen stomach-of the tick as close to the surface of the skin as possible, then pull it straight out. There is no cause for alarm if a piece of the head stays in the skin. Do not use your fingers as bacteria can penetrate the skin. After removing the tick thoroughly wash the area with soap and water and then apply an antiseptic or rubbing alcohol. Wash your hands well. If you think the tick might be infected, save it and call your physician. For the next several weeks, watch for symptoms of Lyme disease.

Measles (red, seven day or ten day)

DEFINITION:

Measles is a highly contagious viral disease that is now considered preventable due to the availability of a vaccine. It attacks the respiratory system and causes a rash. A significant number of people still contract this illness which, in some instances, can be fatal or have serious complications.

The incubation period for measles is between 7 and 14 days. Measles is considered a childhood disease; however, adults also are susceptible. The peak incidence of measles is in preschool or early school years. Measles usually lasts from 4 to 7 days and most often occurs in temperate climates during the winter and early spring months.

Public health services are attempting to completely eradicate measles in the United States. It is considered the most serious of the preventable childhood diseases. In developing countries, measles is still common and accounts for more than 1 million deaths per year. One attack of measles usually provides lifelong immunity.

CAUSES:

Measles is spread by droplets (coughing or sneezing) which come from the mouth or throat of infected individuals. It can also be spread by coming in contact with articles that have been soiled by infected secretions. The virus can be spread 3 to 6 days before the rash appears. After exposure, symptoms will begin to show within 8 to 12 days.

SYMPTOMS:

Physical: The following symptoms usually appear 3 to 5 days prior to the outbreak of the rash: fever, weakness, dry barking cough, sneezing, runny nose, swollen lymph glands, eyes that become red, itchy and light-sensitive, and white spots that appear on the inside of the mouth (Koplik's spots).

After 3 to 5 days you can expect to see pink, flat blotches that appear around the hairline, on the face, neck, and behind the ears. An abrupt rise in temperature usually accompanies the rash and can go as high as 105 degrees Fahrenheit.

Early in the disease the rash will fade if pressure is directly applied to the skin. In time, the rash may darken and become larger patches as it spreads to the chest, abdomen and the limbs. Mild itching may accompany the rash, which sometimes becomes browner in color as the disease matures. As the rash subsides, the fever will diminish. Abdominal pain, vomiting, chills and diarrhea can also accompany the other symptoms of measles.

If you suspect your child has the measles, notify your physician. He will be aware if a local outbreak of the disease exists.

MEDICAL ALERT:

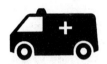

German measles (rubella) is a variety of measles that, if contracted in the first four months of pregnancy, can cause serious birth defects. Women of childbearing age who have not been previously immunized for rubella and who are either not pregnant or will avoid becoming pregnant for at least three months should be immunized to prevent the possibility of birth defects. If you are not sure whether you had rubella as a child and are immune, a blood test can confirm immunity.

Possible complications of measles: Sore throat, ear infection, conjunctivitis, bronchitis, croup, pneumonia, and encephalitis. Children who are at special risk for developing secondary infections are infants under 1 year old, children who take steroids, and children who suffer from any long-term disease, such as diabetes, asthma, or cystic fibrosis.

Note: Severe cases of both measles and whooping cough can cause patches of discoloration on the teeth.

STANDARD MEDICAL TREATMENT:

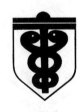

Once measles is diagnosed by your doctor, he will recommend medications such as Tylenol to relieve symptoms. Bed rest and increased fluids will also be suggested. In some cases, cough medicines and decongestants may be prescribed to help control the respiratory symptoms that accompany measles. Antibiotics are useless in the treatment of measles, unless a secondary infection has occurred.

Success rating of standard medical treatment: fair. As in the case of most viral infections, standard medical treatment can only help control the discomfort the disease causes.

HOME SELF-CARE:

WARNING: Do not give children (anyone under 21) aspirin. Giving aspirin when a viral infection is present can increase the risk of Reye's syndrome, a potentially fatal disorder (see the chapter on Reye's syndrome).

◆ Use a cool mist vaporizer to help control the dry, brassy cough that accompanies measles.

◆ Keep the light levels dim. Bright sunlight or glare can be very disturbing to light-sensitive eyes. Reading or watching TV may also further irritate the eyes. While light is bothersome to people suffering from measles, it does not cause any physical damage to the eyes.

◆ Keep fingernails short on young children to prevent irritation from scratching the rash that accompanies measles. Putting gloves or socks on small children at night may be helpful.

◆ A cool cornstarch bath can help quiet the itchy rash.

◆ Wear sunglasses while the eyes are light-sensitive.

◆ To keep runny nose discharge from causing skin irritation, place a thin layer of petroleum jelly or menthalatum between the nose and the upper lip.

◆ Use acetaminophen or ibuprofen for fever.

NUTRITIONAL APPROACH:

◆ Do not be overly concerned if a child suffering from measles refuses solid food. Increase fluid intake using water, fruit and vegetable juices, broths and herb teas.

◆ *Calcium/magnesium:* Helps to promote tissue repair and can be taken in liquid or powder form during infections and fevers.

◆ *Vitamin A and E:* Boost the immune system in fighting viral infections

◆ *Vitamin C:* Good for controlling fever and infection, and has antiviral properties. Have the child take chewables or use a vitamin C powder which can be mixed into liquids.

◆ *Vitamin B complex:* Can become depleted quickly during illness and fever

◆ *Zinc:* Can be taken as throat lozenges. Strengthens the immune system and contributes to cell and tissue repair.

HERBAL REMEDIES:

◆ *Catnip or chamomile tea:* Good for reducing the fever which usually accompanies measles.

◆ *Garlic:* Fights both viral and bacterial infection and can be taken on odorless capsule form

◆ *Warm or cool ginger baths:* Add strong, steeped ginger tea to bath water.

◆ Echinacea: An a natural antiviral herb that boosts the immune system.

- *Yarrow:* Acts a blood cleanser and can help to eliminate toxins released by the virus.
- *Golden seal:* Helps to relieve itching and is considered an herbal antibiotic.
- *Hops:* A natural nervine and relaxant that also helps to reduce fevers.
- *The following herbs in combination may be useful:* Golden seal, echinacea, yarrow, capsicum, myrrh.

PREVENTION:

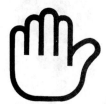

- Immunization against measles is the most effective way to prevent the disease. The measles vaccine should not be given to children under the age of 1 or to those with risk factors for vaccination. This vaccine is usually given in combination with the mumps and rubella vaccine and its side-effects are generally mild. Check with your doctor on any risks associated with the vaccine.
- There are several parents who are concerned about the possible side-effects and risks of vaccines. Educate yourself on the facts concerning the benefits and potential hazards of viral vaccines. Recently, two of three available measles, mumps and rubella vaccines have been withdrawn from the market in London. Cases of mild, viral meningitis have been reported as side-effects of the vaccine. The withdrawal affected Smithkline Beecham's Pluserix MMR and Merieux UK Immravax vaccines. These cases of viral meningitis occurred around three weeks after the vaccine was administered.

Menopause

DEFINITION:

Going through "the change of life" has become a dreaded event by both women and their male companions, who have been inundated with horror stories about its frightening transformations. The Dr. Jekyll/Mr. Hyde attitude toward the perils of menopause does little to educate the public on its true nature. Getting the right facts is the best way to deal with this particular female phenomenon.

Menopause is a medical term referring to the end of the menstrual cycle which includes the cessation of ovulation and menstrual periods. This term is commonly used to described the months or years which come before and after the end of the cycle. A woman can experience her last period sometime between the ages of 40 and 50, although in some cases, menopause can happen as late as age 60. The average age for menopause is 51.

The years which lead up to menopause are characterized by disruptions in the menstrual cycle and in the nature of the periods themselves. It is important to remember that many women experience menopause with little or even no discomfort. A woman is considered post-menopausal when she is past 45 and has had no periods for six months.

CAUSES:

Menopause occurs because the production of estrogen and progesterone in the ovaries greatly decreases. Without the presence of sufficient estrogen, the uterine lining which is shed in menstruation cannot form. This can occur quite suddenly and can initiate a variety of physical and emotional symptoms. Contrary to some popular notions, the loss of estrogen experienced during menopause does not redistribute fat, contribute to a loss of muscle tone or cause wrinkles to appear.

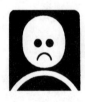

SYMPTOMS:

Physical: Half of all women experience some symptoms associated with menopause and 25 percent of women consider the symptoms distressing. Symptoms may include hot flashes, flushed face, vaginal dryness, sweating, palpitations, irregular periods, joint pains and headaches. In addition, osteoporosis, a thinning of the bones, can also begin with menopause.

Psychological: Menopause can cause depression, anxiety, irritability, lack of concentration, mood swings, sleep disorders, lack of confidence, increased emotional sensitivity, crying for no apparent reason, forgetfulness and social withdrawal. The mood changes that accompany menopause are not all necessarily negative. For example, an increase in energy and motivation may result from the hormonal changes typical of menopause.

Both the physical and psychological symptoms of menopause can last from a few months to up to five years. The average length of menopausal symptoms is a year to two years.

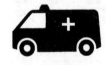

MEDICAL ALERT:

Bleeding between periods, or prolonged or excessive menstrual bleeding may indicate the presence of a uterine tumor. Bleeding after menopause is not normal and should be investigated by a doctor as soon as possible.

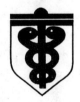

STANDARD MEDICAL TREATMENT:

Hormone replacement therapy is the usual treatment for menopausal symptoms. Hormones may be a combination of progesterone and estrogen or estrogen alone.

These hormones can be taken in tablet form, vaginal creams, or as surgically placed implant patches.

In addition, tranquilizers, antidepressants and sleeping pills are also routinely prescribed by doctors for emotional and psychological disturbances typical of menopause.

Side-effects: Hormonal Therapy: Estrogen: can increase the risk of uterine cancer. Other possible side-effects include water retention and headaches. Any hormonal therapy comes with a whole host of possible side-effects and should be discussed in length with your physician.

Note: Recent evaluation of hormone replacement therapy has concluded that the value of estrogen outweighs its possible risks. Estrogen therapy can help slow osteoporosis, and actually reduce a woman's risk for heart attack. Cardiovascular disease is the leading killer of women.

Recent studies indicate that the death rate from heart disease among women who take post-menopausal estrogen is significantly lower. The addition of progesterone with estrogen has helped to decrease some side-effects. Hormone replacement therapy should be discussed thoroughly with your doctor. Not all health care providers approve of hormone therapy.

HOME SELF-CARE:

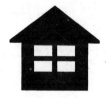

◆ Use a vaginal lubricant (Lubifax, K-Y) for vaginal dryness and itching. Other preparations that might be helpful are unscented creams such as Albolene and Lubrin.

◆ For hot flashes, particularly at night, wear light cotton fabrics which have "breathability."

◆ Drink plenty of water to help with hot flashes.

◆ Carry of packet of premoistened towelettes with you to cool off your face. Small battery operated fans are also available.

◆ The value of regular aerobic exercise to help combat both the physical and psychological symptoms of menopause cannot be overstressed. Regular exercise can increase the secretions of certain brain chemicals which can elevate moods and counteract depression. Walk, swim, climb stairs, or join a spa. Weight bearing exercises have been found to function especially well in preventing the onset of osteoporosis.

◆ Having regular sexual intercourse seems to discourage both vaginal dryness and hot flashes.

◆ Do not smoke: Smoking is lethal regardless; however, when combined with hormone replacement therapy it can cause an interaction which dramatically increases the risk of stroke, high blood pressure and heart disease.

◆ Use relaxation techniques such as yoga or breathing exercises to combat anxiety or nervousness.

◆ Discussing your menopause with an understanding partner goes a long way. Knowing that certain symptoms are perfectly normal and temporary can be extremely valuable.

◆ View menopause not as a tragic end to your youth and sexuality, but rather as a natural transition.

◆ If you need a support group, call your local women's center or start one by placing an ad in the newspaper.

NUTRITIONAL APPROACH:

◆ Avoid alcohol and caffeine, which can aggravate hot flashes.

◆ Eat a diet high in raw foods and low in red meats, sugar and dairy products. Emphasize the following foods: whole grains, sesame seeds, sunflower seeds, almonds, fresh vegetables and fruits, garlic, beans and whole grain pastas.

◆ Eating frequent light meals is preferable to three heavy ones. Doing this seems to discourage hot flashes.

◆ Avoid the following foods: rich dairy products, sugar, fatty greasy foods, red meats, coffee, tea, alcohol and nicotine.

◆ *Calcium/magnesium:* Very important in helping to prevent osteoporosis, which can begin with menopause when estrogen levels drop. This combination is also very beneficial is helping nervous disorders and mental anxiety.

◆ *Potassium:* Can easily be lost in sweats and hot flashes. Important for calcium assimilation.

◆ *Selenium:* Involved in maintaining hormonal balance in the body.

◆ *Vitamin C:* Also recommended for hot flashes and is easily lost through perspiration.

◆ *Vitamin E:* Can help control hot flashes, increase the production of hormones, and combat vaginal dryness.

◆ *Lecithin:* Acts as an emulsifier and can help in assimilating vitamin E.

◆ *Vitamin B complex:* Helps with water retention and is good for emotional or mental disturbances. Vitamin B5 and B6 injections have been known to reduce hot flashes and minimize nervous disorders.

◆ *Acidophilus:* Can help combat vaginitis and cystitis. Some post-menopausal women are more susceptible to bladder infections.

◆ *Primrose or black current oil:* Contributes to estrogen production and works as a sedative and a diuretic. Is also recommended for hot flashes.

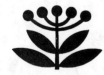

HERBAL REMEDIES:

◆ *False unicorn root:* Stimulates ovarian hormones and is helpful especially in stages of early menopause. This herb contains hormonelike saponins.

◆ *Motherwort:* A uterine stimulant which also helps with heart palpitations and feelings of anxiety.

- *Ho shou wu:* A Chinese herb used to treat the symptoms of early menopause.
- *Chaste-tree:* Helps to normalize hormonal function and balance. Some university studies indicate that chaste-tree appears to stimulate the pituitary gland to balance estrogen and progesterone.
- *Black cohosh:* Helps to stimulate natural estrogen production and is also a nervine tonic.
- *Ginseng:* Helps with depression and in the production of estrogen.
- *Damiana, dong quai and chaparral* taken in combination can help with hot flashes.
- *Licorice:* Can help to stimulate estrogen production.
- *Sarsaparilla:* Contains progesterone and cortin to help achieve glandular balance.
- *Gotu-kola and dong quai:* Help to relieve vaginal dryness and depression.
- *The following herbs in combination may be useful:* Black cohosh, licorice, false unicorn, Siberian ginseng, sarsaparilla, squaw vine, blessed thistle

PREVENTING OR MINIMIZING MENOPAUSAL SYMPTOMS:

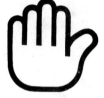

- Exercising regularly, eating a nutritious diet and leading a happy, full life can greatly help to minimize psychological and physical menopausal symptoms. Regular exercise has been chosen as the most significant tool against the negative symptoms that can accompany menopause.
- Keep involved and active. Finding something that you love to do can help you through menopause. Join a bowling league, walk with someone, try a new hobby, or take a class.

Menstrual Cramps (dysmenorrhea)

DEFINITION:

For years, menstrual cramps have been viewed by some men, including some doctors, as an exaggerated female affliction that was used more as a ploy for sympathy than anything else. Thank goodness the myths of menstrual cramps have finally been laid to rest. Today, doctors recognize the reality of these miserable monthly pains. In addition, several treatment options exist to help decrease the intensity of these cramps.

Menstrual cramps accompany menstruation in a large percentage of women. As mentioned above, just a few decades ago, they were considered more psychosomatic than physical. Today, the involvement of hormones called prostaglandins explain the presence of menstrual cramping. Most women experience menstrual cramps several times before they reach menopause. Menstrual cramps usually begin two to three years after the first period once ovulation becomes established.

Menstrual discomfort occurs in at least half of all adolescent females and is the leading cause of school absences. In some cases, cramping will decrease after the age of 25 or after childbirth. Menstrual cramps are characterized by intermittent aching pains located in the lower abdomen or lower back region, which can radiate down the thighs.

Cramps can begin before the actual onset of bleeding and in some cases dramatically decrease by the second day of the period. The existence of cramps has no relationship with the amount of flow. Approximately 10 percent of women have menstrual cramping severe enough to interfere with their daily routine.

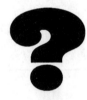

SYMPTOMS:

Physical: Pains in the lower abdomen or back that can come and go in a wavelike pattern and sometimes radiate down the thighs typify menstrual cramps. Menstrual cramps typically begin shortly before the onset of a period and generally last for 12 hours. Cramps can be accompanied by nausea, vomiting and anxiety.

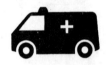

MEDICAL ALERT:

If menstrual cramps are intense see your doctor to make sure that endometriosis or a pelvic infection is not present.

Note: Menstrual discomfort that begins at an early age should be mentioned to a physician.

CAUSES:

Following ovulation, progesterone stimulates the uterus to produce prostaglandin, which forces muscle contraction in the uterus. This contraction combined with the constricting of blood vessels that cut off blood supply to the uterine lining so it will be shed monthly can also cause discomfort.

Excessive production of prostaglandins or a hypersensitivity to them may be responsible for severe cramps. Heredity does not seem to be a significant factor.

Note: Some factors seem to increase the severity and incidence of menstrual cramps. These include:
- Being overweight.
- Having regular periods rather than irregular ones.
- Having a flow that lasts longer than three days.

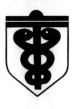

STANDARD MEDICAL TREATMENT:

Prostaglandin inhibitors will be recommended by your physician. Ibuprofen based preparations are the most effective (Motrin, Rufen, Nuprin, Medipren, Advil). Non-steroidal anti-inflammatory drugs function in the same way (Naprosyn, Anaprox, Clinoril, Feldene); however, they require a prescription and are costly. Aspirin is considered an antiprostaglandin, although it is not as effective as ibuprofen. Acetaminophen based products (Tylenol, Anacin-3, etc.) are not antiprostaglandin. They do not have a significant effect on the mechanism that causes menstrual cramps.

In more severe cases, birth control pills are sometimes prescribed to suppress ovulation which, in turn, minimizes the intensity of menstrual cramps. Non-contraceptive hormones may also be prescribed.

Success rating of standard medical treatment: fair to good. In most cases, the severity of cramps can be controlled. They are rarely, if ever, totally eliminated.

Side-effects: Ibuprofen. Upset stomach, dizziness, headache, drowsiness, ear ringing, heartburn, nausea, vomiting, bloating, nervousness, rash, abnormal heart rhythm, lowered blood sugar, and kidney damage.

Warning: While ibuprofen has not been associated with birth defects or other problems among breast-fed infants, if you are pregnant or nursing, do not take it without your doctor's approval.

Side effects: Oral contraceptives. Oral contraceptives can increase the incidence of heart attack, especially if combined with smoking. Other possible side-effects include nausea, abdominal cramps, bloating, vaginal bleeding, change in menstrual flow, breast tenderness, weight change, headaches, rash, vaginal itching and infection, change in sex drive, nervousness, cataracts and loss of hair.

Warning: Do not use oral contraceptives if you might be pregnant, have a history of stroke, high blood pressure, liver, breast or reproductive organ cancer, or blood clots. Using oral contraceptives is not recommended if you have irregular or scanty periods. There are a number of other physical disorders which may pose a health risk if taking oral contraceptives, and any existing condition should be discussed with your doctor.

HOME SELF-CARE:

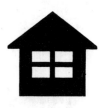

◆ Take ibuprofen immediately at the beginning of cramping and repeat according to drug directions. Waiting to use these medications until cramping is severe is less effective. Do not take this medication on an empty stomach.

◆ Engage your body in a number of stretches. A yoga routine can also be quite effective in minimizing pain. Yoga exercises that should be investigated are shoulder stand, plow, fish, uddiyana, cobra, and posterior stretch. Lunging to the side with

your feet spread apart and one knee bent is also recommended to relieve pain.
- ◆ Reflexology or acupressure may offer some beneficial results. Regular foot massages may help alleviate pain caused by uterine muscle contraction.
- ◆ Take a good brisk walk and breathe deeply as you walk. Do not overexert yourself. Make it a pleasant walk and pace yourself. Walking can help reduce muscle tension and helps release brain chemicals which can actually elevate your mood.
- ◆ Use a hot water bottle or heating pad on the small of your back or on your abdomen. Taking a long, leisurely hot bath can also help with menstrual pain. Some women apply heat to the small of their backs before they anticipate having cramps and find that this minimizes menstrual discomfort.
- ◆ For some women, applying a soft ice pack to the abdomen helps to reduce pain.
- ◆ Drink plenty of hot herbal teas such as raspberry leaf tea.

NUTRITIONAL APPROACH:

- ◆ Avoid taking diuretics, which can deplete your body of essential minerals that help to control menstrual cramping.
- ◆ Avoid salt, caffeine, junk foods and refined sugars. Sometimes the hormonal changes experienced during a period can create food cravings for salty, fatty, or sugary foods. Learn to replace those foods with fruit, steamed vegetables, whole grain pretzels, and fruit.
- ◆ Drink plenty of water and fruit juice to keep your system well hydrated.
- ◆ Emphasize fresh fruits and vegetables, whole grains, chicken and fish.
- ◆ Do not drink alcoholic beverages. Alcohol can increase water retention.
- ◆ *Calcium/magnesium chloride:* An excellent supplement to help alleviate cramping and muscle spasms. It helps to maintain good muscle tone. Magnesium increases the absorption of calcium in the body. Calcium/magnesium may also help in reducing breast tenderness. Some women have found that chewing calcium supplements during their period helps with pain control.
- ◆ *Vitamin E:* Good for reproductive organ health and function.
- ◆ *Vitamin B complex:* Helps to reduce premenstrual tension. In some instances, taking brewer's yeast has decreased the severity of menstrual discomfort, including depression. Some research suggests that menstruation may cause a functional deficiency of vitamin B6.
- ◆ *Vitamin C with bioflavonoids:* Help to strengthen blood vessels and capillary walls in the uterus.
- ◆ *Iron:* Make sure if you suffer from heavy periods that you are not suffering from an iron deficiency.

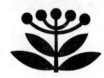

HERBAL REMEDIES:

- ◆ *Dong quai:* Good for a variety of menstrual discomforts including cramps, water retention and mood shifts. Can usually be found in Chinese herb shops.

- *Cramp bark:* Can be taken in tincture form mixed with water and is a traditional herbal treatment for female complaints.
- *Ginger root tea:* Helps to reduce menstrual pain.
- *Squaw vine:* A natural sedative that minimizes uterine spasms.
- *Pasque flower:* Good for all pain including uterine.
- *Black haw:* An antispasmodic especially good for uterine spasms.
- *Blue cohosh:* An antispasmodic that also has a steroidal component. This herb has been used by North American Indian women for generations to relieve menstrual cramping.
- *Black cohosh:* Helps with a number of uterine disorders.
- *Raspberry leaf tea:* Helps to regulate muscle contraction in the uterus.
- *The following herbs in combination may be useful:* Cramp bark, squaw vine, false unicorn root.

PREVENTION:

- Don't become overweight. Women who are overweight suffer more from menstrual cramping.
- Exercise regularly. Women who are physically fit have a lower incidence or severity of menstrual cramps.
- Take a good vitamin and mineral supplement all month long, and prior to your period increase your intake of calcium and magnesium.

Migraine Headache

DEFINITION:

The migraine is the "granddaddy" of all headaches and can literally knock its victims off their feet. Sufferers of migraines typically become totally incapacitated by the agonizing symptoms which result from this headache phenomenon.

The word "migraine" is derived from the French and Greek and means "half a head," referring to the fact that most migraines attack one side of the head. Migraine headaches are surprisingly common and affect 15 to 20 percent of men and 25 to 30 percent of women. Migraines most frequently afflict people between the ages of 20 and 35. Seventy percent of migraine sufferers are women.

The nature of migraines can vary significantly with each individual. Migraines can last up to 18 hours. There is some speculation that unexplained recurring abdominal distress in children can be an indicator that they may be susceptible to migraines later in life.

In some individuals, migraines stop after age 40. Migraine headaches have been associated with a variety of factors. A true migraine can be a debilitating and extremely painful disorder and can significantly hamper the quality of life.

CAUSES:

Specific causes for migraine headaches remain unknown. The physical mechanism which occurs in a migraine involves a defect in the blood flow system, in which arteries become constricted and then dilate, which brings on the headache itself. Other possible contributing factors include alcohol consumption, (especially red wine), nitrates, monosodium glutamate, emotional stress, and hormonal changes common to menstruation, childbirth, and menopause. Using birth control pills has been linked with migraines in some women.

Fatigue, exhaustion, chocolate, cheese, or cured meats, barometric pressure changes, and exposure to the sun or to glare may also be connected to migraine headaches. Using nitroglycerine and the withdrawal from certain drugs such as caffeine and ergotamine may also initiate a migraine headache.

TMJ syndrome, a lack of exercise, environmental pollutants, and constipation have also been linked with the disorder. Heredity plays a significant role. More than half of people who suffer from migraines have a family history of the disease.

SYMPTOMS:

Physical: Typically, the initial stage of a migraine, called an aura, is characterized by a feeling of fatigue and in some cases, by visual disturbances such as seeing sparks, flashes or geometric shapes. This sensation may be followed by nausea and vomiting and occasionally, diarrhea. A sensitivity to light is also common at this point.

Sometime after these symptoms, an intense, gripping headache will occur. The pain commonly begins on one side of the forehead and gradually spreads, causing the entire head to throb and ache. During this stage, it is common to have bloodshot eyes, pale skin, and a runny nose or weepy eyes.

Other possible symptoms include numbness, tingling, dizziness, ear ringing and mental confusion. The length and frequency of migraines is unpredictable.

Psychological: Migraine headaches can be related to mental illness. They have also been linked to perfectionist type personalities who demand a great deal from themselves.

MEDICAL ALERT:

Any severe and persistent headache should be reported to your physician. If you are suffering from a migraine headache, do not drive or operate machinery.

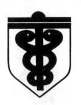

STANDARD MEDICAL TREATMENT:

Most doctors can diagnose migraines from a family history and physical examination. In some cases a full neurological examination may be required to exclude the possibility of a brain tumor.

Your doctor may advise taking aspirin plus an antiemetic drug for simple migraines. If this combination is not effective, ergotamine is usually prescribed. In a drug called Cafergot, ergoramine is combined with caffeine. The effect of this drug is to stiffen blood vessels in the brain to avoid constriction and dilation, and it can be taken in pill or suppository form when a migraine is first coming on. Propranolol (Inderal) is a drug used to treat high blood pressure which is also used for migraines. This drug can significantly decrease sex drive.

Inhalers or sublingual pills are also available and work faster. Some doctors will prescribe pain medications such as Darvon or Tylenol with codeine, which are not effective treatments for a true migraine headache. Doctors routinely prescribe fiorinal for migraines. It is often ineffective and can become addictive.

Side-effects: Ergotamine. This preparation can have some very unpleasant and powerful side-effects on the gastrointestinal system. It also has addictive properties. These potential side-effects should be discussed with your doctor.

Success rate of standard medical treatment: fair. Migraines are treated with strong drug therapy which can significantly reduce pain; however, the side-effects of these drugs must be considered. Frequently, migraines are incorrectly treated by doctors who routinely give out strong pain-killers which are not considered effective against migraines. Ergotamine is the only preparation that has shown significant success in treating true migraines.

OTHER ALTERNATIVE TREATMENTS:

◆ Chiropractic manipulation: there is some indication that while chiropractic treatments do not necessarily reduce the occurance of migraines, they may help with pain reduction during an attack.
◆ Relaxation and biofeedback: Several studies suggest that electrothermal biofeedback may reduce the frequency and severity of migraines and should be investigated.
◆ TENS (transcutaneous electrical stimulation): If TENS is appropriately administered is has been found to significantly reduce migraines and other headaches which are the result of muscle tension.
◆ Acupuncture: There is some evidence to suggest that acupuncture may reduce the frequency of migraine headaches and should be investigated as a possible treatment. After traditional acupuncture treatments, migraine victims can learn

to use acupressure to stop the onset of a migraine. It is an alternative which, unlike drugs, has no side-effects and may prove valuable.

MEDICAL UPDATE:

◆ Taking too many analgesics (painkillers) is now considered an often unrecognized cause of chronic headaches. In several cases, when barbiturates, acetaminophen and narcotics were discontinued, headaches decreased dramatically. This particular phenomenon is referred to as analgesic rebound and may contribute to aggravating migraines also.

◆ One of the newest drugs out for the treatment of migraines is sumatriptin succinate (Imitrex) and its use should be discussed with your doctor.

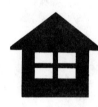

HOME SELF-CARE:

◆ Keep track of what you were doing or eating before your migraines occur to see if there is any connection with ingesting chocolate, cheese or other foods.

◆ If your migraines seem related to taking birth control pills, notify your doctor. Changing the type of oral contraceptive may eliminate the headaches.

◆ At the very first indication that a migraine is coming on, take aspirin, apply a cold compress to your face, a soft ice bag to your head and lie in a quiet dark room for 2 to 3 hours. Listen to music or try breathing exercises or visualization therapy, but do not read during this time.

◆ A rather unusual treatment for migraines which has been successful with some people is to place their heads under a bonnet type hair dryer at the first sign of a headache to the warm or hot setting. The use of heat to treat migraines has not been scientifically explained.

◆ Try getting a neck and head massage to see if this aggravates or alleviates your symptoms.

NUTRITIONAL APPROACH:

◆ There have been significant studies done which suggest that some migraines may be caused by food allergies. Foods most commonly found to induce migraine headaches in some people are all dairy products, wheat, chocolate, eggs, oranges, tomatoes, rye, and beef.

◆ Especially avoid chocolate, cheese, citrus fruits, shellfish and alcohol. These foods contain vasoactive amines such as tyramine, which can cause brain vessels to constrict and are also common food allergens. Some people who suffer from migraines are deficient in platelet enzymes which normally break down these amines. Other foods which contain these amines are avocados, bananas, cabbage, eggplant, pineapple, potato, canned fish, aged meats and yeast extracts, yogurt, canned figs, onions and peanut butter.

◆ Avoid aspartame found in NutraSweet. This particular chemical has been implicated in various studies as a migraine inducer.

◆ Do not consume MSG. This substance may trigger migraines in some people.

◆ Eating several small meals may help inhibit blood sugar swings.

◆ Nitrates and monosodium glutamate are considered migraine inducers. Check ingredients of food items, even in restaurants.

◆ *Quercetin:* This bioflavonoid is an anti-inflammatory that may help to protect against headaches caused by food sensitivities.

◆ *Vitamin C:* An antistress vitamin which also contributes to healthy blood vessels.

◆ *Niacin:* A natural vasodilator that has been traditionally used for migraine. Niacin helps to increase blood flow to the brain. Niacin is not recommended if the migraines are the cluster type.

◆ *Brewer's yeast:* Contains B complex vitamins.

◆ *Magnesium:* Magnesium is important in collagen production, which may affect blood vessel function and strength. Some studies indicate that migraine victims may be suffering from a magnesium deficiency in brain cells. Magnesium can help relax muscles.

Herbal remedies:

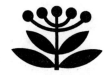

◆ Herbal therapies have been used for generations to treat migraine headaches.

◆ *Evening primrose oil:* Unsaturated fatty acids are needed for healthy brain cells and for the proper utilization of fat.

◆ *Feverfew:* Research has indicated that a number of patients who did not respond to conventional treatment for migraines found some relief by taking feverfew on a daily basis. The herb helps to decrease blood vessel response to vasoconstrictors and also helps to control the nausea associated with migraines. Do not take this herb if you are pregnant or if you show any signs of an allergic reaction.

◆ *Capsicum:* Cayenne pepper has a long history for its use in the treatment of all kinds of pain, and may also have some effect in preventing migraines.

◆ *Valerian root:* A strong natural sedative with anti-spasmodic properties.

◆ *Jamaican dogwood:* Treats pain that is linked to nervous tension.

◆ *Ginkgo:* Helps to promote proper cerebral circulation.

◆ *Lavender:* An herbal analgesic with antispasmodic properties. Can be massaged into the temples and taken internally as well. The fragrance of lavender can also promote overall relaxaton.

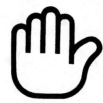

PREVENTION:

◆ Avoid any trigger factors such as culprit foods, loud, noisy environments, bright lights, etc.

◆ For patients who suffer from severe and persistent migraines, certain drugs that are thought to prevent migraine headaches may be prescribed. Some of these are high blood pressure drugs, some antidepressants, nonsteroidal anti-inflammatories, and some antihistamines. Any ongoing drug therapy has negative side-effects which should be carefully evaluated.

◆ Some doctors recommend the use of steroid drugs to help prevent migraines. This approach is not recommended. The dangers of steroids outweigh any possible benefits.

◆ Taking aspirin every other day has also been found to help cut the incidence of migraine attacks in people who are susceptible to the headaches. Always check with your physician before initiating any kind of ongoing drug therapy. Do not give aspirin to anyone under 21.

◆ Watch for analgesic rebound if routinely using painkillers such as acetaminophen.

◆ Use biofeedback techniques regularly to learn to relax muscles and even to control blood vessels. Biofeedback has been found to be especially helpful for headache sufferers.

◆ Taking regular naps, keeping fit through exercise and avoiding unhealthy foods can help reduce both the physical and mental stress associated with migraines.

◆ Take time to relax every day through yoga, massage etc. People who operate under stress and tension for prolonged periods of time and then relax may be prone to experience a migraine. Learn to relax on a regular basis.

Mononucleosis

DEFINITION:

During the 60s and 70s, mononucleosis, more commonly known as "the kissing disease," received a great deal of publicity, especially among teenage circles. Today the disease is still prevalent; however, its connection to kissing has been somewhat downplayed.

Infectious mononucleosis is an acute viral disease caused by the Epstein-Barr virus, which is believed to also cause chronic fatigue syndrome. It affects the respiratory system and the lymph glands, and can be mistaken for influenza. Approximately 90 percent of the American population has been exposed to the Epstein-Barr virus by the time they reach the age of 21.

Mononucleosis usually affects young adults and is rarely seen after the age of 35. Most cases occur between the ages of 15 and 17. The onset of the disease can be sudden or gradual and most victims recover with no complications. The illness usually lasts between one and four weeks; however, it can persist for up to 3 months.

Most victims recover without medications. Exactly how the disease spreads is not known. There is some evidence that anyone who has lowered immunity due to malnutrition, excessive fatigue, or who has had recent surgery is more vulnerable to the disease.

CAUSES:

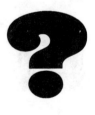

Mononucleosis is caused by the Epstein-Barr virus, a member of the herpes family that is also believed to cause chronic fatigue syndrome. Once in the body, the virus multiplies in the lymph system and causes the spread of white blood cells, which explains why victims of this disease have an elevated white cell count.

SYMPTOMS:

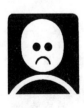

Physical: mononucleosis can cause flulike symptoms including sore throat, headache behind the eyes, fatigue, malaise, fever, muscle aches and swollen lymph glands in the neck, under the arms and in the groin area. In addition, depression, spleen enlargement, loss of appetite, a measles like rash, yellowing of the skin, and a loss of taste for cigarettes can occur with the disease.

In some cases, mild liver damage develops. If the tonsils become swollen, breathing may become obstructed. If spleen enlargement is present, precautions should be taken during any activity to protect that area of the body from injury. For months after recovering from mononucleosis, certain symptoms such as depression, lack of energy, and malaise can persist.

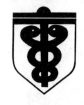

MEDICAL ALERT:

Infectious mononucleosis can be confused with acute leukemia in that the two conditions share many of the same symptoms.

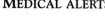

STANDARD MEDICAL TREATMENT:

Diagnosis is made by testing the blood for an increase in certain white blood cells and antibodies. Your doctor will prescribe rest for at least a month to allow the immune system to destroy the virus. In some cases, when the inflammation is severe, corticosteroid drugs may be recommended.

NOTE: Mononucleosis is a viral disease and does not respond to antibiotics. Using steroids to treat the disease should be avoided unless specific conditions persist, such as chronic fever or tonsil swelling. If ampicillin is mistakingly prescribed it may produce a rash and actually worsen symptoms.

Success rating of standard medical treatment: fair. Because mononucleosis is a viral infection, medical treatment is limited. The use of antibiotic therapy is of no value. Supportive treatments can help with complications; however, bed rest and good nutrition take precedence in most cases.

HOME SELF-CARE:

Adequate rest and good nutrition are essential in the treatment of mononucleosis. While moderate activity is now recommended, taking naps and eating properly are stressed for heightened recovery.

Be patient and realize that it takes a substantial amount of time to recover from mononucleosis. Use this time well. Read, write, learn a new language through instructional tapes and learn to relax while recuperating. Putting life on hold can have its advantages.

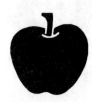

NUTRITIONAL APPROACH:

- Eating nutritous a diet cannot be overemphasized as you recover from this disease. Eat three good meals a day and take a strong vitamin and mineral supplement.
- Eat a diet especially high in raw foods such as raw almonds and raw fruits and vegetables, especially dark green, yellow or orange varieties.
- Drink plenty of vegetable and fruit juices. Vegetable broths are a good source of vitamins and minerals.

- Emphasize the following foods: citrus fruits, baked potatoes with the skin left on, vegetable broths, celery, parsley, onions, garlic, cabbage, baked squash, fish, turkey, chicken, and whole grains.
- Protein supplements that can be mixed into shakes may help to combat fatigue especially if appetite is depressed.
- Avoid foods which are considered immune system depressants such as white sugar, white flour, caffeine, and high-fat/empty-calorie junk foods.
- *High potency vitamin B complex:* Vital in building up the system during times of stress. Investigate the possibility of injections with your doctor.
- *Vitamin A and E:* Needed to build up a healthy immune system and properly oxygenate cells.
- *Calcium and magnesium:* Can help calm the system under times of stress and combat fatigue.
- *Germanium:* Boosts the functions of the immune system.
- *Vitamin C with bioflavonoids:* Considered a virus fighter which also protects the glands and the immune system.
- *Liquid chlorophyll:* Boosts the immune system.
- *Acidophilus:* Replaces friendly bacteria which help fight infection.

HERBAL REMEDIES:

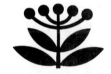

- Burdock, dandelion and chaparral help to protect the liver.
- *Echinacea:* Fights viral infection and promotes glandular function.
- *Garlic:* Recommended in fighting any viral infection. Is considered both antiviral and anti-bacterial.
- *Golden seal:* A natural infection fighter that boosts the body's defense systems.
- *Pau d'arco:* Helps to detoxify the blood and strengthen the liver.
- *Red clover:* Helps to promote a healthy lymph system, which is directly affected by the Epstein-Barr virus.
- *Ginseng:* Helps to build stamina that is typically lost with mononucleosis.

PREVENTION:

- The best way to prevent mononucleosis is to avoid getting run down by eating right, exercising and getting enough rest.
- A diet high in raw foods and low in fat and sugar has been proven to promote good health.
- Immunity can become impaired when the body is under physical and mental stress, making it easier to contract viral and bacterial infections.
- If you know someone who has this disease do not use the same eating utensils, glasses, etc. While the disease is considered contagious, it is not as easily contracted as the common cold or influenza.

Multiple Sclerosis (MS)

DEFINITION:

A diagnosis of multiple sclerosis can be devastating, not only to its victims but to family members as well. Obtaining good information helps to dispel myths which may create feelings of hopelessness concerning this disease. Much of the news about MS is encouraging, and anyone suffering from the disease should be assured that life is far from over.

MS is a progressive, degenerative disease of the central nervous system which usually affects people between the ages of 25 and 40. It is the most common acquired disease of the nervous system in young adults. The incidence of multiple sclerosis in temperate climates is approximately one in every 1000, and more women than men suffer from MS.

Multiple sclerosis can affect several areas of the nervous system by destroying the myelin sheaths, which form a protective covering for the nerves. As a result of this destruction, an inflammatory response occurs.

The severity of MS varies markedly with each individual. In some cases, the disease is characterized by mild relapses called exacerbations, followed by long symptom-free periods. Other victims of MS may experience a series of flairups which may cause some permanent disability. Even in these cases, remission periods be lengthy.

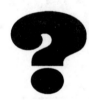

CAUSES:

The causes of MS remain unknown. Multiple sclerosis is thought to be an autoimmune disorder in which the body's immune system attacks myelin as if it were a foreign substance. There is some evidence to support that MS is more likely to occur after periods of stress or malnutrition. Once the disease is contracted and is in remission, the presence of infections, emotional stress or trauma due to an injury can help to trigger an attack. Multiple sclerosis is not hereditary, however, a genetic predisposition exists with the disease. Relatives of affected people are more likely to contract the disease. Environmental factors may also play a role. MS is five times more common in temperate zones than in tropical areas. In Japan, however, the disease is rare at any latitude.

Possible reasons for the geographic distribution of the disease include diet, sun exposure, and genetics. Mainstream medicine has been attempting to link MS with a viral cause, such as the measles virus; however, a substantial amount of research suggests that MS is not virally caused but is, rather, a disorder of the immune system. The association of diet and MS has also been investigated. A diet rich in animal fat and dairy products has been strongly linked to the incidence of MS.

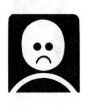

SYMPTOMS:

Physical: Symptoms can vary according to the location of the myelin sheath damage. Possible symptoms include slurred speech, staggering, a tendency to drop things, blurred vision, numbness, tingling, electrical sensations, dizziness, and nausea. In addition, breathing difficulties, weakness, tremors, bladder and bowel problems, incontinence, paralysis, sexual impotency, and paralysis can also occur.

Some victims of MS experience serious debilitating symptoms within the first year. Others may become gradually disabled. Additional problems that victims of MS may have to deal with include painful muscle spasms, urinary tract infections, constipation, skin ulcers, and mood swings which can range from euphoria to depression. Only a limited number of people are crippled by MS.

Psychological: If you have been diagnosed with MS, it is vital realize that a positive attitude toward the disease is invaluable. MS can be a very manageable disorder, and anyone who approaches the condition with a negative or fatalistic attitude which stresses its "incurability" should be avoided. Educating yourself and your family concerning this disease is essential. Even after a particularly severe exacerbation, recovery can be dramatic. Victims of MS can lead productive lives with minimal limitation.

STANDARD MEDICAL TREATMENT:

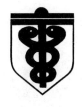

There is no single diagnostic test to confirm the presence of multiple sclerosis. When symptoms of MS are present, your doctor will probably order a spinal tap, along with CT scanning, brain wave tests and an MRI. Corticosteroid drugs such as prednisone may be prescribed to alleviate acute symptoms during an attack.

ACTH and cyclophosphamide may also be recommended by your physician to suppress immune reactions. Muscle relaxants may be prescribed for muscular stiffness or pain and occasionally surgery to relive spasms may be advised. In some cases, antidepressants may be recommended. Physical therapy will be suggested to help strengthen muscles and promote mobility.

Success rating of standard medical treatment: poor to fair. Once a diagnosis is made, medical science has little to offer victims of this disease. Unfortunately, some medical physicians approach the disease with an attitude of hopelessness. Using corticosteroids can provide some symptomatic relief; however, the side-effects of these drugs are significant. A great deal of research promises the emergence of medications which may dramatically improve the prognosis of the disease.

MEDICAL UPDATE:

In some studies, x-ray irradiation of the lymph glands and spleen has halted the progress of MS in a significant percentage of patients treated. However, radiation therapy can depress the immune system and increase susceptibility to infection. Discuss this treatment with your physician.

◆ Some experimentation has been done with a drug called Copolymer 1 in the prevention of MS attacks. Contact the Albert Einstein College of Medicine for further information on this treatment.

◆ The use of spinal injections of human fibroblast interferon is also under current investigation.

◆ The value of acupuncture, acupressure and chiropractic adjustments should be investigated for their potential in helping to control pain and promote mobility.

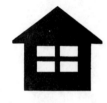

HOME SELF-CARE:

◆ Regular exercise is recommended; however, avoid overexertion and fatigue. Swimming is particularly beneficial. Exercises which can significantly increase body temperature are discouraged.

◆ Avoid extremely hot baths, hot tubs, and hot showers. Abrupt rises in temperature have been associated with triggering MS attacks.

◆ Regular massage is excellent for relieving pain and improving muscle tone.

◆ Portable electrostimulator units have been used with some success in controlling pain and increasing mobility. These can be obtained through a physician or physical therapist. Acupuncturists also use these units.

◆ If you are under a physician who has a negative attitude and makes you feel depressed, change doctors.

◆ Avoid emotional stress. Take time every day to relax. Breathing exercises can be quite valuable. Other meditative techniques including music therapy, hypnotherapy, and visualization can help counteract tension.

◆ Be wary of practitioners who claim to have a cure for multiple sclerosis.

NUTRITIONAL APPROACH:

Japan has an unusually low rate of MS even in its temperate zones. Investigations of the Japanese diet reveal that the consumption of marine foods, seeds and fruit oil is high. These foods contain abundant polyunsaturated fatty acids, including omega-3 oils. As a result, there is some speculation that a deficiency of omega-3 oils may interfere with the proper formation of myelin. Victims of MS appear to suffer from a defect in their ability to absorb fatty acids. Eating saturated fats further aggravates that deficiency. There is no question that the role of diet and nutrition in the treatment and prevention of MS is significant.

- Eat a diet low in saturated fats. Several studies support that fact that avoiding saturated fats for a prolonged period of time can retard the process of this disease and reduce the number of attacks.
- Do not eat over 10 grams of saturated fat per day, and eat 40 grams of polyunsaturated oils per day. Oils that can be used sparingly are extra virgin olive oil, canola oil, safflower and sunflower oils.
- Do not eat margarine, shortening, or hydrogenated oils.
- Take 1 tsp. of cod liver oil daily. Taking black current oil on a regular basis is also recommended. Evening primrose oil is also beneficial.
- Consume fish abundantly. Fish provides an excellent source of omega-3 oils. These oils are essential to normal nerve cell function and myelin sheathe production. Sardines are also a good source of omega-3 oils.
- Eat plenty of legumes, grains, vegetables and fruits.
- Increase the fiber content of your diet to avoid becoming constipated. Taking acidophilus culture and psyllium is recommended.
- Drink plenty of fresh vegetable and fruit juices. A mixture of carrot and green pepper is highly recommended.
- Avoid: sugar, coffee, chocolate, salt, dairy products, meat, highly seasoned foods, processed foods, caffeine, alcohol, nicotine and saturated fats.
- *Linoleic acid:* Sunflower seed, safflower and soy oil contain linoleic acid and may help protect the nerves against inflammation.
- *Pantothenic acid:* Helps to protect the myelin sheath.
- *Flaxseed oil:* Contains both linoleic acid and alpha-linolenic acid, which are readily incorporated into brain lipids and thought to help normalize immune function.
- *Selenium and vitamin E:* Both of these supplements contribute to better lipid assimilation.
- *Vitamin B complex:* Essential for tissue repair and the proper functioning of the immune system. A vitamin B deficiency can result in further nerve damage.
- *Coenzyme Q10:* Helps provide oxygen to tissues and cells.
- *Calcium/magnesium:* Essential to prevent muscle cramping and nervous disorders.
- *Magnesium:* A magnesium deficiency can produce MS-like symptoms.

Herbal remedies:

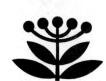

- *Hops:* Considered a tonic for the nerves and a natural tranquilizer.
- *Lady's slipper:* Works to promote the proper function of brain and nerve cells.
- *Lobelia:* Helps to calm and soothe the nerves and helps with sleep difficulties.
- *Saffron:* Helps with the normal digestion of fats.
- *Safflower:* Contains linoleic acid, which helps with the assimilation of fats.
- *Skullcap and valerian:* Considered nervines, which calm the nerves.

PREVENTION:

◆   Avoiding a diet high in animal fats may help to prevent a susceptibility to the disease, although there is no scientific evidence to support this.

Muscle Aches (fibromyalgia)

DEFINITION:

Most people have never heard of the term "fibromyalgia" and unfortunately, even some physicians are not familiar with the disorder. If you have suffered the unexplained muscle aches that are typical of the disease, you may have gone from doctor to doctor looking for answers.

Fibromyalgia is one of the most common disorders seen by rheumatologists, and yet it is probably one of the least familiar and understood conditions. Victims of this disorder, who are mainly women, are often unaware that they are suffering from a specific ailment. Fibromyalgia belongs to a family of disorders that are characterized by an overreaction to what is considered a normal stimulus. Some of these also include insomnia, irritable bowel syndrome, and migraine headaches.

Not too long ago, this particular disorder was considered to be a psychosomatic illness, which was particularly troubling to its victims. Fibromyalgia is another in a long line of disorders that is considered to be a by-product of Western life-style and is rarely seen in underdeveloped countries.

CAUSES:

While the specific causes of this disorder are unknown, EEG tests showed that victims of fibromyalgia had a specific type of disruption in their brain wave patterns while they were asleep. The meaning of this brain wave abnormality as it relates to the disease remains inconclusive. Other possible causes include tension, viral infections, trauma, unusual exertion, nutritional deficiencies, and in rare instances thyroid disease.

SYMPTOMS:

Physical: Fibromyalgia typically causes stiff or sore shoulders, hip, neck or back muscles, inability to sleep well or non-restful sleep, persistent fatigue, and tenderness in the elbows and knees. Fibromyalgia can be very bothersome and create in its victims a feeling of discouragement and frustration. Frequently victims of this disorder assume they must have some form of arthritis.

Psychological: Unless you find a physician who is familiar with this disorder, your symptoms may be considered psychosomatic. If you feel you are suffering from this ailment and it has not been recognized by your doctor, bring it to his or her attention.

MEDICAL ALERT:

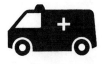

If persistent muscle pain is accompanied by fever or weight loss, see your physician.

STANDARD MEDICAL TREATMENT:

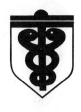

If the disease is recognized and diagnosed correctly, the best medical therapy appears to focus on exercise and the use of antidepressants. For reasons not totally understood, low-level doses of antidepressants such as amitriptyline (Endep, Elavil) and imipramine (Tofranil, Janimine) are effective in treating the sleep disturbances that accompany fibromyalgia. The use of these drugs should be discussed with your physician. Oral corticosteriods should not be used for this condition.

It is interesting to know that doctors often disagree on what exactly to call this disorder. It may be referred to as psychogenic rheumatism, fibrositis, non-articular rheumatism, or chronic muscle-contraction syndrome. If you suspect you have this disorder, see a rheumatologist who will be more familiar with effective treatment.

Side-effects: Amitriptyline (Elavil, Endep) and imipramine (Tofranil, Janimine): Blood pressure changes, abnormal heart rates, heart attack, confusion, hallucinations, disorientation, delusions, anxiety, restlessness, excitement, numbness, tingling in the extremities, lack of coordination, muscle spasms or tremors, seizures, dry mouth, blurred vision, and constipation are just a few of the known side-effects of this drug.

Warning: Do not take this drug if pregnant or nursing. Amitriptyline may cause birth defects and passes through breast milk.

Success rating of standard medical treatment: very poor. Unfortunately, this disorder is easily misdiagnosed. As a result, doctors will routinely prescribe anti-inflammatory drugs such as Naprosyn and Motrin, which do not effectively treat muscular ailments resulting from spasms rather than inflammation. Frequently, tranquilizers and sleeping pills will be prescribed which further diminish the quality of sleep and can make things worse. On the whole, medical treatment is not particularly helpful to victims of this disorder.

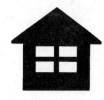

HOME SELF-CARE:

Regular low-impact exercise can go a long way to strengthen muscle tone and discourage the spasms which create the aches. Walking, low-impact aerobics, swimming, etc. are all recommended. Regular exercise also helps to promote better sleep. Make sure to warm up and stretch before beginning any exercise. Taking a hot shower or bath before exercising has been suggested by some professionals.

Have a professional massage on a regular basis. The regular manipulation of muscle groups can help alleviate pain and improve tone. Massaging muscles can also help remove the lactic acid which causes muscles to feel sore after exercising.

Acupressure and acupuncture should be investigated. Often, with these types of disorders, these methods of treatment can offer pain relief; however, it is usually only temporary.

Stretching exercises characteristic of yoga are recommended for their pain relieving results. Yoga can also promote overall relaxation, which can promote better sleeping. Stretching all muscle groups while lying in bed is a great way to relax before sleeping and upon rising.

◆ Chiropractic manipulations may offer some relief.

◆ Physical therapy, including electrical muscle stimulation, should also be investigated for it potential benefits.

◆ Use the hot tub, whirlpool or bathtub to discourage muscle spasms. Moist heat is recommended for most muscle spasms.

◆ Sleep in roomy pajamas and do not weigh your body down with heavy blankets.

◆ Use padded shoe soles if you have to stand for long periods of time.

◆ If you must sit at a desk while working, make sure your chair offers the proper back support.

◆ If this problem seems to significantly improve while on vacation, stress and tension may be significant causal factors and should be addressed.

NUTRITIONAL APPROACH:

◆ Avoid red meats, fatty foods and acidic foods such as tomatoes and vinegar. Acidic foods can interfere with the body's absorption of calcium, which can cause muscle spasms.

◆ Drink plenty of fluids, especially freshly squeezed vegetable and fruit juices. Carrot juice is highly recommended.

◆ Eat plenty of green leafy vegetables. Kelp and chlorophyll supplements are also recommended.

◆ *Calcium/magnesium:* Very important for proper muscle contraction and nerve function and should be taken as a supplement daily. A calcium deficiency can actually cause muscle cramping. Good sources of dietary calcium are yogurt, skim milk, and low-fat cheeses. In the case of fibromyalgia, calcium/magnesium supplements may be more effective. Magnesium increases the body's absorption of calcium. Taking a calcium/magnesium supplement at bedtime may help reduce pain and promote sleep.

◆ *Potassium:* Vital to proper muscle functioning and, like calcium, can cause muscle pain if levels get too low. Potatoes, bananas, dried peaches and prunes are good natural sources of potassium. If you exert your muscles routinely, take a potassium supplement.

◆ *Silicon:* Also helps promote calcium absorption.

◆ *Vitamin E:* Improves overall circulation. A deficiency of vitamin E has been linked to muscular aches and cramping.

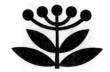

HERBAL REMEDIES:

◆ *Passion flower:* An antispasmodic that also helps to induce sleep.

◆ *Wild yam:* Useful in that it helps relax muscle fiber.

◆ *Peppermint tea:* Helps to control muscle spasms.

◆ *Blue cohosh:* An antispasmodic which contains calcium, magnesium and potassium.

◆ Crampbark, mistletoe and lady's slipper are all considered natural muscle relaxants.

◆ *Skullcap:* An antispasmodic and natural sleep inducer.

◆ *Chaparral:* Works to help alleviate leg cramps.

◆ *The following herbs in combination may be useful:* Valerian root, lobelia, skullcap, and myrrh gum.

PREVENTION:

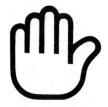

◆ This is one of several disorders in which specific causal factors remain unknown.

◆ Keeping fit through regular exercise and eating a diet high in calcium and magnesium is recommended. In addition, staying at an ideal weight puts less strain on muscle groups.

◆ Employing a daily relaxation regimen can also keep muscles from tensing up and causing stress-induced pain.

Nicotine Dependency

DEFINITION:

Kicking the nicotine habit is an extremely difficult thing to accomplish, and yet it is done by thousands of people yearly who refuse to write their own death sentences. Nicotine, which is the main substance in cigarettes, is considered as addictive as heroine. Like any other addictive substance, the feeling of well-being and satisfaction created by nicotine requires a larger and larger dose to maintain. A truly nicotine-dependant person may require a cigarette every half hour in order to feel good.

Nicotine causes the brain to release catecholamines and stimulate adrenalin release. As a result, heart rate and blood pressure rise, creating a lift for the smoker. Withdrawing what has been a continuous supply of nicotine from the body can cause significant physical and emotional distress. While giving up cigarettes is not easy, it is unquestionably worth it. Withdrawal symptoms are temporary and every tobacco user, no matter how addicted, can stop smoking.

SYMPTOMS OF NICOTINE WITHDRAWAL:

Nicotine withdrawal causes irritability, anxiety, confusion, insomnia, nausea, headache, constipation or diarrhea, a decrease in blood pressure and heart rate, fatigue, drowsiness and the inability to sleep. Withdrawal symptoms are usually intense for the first two weeks after giving up smoking and commonly require support in order to stem a reversal.

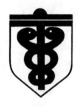

STANDARD MEDICAL TREATMENT:

In addition to behavioral intervention programs, your doctor may choose to prescribe nicotine gum, which must be chewed infrequently and not be allowed to touch any mucous membranes within the mouth. This treatment slowly weans the tobacco-addicted person off smoking. A nicotine patch is also available which releases small amounts of nicotine into the body. Your doctor may also recommend clonidine therapy which involves using a high blood pressure drug to help to block the symptoms of nicotine withdrawal.

Side-effects: Nicotine gum: Nausea, jaw irritation, and heartburn.

Side-effects: Clonidine (Catapres): Dry mouth, drowsiness, sedation, constipation, dizziness, headache, and fatigue.

Warning: This drug should not be taken by pregnant women or nursing mothers.

Success rating of standard medical treatment: Most treatments have varying levels of success. Nicotine gum has worked well for some people and not at all for others. Of the 2 million Americans who quit smoking each year, 95 percent do it without medical intervention.

MEDICAL UPDATE:

◆ A new mouth spray which, produces an unpleasant taste when mixed with tobacco smoke may be helpful for some people who are trying to quit. The spray consists of silver acetate, and its success depends on the willingness of the person who smokes to use it frequently.

◆ Three new reports conclude that nicotine replacement products such as nicotine gum and the nicotine patch do contribute to helping smokers abstain. According to investigations at the Radcliff Infirmary in Oxford, for some people, using these aids can significantly raise their chances of success in becoming tobacco-free.

HEALTH BENEFITS OF QUITTING:

◆ Smokers who quit and stay nicotine free for 10 to 15 years can dramatically decrease their risk of a shortened life expectancy.

◆ The risk of getting cancer of the lungs, larynx and mouth becomes close to that of non-smokers after 15 years of a smoke-free environment.

◆ After seven years of not smoking, the risk for bladder cancer decreases to that of a non-smoker.

◆ Immediate benefits include decreasing the risk of coronary and heart disease, an immediate improvement in breathing and a decline in the rate of lung deterioration.

◆ Other benefits are improved stamina, no morning cough, fresher breath, better environment for your family and more money in your pocket.

HOME SELF-CARE:

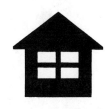

◆ Plan your strategy, talk to someone who has succeeded and follow their advice.

◆ Get rid of anything that is smoking-related from your environment, both at work and at home.

◆ Keep a supply of hard candy and gum available to help stifle cigarette cravings.

◆ Increase your exercise routine while withdrawing from nicotine. Plan to go the spa everyday or meet someone for jogging. Every time you get the urge to light up, take a walk.

◆ The urge to smoke usually lasts only three to five minutes. Wait it out and it will get easier to go without a cigarette.

◆ Drink a glass of water to which you have added 2 tablespoons of bicarbonate of soda if you are not on a sodium-restricted diet.

◆ Reduce or eliminate caffeine and alcohol consumption. The effects of both of these substances intensify when you stop smoking.

◆ Hypnosis has been shown to be quite effective in helping motivate individuals to succeed in their attempts to quit smoking. This approach usually includes self-hypnosis and interpersonal support. The success of this option relies on the hypnotizability of the individual, which can be assesses by a qualified hypnotherapist.

◆ Other support strategies that not only help in quitting the habit, but also in staying nicotine-free include social support intervention groups, buddy systems, and telephone networks etc.

◆ Make a personal list of your reasons for quitting and if you are tempted to light up, consult the list.

◆ Calculate what you have spent on cigarettes over the last five to ten years.

◆ If you feel you cannot go cold turkey, then give yourself so many cigarettes per day and only smoke them halfway down. Decrease the number of cigarettes gradually until you have completely stopped.
    NOTE: The majority of those who quit smoking say that going cold turkey is better and more effective than gradually cutting down.

◆ Acupuncture and controlled breathing exercises are of value in helping to reduce withdrawal symptoms.

NUTRITIONAL APPROACH:

◆ Stock your pantry and refrigerator with a large assortment of low-calorie snacks such as fresh veggies, cut-up fruit, low calorie crackers and cheese, yogurt, pretzels, etc. Smoking dulls and the appetite; consequently, many people experience a new hunger for food. Don't worry about possible weight gain at this time. What is vital is to stop a potentially life-threatening habit and then go on to issues like weight.

◆ Drink plenty of fluids to facilitate nicotine removal from the body. Fresh fruit juices and carrot juice in particular are recommended.

◆ *Vitamin B complex plus added B12:* Important when the body is under stress. Helps the liver to detoxify the system of nicotine.

◆ *Calcium/magnesium:* Works to calm the central nervous system and can help to control the tremors that often accompany any drug withdrawal.

◆ *GABA:* Can help to decrease nicotine cravings and also acts as a relaxant.

◆ *L-glutathione:* An amino acid that helps the body detoxify poisons like nicotine.

◆ Take a good protein supplement to fortify the body and build stamina during the withdrawal process.

◆ *Vitamin C:* Helps to detoxify tissues and can also work to decrease cravings.

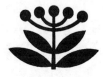

HERBAL REMEDIES:

◆ *Barley juice powder:* Take as a supplement while in withdrawal. Barley juice helps to cleanse the cells and can help to neutralize the toxic effects of nicotine as it leaves the body.

◆ *Catnip:* Calms the stomach and soothes the nerves. This herb can help to counteract many symptoms that are associated with nicotine withdrawal.
◆ *Siberian ginseng:* Has been used to help combat cocaine-withdrawal symptoms.
◆ Burdock and echinacea help purify the blood of nicotine.
◆ *Skullcap, lobelia and vervain:* Help to calm the jittery nerves and restlessness that can accompany nicotine withdrawal.
◆ Some herbal combinations which contain lobelia are specifically designed to help control the symptoms of nicotine withdrawal.

PREVENTION:

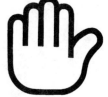

◆ Don't start smoking.

American Cancer Society
7-Day Quitter's Guide
1599 Clifton Road NE
Atlanta, Georgia 30329

Nosebleeds

DEFINITION:

Nosebleeds are notorious for interrupting a romantic dinner conversation, complicating a visit to the theater or just causing general embarrassment. They usually create a social predicament regardless of when or where they choose to inconveniently occur. A nosebleed is a common occurrence experienced by almost everyone at one time or another.

In the vast majority of cases, nosebleeds are not serious and are easily taken care of. Most nosebleeds originate from the front part of the nose. The nasal membranes of the nose are full of blood vessels which are susceptible to damage and can easily burst.

On rare occasions, more serious nosebleeds can occur from the posterior or back of the nose, which causes the flow of blood to run down the back of the throat. This type of nosebleed usually requires medical attention because it is more difficult to control. Elderly people who suffer from high blood pressure may be more prone to posterior nosebleeds.

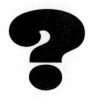

CAUSES:

Nosebleeds can be caused by a blow to the nose or other trauma; lack of humidity which causes nasal membranes to crack, crust over and bleed; blowing the nose too hard; viral irritation; a sudden change in atmospheric pressure; allergic rhinitis; and picking the nose.

More serious causes of nosebleeds can be high blood pressure, hemophilia, thrombocytopenia, alcoholism, a tumor, heart disease, kidney disease, skull fracture or leukemia. Certain drugs, especially blood thinners such as Coumadin, Heparin or aspirin may also cause nosebleeds.

Oral contraceptives may also increase the risk for nosebleeds. Nosebleeds can often follow upper respiratory infections, especially in children. The presence of a fever can dry out nasal membranes, which can make them more susceptible to nosebleeds.

NOTE: There is some question among physicians whether high blood pressure causes nosebleeds. The general consensus is that if you suffer from high blood pressure and are experiencing nosebleeds, have your blood pressure checked.

Attention: Taking oral contraceptives can change the production of mucus in the body and may initiate nosebleeds. If you have a problem with nosebleeds, tell your doctor before taking oral contraceptives.

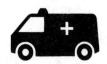

MEDICAL ALERT:

If nosebleeds occur frequently or are unusually hard to control, see your physician. If you are experiencing a nosebleed than cannot be stopped by following the instructions below and you can feel blood running down the back of your throat, see a physician immediately.

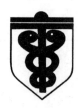

STANDARD MEDICAL TREATMENT:

For difficult nosebleeds, packing the nose with petroleum jelly and gauze may be required. Postnasal packing is sometimes required for posterior nosebleeds and is rather uncomfortable. Nose packing with gauze has its drawbacks and should be avoided if possible.

Your physician may also choose to cauterize the site of the bleeding with electrocautery or silver nitrate. If nosebleeds keep occurring, a physical examination will be done and blood-clotting tests may be ordered. Checking to see if anemia has resulted from recurring nosebleeds may also be done through a blood test.

HOME SELF-CARE:

The simplest method of controlling a nosebleed is to blow your nose and then grasp and pinch the fleshy part of the nose for 5 minutes in order to promote clotting. Stay in a sitting position to discourage the flow of blood down the back of the throat. Almost all nosebleeds can be controlled this way if the nose is pinched long enough.

◆ Ice packs may also be applied to the bridge of the nose, neck and cheek area.
◆ If the nose continues to bleed after being pinched for 5 minutes, cover a piece of gauze with petroleum jelly, insert into the nose and pinch again for 10 minutes.
◆ Soaking a piece of gauze with witch hazel and placing in the nose is also recommended. Using a cotton ball soaked with white vinegar can have the same mild cauterizing effect.
◆ After the nosebleed has stopped, rest briefly and do not blow your nose for the next couple of days.

NUTRITIONAL APPROACH:

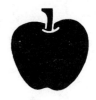

◆ Avoid alcohol: Alcohol dilates blood vessels and because the mucous membranes of the nose have relatively large vessels which are exposed to injury, spontaneous bleeding can easily occur.
◆ If you are prone to frequent nosebleeds avoid ingesting substances that contain salicylate such as coffee, tea, almonds, apples, apricots, berries, green peppers, tomatoes, peaches, plums, cucumbers and pickles.
◆ *Vitamin K:* Vital to the normal clotting of blood and can be found in green leafy vegetables such as kale, spinach etc.
◆ *Vitamin C and B complex:* Necessary for the formation of collagen and the maintenance of mucous membranes. Vitamin C also strengthens the capillary walls of the nasal passages.
◆ *Calcium:* Helps to tone fragile capillaries.
◆ *Iron:* Helps to replace the body's blood supply and is especially important if you have recurring nosebleeds.
◆ *Liquid chlorophyll:* Helps to build up hemoglobin in blood cells.

HERBAL REMEDIES:

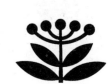

◆ Aloe vera ointment or gel can be placed in the nose to help alleviate dryness.
◆ *Comfrey:* Can also be used as an ointment to lubricate the nose.
◆ *Yarrow:* Encourages clotting and can be taken in capsule form.
◆ *Amaranth:* High in iron and vitamin C, it helps to control excessive bleeding.
◆ *Horsetail:* Helps to promote blood coagulation.
◆ *Cayenne and golden seal:* Taken internally, these herbs help to stop excessive bleeding and promote clotting.

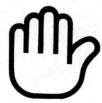

PREVENTION:

- Use a humidifier if air is dry and lack humidity.
- Keep your house cool at night. During the winter months, running the heater all night may have a very drying effect on the nasal membranes.
- Keep fingernails short on children to prevent internal nose injury.
- Use a saline spray regularly to keep your nasal passages moist. Saline spray can be made by adding 1 teaspoon of table salt to 1 pint of water.
- Aspirin can increase bleeding and should not be given to children.
- Blow your nose gently.
- Don't smoke: Smoking drys out the nasal membranes.
- Eat a diet high in vitamin K, vitamin C and calcium.

Obesity

DEFINITION:

Being on a diet has become an American way of life. Oddly enough, no matter how ineffective most weight loss schemes are, the latest diet fad has us all running to the bookstore to get a firsthand look. Today, we know better than ever before the truth about obesity and weight loss. Unfortunately, that doesn't mean that we won't continue to fall prey to get-thin-quick diets that can end up making us fatter than we were when we started. There is no denying that obesity is a serious problem in this country; however, it must be confronted with sound and effective strategies.

Technically, obesity refers to a weight condition which is defined as being 20 percent over the prescribed weight for a particular age, build or height. Estimates assessing the extent of obesity in the United States range from 10 percent to 50 percent of the overall population. The number of obese children in Western countries has dramatically increased, nearly doubling between the years of 1965 and 1980. One in every four American children is overweight. One in every five men and almost one in every three women is considered obese.

Simply stated, obesity is an excessive amount of body fat. It is important to remember that weight alone can be a poor indicator of whether you are obese or not. Building muscles adds weight to the body but it does not contribute to obesity.

Obesity is a complex and frustrating problem which involves more than just overeating. Factors which can influence obesity are genetics, cultural background, physical characteristics and social or economic status.

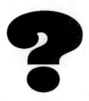

CAUSES:

Overeating and lack of exercise are considered the most common causes of obesity. A diet that is low in fiber and high in refined carbohydrates and fat is believed to be one of the major factors responsible for the high rates of obesity found in Western cultures. Other possible causes are glandular malfunctions, genetic predisposition or defect, emotional relationship with eating, malnutrition, and boredom.

Complications of obesity: Obesity increases the risk for kidney disease, heart trouble, stroke, gall bladder disease, certain types of cancer, hemorrhoids, varicose veins, diabetes, high blood pressure, problems in pregnancy, liver damage and psychological disorders.

SYMPTOMS:

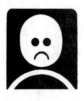

Physical: The most obvious sign of obesity is an increase in body weight due to a rise in the fat percentage of total mass. Other symptoms of obesity are increased foot problems, back problems, reduced physical endurance, labored breathing, and sleep difficulties (especially sleep apnea).

Psychological: Obesity carries with it a significant societal stigma. Discrimination is routinely experienced by obese individuals. As a result, these people often adopt self-defeating and self-degrading attitudes such as low self-esteem and depression; consequently, overeating may occur.

Counseling can afford the obese person an opportunity to change attitudes and improve self-esteem. Initial counseling prior to any weight-loss program has been found to increase the rate of success.

STANDARD MEDICAL TREATMENT:

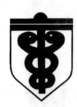

Obesity is extremely difficult to successfully treat. Most physicians will suggest a diet that will usually lower caloric intake to 1,500 calories per day combined with 15 to 20 minutes of aerobic exercise for at least three to four times weekly. Gradual weight loss is recommended (1/2 pound to 1 pound per week). Diets are usually designed to take advantage of all five food groups recommended for overall good health.

Antiobesity drugs such as nonamphetamine appetite suppressants are prescribed by some physicians; however, their use is discouraged due to their negative side-effects. Drugs which are designed to increase the body's energy requirements are currently being tested.

Wiring the teeth together to prohibit eating is another possible medical treatment for obesity. The treatment is uncomfortable and while it may produce results, weight loss is usually temporary and has nothing to do with modifying poor eating habits. In addition, wiring the jaw may promote tooth decay and mouth infections.

Warning: The drug dimitrophinol which is prescribed by some physicians for weight loss may cause cataracts.

Side-effects: Many non-amphetamine appetite suppressant drugs have similar side effects as amphetamines which include nervousness, restlessness, sleeplessness, palpitations, high blood pressure, drowsiness, dizziness, headache, tremors and over stimulation.

Surgical options:

Liposuction: Involves an incision through which a tube is placed which makes it possible to suck out fat cells. The procedure is extremely traumatic to surrounding tissue and causes a considerable amount of bruising and pain. The possibility of developing a blood clot exists from this procedure, which could be potentially life-threatening.

Colectomy: This type of bypass surgery reduces the area of intestine through which food can be absorbed. It can also decrease appetite. This is considered a major surgical procedure and carries with it the risk of serious complications or death. The proper assimilation of vitamins and minerals is also impaired. The use of this surgery has declined due to its adverse effects.

Stomach stapling: Reduces the size of the stomach therefore limiting the amount of food which can be ingested at one time. This also is a major surgical procedure which carries with it serious complications or the risk of death. In several instances, the staples do not hold and the surgery has to be repeated. Eating disturbances such as involuntary regurgitation can result from this procedure.

NOTE: A high percentage of people who use drastic surgical procedures to lose weight eventually gain it back.

Success rate of standard medical procedure: very poor. Traditional medical treatment of obesity has proved to be rather frustrating for both patient and doctor. Using drugs or drastic surgical procedures has a poor success rate and comes with a number of negative side-effects.

MEDICAL UPDATE:

Experts at the University of Florida have concluded through their research that people who are extremely obese may be victims of the Prader-Willi syndrome which is caused by a defective gene which causes them to store fat abnormally. These people have to reduce food intake to below normal levels just to maintain their weight.

A 12 week study in Rome has recently studied the effects of an experimental appetite suppressant for obese individuals that shows promise. Oral hydroxytryptophan (5-HTP) was administered without any dietary restriction and weight loss averaged 4 pounds per week. The drug is a serotonin precursor and inhibits the desire to eat.

Anti-depressant drugs such as Prozac are also being investigated for their possible role in weight loss.

HOME SELF-CARE:

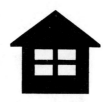

Traditionally it has been accepted that in order to lose weight, you must help your body use up more calories than you consume, or you must create an energy deficit. Recently, there has been more emphasis placed on counting fat grams rather than calories, implying that the type of calories we consume may be more important than the actual number. In any case, the role of regular exercise cannot be overly stressed. Exercising not only burns calories but can suppress the appetite and increase the overall metabolic rate of the body. This means that if you participate in regular aerobic exercise every day, you can get away with eating more without weight gain.

Exercise regularly. Exercise is considered by far the best method to control weight. Begin slowly. Take a 10-to 15-minute walk every day and then slowly increase your distance and your pace. Light exercise right after eating is recommended and can help to burn calories that have just been consumed. Don't make the mistake of overexerting yourself, which usually results in giving up the entire practice. You've got plenty of time. Build up your stamina and endurance slowly.

◆ Don't become constipated. Drink 6 to 8 glasses of water per day.

◆ Don't chew gum: Chewing gum can activate the flow of gastric juices and make you feel like eating.

◆ Eat only when you are truly hungry. Often thirst can be mistaken for hunger. Drink when you feel the urge to eat.

◆ Avoid the following bad habits:

• Eating when you are anxious, bored or frustrated. Find something else to do when you feel inclined to eat under these circumstances.

• Eating while reading or watching TV. As fun as this might be, it promotes inactivity and weight gain. If you have to eat during these activities, munch on raw veggies. Television watching, video games, etc. have greatly decreased the amount of physical activity children pursue. These sedentary activities have been strongly linked to obesity.

• Nibbling after the meal is over. Mothers are particularly susceptible to this. While they may eat sensibly during the meal, picking at leftovers while putting dishes away can significantly contribute to weight gain.

• Don't use food as a reward.

◆ Keep all high-calorie foods on high shelves or on the back shelves of the refrigerator and low calorie foods easily accessible.

◆ Eating too fast or improper chewing can also result in the consumption of more calories during a certain period of time. Eating a diet that is high in fiber can automatically increase chewing time and slow the eating process. People who eat too fast often become hungry again soon after eating. Listen to calm, soothing music while you eat and chew slowly.

◆ Don't eat when you are depressed, lonely or angry.

◆ Avoid fad diets, which can make your body feel as if it's starving and actually lower your metabolism, which slows the burning of fat stores.

◆ Do not use diuretics or laxatives to induce weight loss. These can be potentially hazardous to your health and result in temporary weight loss only.

◆ Join a support group like Weight Watchers which takes a sensible and healthful approach to losing weight. Be wary of diet organizations that are costly or limit you to their own foods.

◆ Be patient. More permanent results will be obtained if weight loss is gradual. Remember that it takes time for the body to readjust to its new programmed weight set point.

NUTRITIONAL APPROACH:

Research supports the fact that the amount of calories consumed is not as important as what those calories are made of. Eating a diet that is high in fiber, complex carbohydrates, fresh vegetables, and fruits and low in fat is the winning combination. In addition, raising your caloric intake of non-fatty foods seems to enhance weight loss. Cultures that routinely eat high-fiber diets have a very low incidence of obesity and they probably don't count calories. High-fiber diets improve the excretion of fat in the feces, improve glucose tolerance, and provide a feeling of satisfaction and fullness. In addition, studies support that if we eat a diet that is nutritious we do not experience food cravings, which can result in overeating the wrong things.

Some studies indicate that when there is an inadequate intake of essential nutrients, fat is not burned efficiently, which may contribute to obesity.

Sugar in the form of soda pop, candy, cookies, cakes, ice cream and pastries is responsible for much of childhood obesity. Salted snack foods such as potato chips and corn chips are as much as 40 percent fat. Making these foods unavailable to family members can go a long way to fight obesity. Note: Many breakfast cereals are up to 60 percent sugar.

EMPHASIZE THE FOLLOWING FOODS:

Lentils, beans, plain baked potatoes, baked squash, brown rice, whole grain breads (low fat or no fat), white fish, white chicken, skim milk, low- or no-fat cottage cheese, no-fat yogurt, and turkey, fresh fruits and vegetables. Restrict your intake of the following: avocados, figs, bananas, white rice, sweet potatoes, coconut and corn. Beans are especially beneficial to anyone trying to shed a few pounds. You can buy precooked beans in cans that have no additives. Beans are tasty and satisfying and provide an excellent source of fiber.

Avoid the following foods: cheese, sour cream, ice cream, butter, whole milk, rich dressings, soda pop, mayonnaise, fried foods, red meats, gravies, custards, pastries, cakes, peanut butter, and junk foods.

Do not eat too little. At least 1,200 calories per day are critical for the maintenance of good health and the promotion of permanent weight loss. In addition, all diets should contain some percentage of fat, which can be ingested in the form of olive, evening primrose or safflower oil. Supplementing your diet with 1 to 2 teaspoons per day of these oils is thought to actually improve the body's ability to burn fat.

◆ Do not consume alcohol: All alcoholic beverages are high in calories.
◆ Fiber supplements can be taken in the form of guar gum or glucomannan.
◆ Avoid artificial sweeteners. There is some evidence that artificial sweeteners can actually increase appetite and result in weight gain.
◆ Barley malt sweetener can be used instead of sugar.
◆ Omit all substances which are thought to be appetite stimulants such as salt, hot spices, coffee, tea, tobacco and sugar.
◆ Avoid any fad diets that are designed around a high protein, low carbohydrate regimen. This combination, if eaten over a long period of time, poses some significant health hazards.
◆ *Glucomannan:* Helps to control blood sugar fluctuations.
◆ *Primrose oil:* Supplies essential fatty acids.
◆ *Lecithin:* Helps to emulsify and break down fat stores.
◆ *Vitamin E:* Plays a role in the metabolism of fat.
◆ *Vitamin B complex:* Helps control the appetite
◆ *Chromium picolinate:* Helps regulate blood sugar, which can influence appetite.
◆ *L-methionine:* An amino acid which can act as an appetite suppressant. Check with your doctor before taking any amino acids.
◆ *Pancreatin:* Can help decrease appetite and has been shown to promote weight loss in animals.

Herbal remedies:

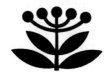

◆ Ma huang, cola nut and green tea have traditionally been used to stimulate the burning of fat. These herbs contain caffeine and other alkaloids, which can also cause insomnia or restlessness.
◆ *Glucomannan:* High in fiber, this herb can help normalize blood sugar, and break down fat.
◆ *Dandelion root:* Has a long history of use as a weight loss aid. Dandelion is considered a liver tonic. There is evidence to support that fact that improper liver function is found in a large percentage of overweight individuals.

- Gotu kola and ginseng: help to provide energy and stamina for exercising.
- Sassafras and burdock: good for appetite control.
- *Kelp:* Helps to promote good glandular health and body metabolism. It also contains small amounts of lecithin, which helps to burn fat.
- *The following herbs in combination may be useful:* Juniper berries, uva ursi, chickweed, gotu kola, dandelion, and licorice root.

PREVENTION

- Weigh yourself regularly and record your weight on a chart. If you go up three pounds from your ideal weight, adjust your diet and exercise to lose those three pounds. It is much easier to lose three pounds than to lose twenty.
- Stay off the diet rollercoaster of overeating and then crash dieting. Keep a consistent healthy life-style centered around sensible eating and regular exercise.
- Keep your kitchen stocked with healthy low-fat, low-sugar snacks.
- Accept the fact that maintaining an acceptable weight cannot rest on temporary diets and must come from permanent life-style adjustments.

Osteoporosis

DEFINITION:

Osteoporosis has received a great deal of attention over the last few years. To some extent, it is considered a natural part of aging, and occurs when bone density is lost, making bones more brittle and easily fractured. By age 70, it is estimated that the density of the skeleton has decreased by approximately one-third. Osteoporosis literally means porous bones. For hormonal reasons, osteoporosis is much for common in women than men. Twenty-five percent of all postmenopausal women have the disorder.

Bones that are affected by osteoporosis can become thin and porous, which makes them vulnerable to fractures. The most common sites of bone loss are in the spine, hips, and ribs. Osteoporosis affects over 15 million people in the United States and is estimated to cost over 3.8 billion dollars annually. Approximately 650,000 fractures occur annually in the United States as a result of osteoporosis. The good news is that osteoporosis can be slowed or even reversed if certain steps are taken.

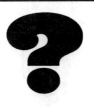

CAUSES:

After menopause women are particularly vulnerable to osteoporosis due to the decrease of estrogen, which helps to maintain bone mass. Other possible causes of osteoporosis are lack of calcium in the diet, removal of the ovaries, Cushing's syndrome, lack of mobility, or the prolonged use of corticosteroid drugs. Smoking and alcohol consumption are also associated with a higher incidence of this disorder. Women who have mothers who suffered from osteoporosis are more likely to develop the disorder.

The risk of osteoporosis increases with age. Certain drugs can result in a calcium loss from the body. A few of these are diuretics (Furosemide), blood thinners (Heparin), some anticonvulsants, and especially some thyroid medications (L-thyroxine).

Certain factors increase the risk for developing osteoporosis. Some of these are consuming alcohol and caffeine, smoking, never having been pregnant, a fragile frame and fair skin, being underweight, sedentary life-style, low intake of calcium, a high-protein diet, too much iron, and the presence of digestive disorders. In addition, early menopause and a family history of the disease raise the risk of osteoporosis.

People who suffer from diabetes, chronic pulmonary disease, rheumatoid arthritis and Cushing's syndrome are also more susceptible to this disorder.

SYMPTOMS:

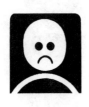

Physical: Osteoporosis can begin at menopause and go without any significant symptoms for a long period of time. Often the first symptom of the disease is discovered when a minor fall causes a fracture. Typical sites for these fractures are above the wrist and the top of the femur. Fractures of one or several vertebrae can also occur and result in a progressive loss of height and a curvature of the spine.

In these cases, compression of the spinal cord may cause chronic pain. Osteoporosis can also cause a backache if it is occurring in the vertebrae.

MEDICAL ALERT:

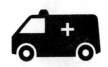

If you develop a sudden and extremely severe attack of back pain see your physician. A spinal fracture can occur in osteoporosis and could result in paralysis.

Note: Women who are approaching menopause and are at risk for developing osteoporosis should consult their physician about a bone density study to evaluate their skeletal status. Some doctors dispute the value of this type of diagnosis. Discuss its advantages with your doctor.

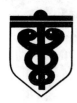

STANDARD MEDICAL TREATMENT:

Osteoporosis is diagnosed from bone x-rays, blood tests and in some cases, a bone biopsy. Unfortunately, x-rays do not usually detect the disorder until a 30 to 50 percent bone loss has already occurred. Calcitonin, a prescription drug recently approved by the FDA, can help to prevent bone loss in a large percentage of patients with osteoporosis. It has had a very positive effect in treating the disease and should be discussed with your doctor.

The use of estrogen replacement therapy may also be recommended by your doctor and its pros and cons should be carefully discussed and evaluated.

NOTE: If you have trouble with kidney stones, drugs like calcitonin and other calcium supplements may be problematic. Discuss this with your doctor.

Success rating of standard medical treatment: fair to good. Traditional treatments of osteoporosis are sometimes too late to make a significant difference. Prevention should be stressed more in the medical community and women need to educate themselves on preventive measures. Hormone replacement therapy has had some good success within the medical community and should be investigated upon reaching menopause.

MEDICAL UPDATE:

◆ Recent studies have shown that women who take synthetic thyroid hormones run a much greater risk of developing osteoporosis; however, if they also take estrogen, they can significantly lower their risk of bone loss. Reports in the Journal of the American Medical Association disclosed that women taking estrogen with Sinthroid or with Corticosteroid showed less bone loss from these drugs. For more information of this subject in a free booklet write to:

Medications and Bone Loss
NOF
1150 17th Street, NW, Suite 500
Washington, D.C. 20036

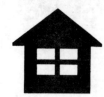

HOME SELF-CARE:

◆ Keeping your body active by exercising regularly can help to minimize calcium loss, which causes osteoporosis. Even if calcium is present in the body it cannot be used properly unless you exercise. In addition, exercise can slow the effects of osteoporosis and help to reverse some of its symptoms to some extent. A brisk daily walk is recommended. Mini-trampolines are also good in that they do not put as much impact stress on the skeletal frame. Some studies indicate that some weight-bearing exercises can also block the usual loss of calcium that occurs

after menopause.
◆ Do not smoke, drink alcohol or consume caffeine. All three of these activities have been linked to an increase in bone loss.
◆ Take precautions to avoid falls. Remove possible hazards such as loose rugs or electrical wires. Keep your house well lit at night.
◆ If you need to, use a cane to avoid the possibility of falls and fractures.
◆ When you stand, use furniture to help support your body.
◆ Use cushioned soles to prevent injury and stress to the bones of feet, legs and hips.
◆ Don't twist to pick something up off the floor. Fractures can result from sudden motions and twists if you have osteoporosis.

NUTRITIONAL APPROACH:

The current recommendation for post-menopausal women is 1,200 to 1,500 milligrams of calcium per day. Recommended sources of calcium are buttermilk, buckwheat, kelp, founder, nuts, oats, cheese, whole wheat, yogurt, skim milk, and sardines. Some vegetables are also high in calcium but contain oxalic acid which can inhibit calcium absorption. Some of these are broccoli, kale, and turnip greens. Other foods high in oxalic acid are beet greens, almonds, cashews, chard, rhubarb and spinach. Calcium/magnesium supplements are suggested along with dietary sources. Soluble calcium sources are considered better than others for their absorbability.
◆ Take your calcium supplements before going to bed. Calcium can help to calm the nerves and ensure a better night's rest.
◆ Several studies indicate that a high percentage of post-menopausal women are severely deficient in stomach acid, which can dramatically decrease the absorption of calcium ingested. In these cases, calcium carbonate is not recommended as a supplement. Soluble calcium found in calcium citrate, calcium lactate, and calcium gluconate is superior. Calcium citrate also appears to be less likely to cause kidney stones.
◆ Eat a diet high in fruits and vegetables and low in fat and animal protein. Increase your consumption of flavonoid-rich foods, such as dark colored berries and fruits.
◆ Eliminate soft drinks, high-protein animal foods, caffeine, and alcohol. The phosphates contained in these foods can cause calcium to be excreted in excess amounts. Colas and carbonated drinks are often high in phosphoric acid and should be avoided. Several studies confirm that eating a diet high in meats seems to initiate more bone loss than a vegetarian diet. Caffeine has also been linked to calcium loss by causing the excretion of increased amounts of calcium in the urine.
◆ Do not eat too much fiber. A high fiber diet can bind calcium in the stomach

and limit the amount that is absorbed. However, for fiber to be a significant factor in calcium reduction, the amount of fiber would have to be abnormally high.

◆ Avoid salt: Salt, like phosphorus, can cause too much calcium to be excreted in the urine. Check ingredient labels for high-salt foods.

◆ *Calcium/magnesium:* Very important in treating and preventing this disorder. Take magnesium with calcium to ensure adequate calcium assimilation in the body.

◆ *Silicon:* Contains calcium and is easily absorbed in the body.

◆ *Silica, manganese and phosphorus:* Several studies indicate that even if calcium is present in the body, it can be inefficiently utilized by the body. These three minerals significantly increase the uptake of calcium by the bones and are especially important if a fracture has already occurred.

◆ *Boron and copper:* Improve the uptake of calcium and also make up the substance which comprises bone.

◆ *Sulfur:* Helps with calcium absorption and is important for bone and connective tissue strength.

◆ *Zinc:* Also plays a role in calcium assimilation.

◆ *Kelp:* A good source of minerals for proper bone health.

◆ *Vitamin C:* Helps to ensure collagen and connective tissue strength.

◆ *Bioflavonoids:* are excellent for their ability to stabilize collagen tissue, which is the major protein found in bone.

◆ *Vitamin D:* Helps to increase and stimulate the absorption of calcium.

◆ *Vitamin B6, folic acid and vitamin B12:* A lack of these vitamins, which is particularly common in elderly people, can result in a rise of homocysteine, which can contribute to the development of osteoporosis.

◆ *Vitamin K:* necessary to hold calcium within the bones.

HERBAL REMEDIES:

◆ *Alfalfa:* An herb which is high is calcium and vitamin K.

◆ *Feverfew:* Contains silicon and zinc and is also good for pain relief. Feverfew should not be taken by pregnant women.

◆ *Horsetail:* Contains silica and manganese required for calcium uptake and fracture healing.

◆ *Oatstraw:* Contains a high amount of silica which is needed for calcium assimilation.

PREVENTION:

◆ Preventing osteoporosis should begin long before old age. Diet and life-style changes can greatly contribute to a reduced risk of developing osteoporosis. Suggestions are listed below.

◆ Both men and women should make sure that their calcium intake is adequate. Sources for calcium are milk and dairy products, green leafy vegetables, citrus fruits, sardines and shellfish. Calcium/magnesium supplements are recommended. It is important to remember that studies have indicated that even if a high level of calcium is ingested, if the diet is protein-rich, absorption of calcium can be impaired.

◆ Exercise regularly. Exercise helps to build and maintain bone mass. The importance of exercise in preventing osteoporosis cannot be overemphasized. Even if calcium is present in the body, without exercise the bones will not take it up. Studies indicate that a sufficient amount of exercise can maintain bone strength for an indefinite period of time. Exercise is perhaps the best anti-aging activity available.

◆ Hormone replacement therapy at menopause has been shown to help prevent osteoporosis in women. It has cut fractures caused by post-menopausal women by half in the United States. The possible side-effects of this treatment should be carefully discussed with your physician.

◆ A diet that is adequate in protein, calcium, magnesium, phosphorus, vitamin C and vitamin D combined with regular exercise is the best prevention for osteoporosis.

◆ Do not smoke: Smoking accelerates bone loss in both men and women.

Periodontal Disease (gum disorders)

DEFINITION:

The possibility of developing gum disease as we age should motivate all of us to take care of our teeth and gums the way we know we should. Unfortunately, most of us don't spend enough time thoroughly cleaning our teeth and stimulating our gums and sadly enough, we may live to regret it later.

Periodontal disease refers to any disorder which affects the gums or other tissue that surround the teeth. Gingivitis, which is an inflammation of the gums, is considered an early form of periodontal disease. If left untreated, it can progress to pyorrhea, which can result in serious complications. Gum disease is a common condition of middle-aged people that can often require painful and expensive dental treatment.

According to some estimates, the majority of the American public is at high risk for developing periodontal disease. The average senior citizen has only five natural teeth left. Forty percent of all retired people wear dentures of some type. Men are more susceptible to periodontal disease and it is also more common among lower social and economic groups.

CAUSES OF GINGIVITIS AND PYORRHEA:

Gingivitis can be caused by deposits of plaque and bacteria in and around the teeth that can result from poor dental hygiene, food impaction, mouth breathing, tooth grinding, dentures that do not fit properly and faulty dental fillings which can cause gum irritations. In addition, missing teeth and tooth decay can contribute to gum disease.

A diet low in fibrous foods, lack of vitamin C, folic acid, calcium or niacin, chronic illness, blood diseases such as leukemia, anemia, smoking and poor nutrition have also been associated with gingivitis. Certain drugs, some glandular disorders and excessive consumption of sugar and alcohol are also considered significant contributory factors.

Diabetics can be at much higher risk for developing gum disease due to their decreased resistance to infection. Tobacco smoking also increases the risk of gum disease. In addition, pregnant women are more susceptible to periodontal disease.

SYMPTOMS:

Physical: Gingivitis is characterized by gums that are swollen, sore and bleed easily. In addition, the gums can appear red, soft and shiny. Pyorrhea, which is an advanced stage of periodontal disease, is characterized by painful bleeding, receding gum line, swelling in the jaw region, sensitivity to hot and cold, toothaches, halitosis, bone loss in the jaw, and abscesses.

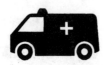

MEDICAL ALERT:

See your dentist as soon as possible if you have any of the following symptoms:
◆ gums that are shrinking away from your teeth
◆ an altered bite so that your teeth come together differently than they did before
◆ the presence of pockets of pus between your teeth
◆ teeth that become loose or fall out
◆ gums that continually bleed and stay sore and swollen

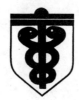

STANDARD MEDICAL TREATMENT:

Your dentist may initially prescribe an antibacterial mouthwash such as Peridex and recommend a routine of good oral hygiene. In severe cases, x-rays will be taken to determine the condition of the underlying bone. Very loose teeth can be anchored, and cementum that has worn away can be replaced with synthetic material.

If pus is present, it will be drained through a root canal. Very meticulous cleaning of the teeth can help prevent further plaque and calculus formation. Scaling and root planing are used to accomplish this. Teeth may have to be extracted. If bone loss is extensive, dentures may be required. Antibiotics are routinely prescribed if infection is severe.

Surgical options: Periodontal surgery may be required if deep pockets of infection have formed.

A gingivectomy is a minor surgical procedure performed in a dentist's office under local anesthesia in which the gums are trimmed. A periodontal pack is used to cover the gums after the surgery. It remains in place for about two weeks, during which healing takes place.

Curettage may be required to remove any diseased lining from gum pockets so healthy tissue can reattach itself to the tooth.

Splinting: This procedure can anchor loose teeth to ones that are still firmly planted.

Osseous surgery: In advanced cases of periodontal disease, surgical corrections of the bone structure of the mouth may be necessary.

Side-effects: Peridex: Contains chlorhexidine, an antibacterial agent which can cause discolored teeth and fillings and a brown film on the mouth. Professional cleaning can remove these stains.

Success rating of standard medical treatment: fair to good. Most of the above treatments are initiated long after gum disease has progressed and can only offer limited success if the disease is advanced. Often teeth are lost, which results in full or partial dentures. Implants offer a better alternative to dentures; however, they are costly and can only be done if bone mass permits.

HOME SELF-CARE:

- Take the time to brush and floss correctly and completely. Good oral hygiene takes time and should not be rushed. Brush your teeth, gums and tongue. Use unwaxed dental floss and be thorough.
- Use a soft, flexible toothbrush. Hard toothbrushes can scratch and puncture gums and they do not get into crevices efficiently.
- Buy oral mouthwashes that contain cetylpyridinium chloride or domiphen bromide which can help reduce plaque. Plax and Listerine are recommended.
- A homemade mouthwash comprised of 3 percent hydrogen peroxide mixed half and half with water can control bacterial growth in the mouth.
- Mouthwashes that contain at least 5 percent zinc solution are also recommended for inhibiting the growth of plaque.
- Brush with baking soda and water to neutralize acid, eliminate bad breath and

clean the teeth. A paste can also be made of water, baking soda and peroxide and left on the gums for long periods of time.

◆ Make sure to brush your gums along with your teeth. Brushing the gums helps to remove hidden food particles and stimulates good circulation, which discourages disease.

◆ Rinse your toothbrush with alcohol after using. Toothbrushes can accumulate bacteria.

◆ Stimulate your gums daily with rubber devices or special wooden sticks which your dentist can recommend.

◆ Stop smoking and drinking alcohol: Both of these habits can deplete the body of nutrients required for the maintenance of healthy teeth and gums.

◆ There are several natural toothpastes available in health food stores which offer alternatives to the regular ingredients offered in standard toothpastes. Some of these natural ingredients to watch for are sea salt, calcium bases, silica, baking soda, and myrrh.

◆ The use of water jet devices such as Waterpic to remove food particles remains somewhat controversial among dentists. Evidence to support their effectiveness is incomplete.

◆ Have your teeth and gums cleaned by a professional dental hygienist twice a year.

NUTRITIONAL APPROACH:

◆ Make sure your diet is high in calcium and magnesium to help prevent jaw bone loss, which can affect the health of teeth and gums. In some studies, even those suffering from advanced periodontal disease showed improvement after taking calcium supplements. Gum inflammation and tooth mobility were both reduced.

◆ Eat plenty of raw vegetables and fruits, which supply vitamin C and minerals and also serve to stimulate and clean the teeth and gums.

◆ Blueberries are especially recommended for their high content of flavonoid.

◆ A high fiber diet is also desirable due to the fact that fiber causes an increase in salivation.

◆ Avoid refined sugar, white breads, pastries, soda pop, candy, gum, and other refined foods. These foods provide an excellent environment for bacterial breeding in the mouth. The Western diet is so high in sugar that it not only increases rates of tooth decay but can depress the immune system as well, which can increase the risk of periodontal disease.

◆ *Vitamin C with bioflavonoids*: Vitamin C is excellent for bleeding gums and should be supplemented daily. Vitamin C is essential in maintaining collagen integrity in the gums and in boosting the immune system. A lack of vitamin C can also result in an increased permeability of the gums to toxins and bacterial invasion. Bioflavonoids are very good in reducing gum inflammation and strengthening collagen.

◆ *Coenzyme Q10*: Has been used to treat gum disease with a good deal of success.

◆ Vitamin A: Promotes healing of mouth and gum tissues. A vitamin A deficiency can predispose one to gum and mouth disease. Beta carotene helps to strengthen gum tissue and is a strong antioxidant.

◆ *Vitamin E and selenium:* Important for cell replacement in gum tissues. Vitamin E oil can be rubbed directly on the gums. Selenium in combination with vitamin E can help deter periodontal disease with its antioxidant properties. Free radicals can be very damaging to gum tissue.

◆ *Folic acid:* Produces a significant reduction in gum inflammation and bleeding and can be used internally and externally in the mouth itself.

◆ *Zinc and copper:* Help to fight bacterial infections, which can promote periodontal disease. When taking calcium, zinc requirement increases. A lack of zinc can greatly increase the risk for periodontal disease.

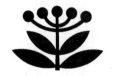

Herbal remedies:

◆ *Golden seal:* Helps to fight infection and promote healthy gums. Make a paste out of the powder and use to brush with. This also makes a good mouthwash.

◆ *Echinacea:* Can be rubbed on the gums in the form of a paste. Helps to fight infection.

◆ *Myrrh tea mouth rinse:* Myrrh has a long history in treating periodontal disease. It helps to tone the gums and remove plaque.

◆ *Aloe vera gel:* Helps to heal the mouth and gums and can reduce some plaque. Brushing with the gel is recommended.

◆ *Chaparral and myrrh:* Have antiseptic actions which inhibit the growth of mouth bacteria that promote tooth decay and gum disease.

◆ *Hawthorne berries:* A rich source of bioflavonoids, which have had remarkable results in studies of gum disease treatment.

◆ *Horsetail:* Contains silica and other minerals which help to control the loss of bone mass.

Prevention:

◆ Good oral hygiene is essential. Taking the time to brush and floss every day is the best prevention for gum disease.

◆ Keep toothbrushes free from bacteria by rinsing them in alcohol after each use.

◆ Keep your immune system healthy. Through proper diet, a healthy immune system can fight the infections which promote gum disease. Eat a diet high in fiber, raw fruits and vegetables and low in sugar and fats.

Pneumonia

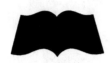

DEFINITION:

Before the discovery of antibiotics, pneumonia was a dreaded and often fatal disease. While it is still considered a serious disease, it is usually only fatal to older segments of the population or to people who have weakened immune systems.

Pneumonia is described as an inflammation of the lung which can be caused by a wide variety of bacteria, viruses and fungi. Most viral pneumonias are mild. A recently discovered form of pneumonia called Legionnaire's disease is caused by a bacteria. This particular type of pneumonia received extensive publicity when it took the lives of several people who were staying in the same hotel. Legionnaire's disease can occur in epidemics.

Pneumonia is the sixth most common cause of death in the United States and is considered an opportunistic infection. It can develop as a common complication of any serious illness. It occurs more often in males during infancy and old age and in people suffering from AIDS or leukemia. Chronic alcoholics are also prone to pneumonia.

Pneumonia generally lasts for about two weeks. Elderly people who contract the disease often fail to respond to treatment, and death can occur due to respiratory failure. Double pneumonia is a term used when both lungs are infected with the disease.

CAUSES:

Pneumonia can develop when bacteria, viruses, fungi or other foreign substances enter the lungs and cause inflammation. When the epiglottis, which forms a protective barrier for the lungs, becomes weakened, as it does in the event of a stroke, surgery, or during a loss of consciousness or seizure, microbe invasion can occur, thereby increasing the risk of infection.

Other factors that raise the risk of getting pneumonia are smoking, malnutrition, kidney failure, asthma, sickle cell anemia, certain cancers, and chronic viral infections of the upper respiratory tract. Pneumonia is a common complication of influenza and AIDS.

Viruses that can cause pneumonia are the adenovirus, the syncytial virus or the coxsackievirus. Bacterial pneumonia is most often the result of the streptococcus pneumoniae. Hemophilus influenzae and legionella pneumophilia can also cause the disease.

Pneumonia can also be caused by inhaling vomitus, or poisonous gases such as chlorine gas. Taking immunosuppressive drugs and steroids can increase one's susceptibility to contracting pneumonia.

SYMPTOMS:

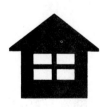

Physical: Pneumonia typically causes fever, headache, malaise, chills, cough, rapid breathing, nausea, vomiting, coughing up rust-colored sputum, sweating, and chest pain. In addition, there may be a bluish tinge to the skin, and occasionally mental confusion or delirium.

The larger the infected area in the lung is, the more severe the symptoms will be. After recovering from pneumonia, it is common to feel fatigued for up to 8 weeks.

MEDICAL ALERT:

Contact your physician immediately if you have shortness of breath, pain upon breathing, or if you cough up blood-tinged sputum.

STANDARD MEDICAL TREATMENT:

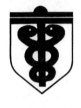

To diagnose pneumonia, listening to the chest will be carefully done by your doctor to check for the presence of fine, crackling noises. If pneumonia is present, tapping the chest will produce characteristic thudlike sounds. Chest x-rays are required to make a definitive diagnosis.

To determine what type of infection is present lab tests will be ordered and sputum samples taken. Antibiotic therapy will be initiated, which can be administered in pill or injection form. For bacterial pneumonia, penicillin and erythromycin will be prescribed. For viral infections, tetracycline is sometimes prescribed if a subsequent bacterial infection occurs. Simple viral infections do not respond to antibiotics.

In severe cases, hospitalization may be required, where oxygen therapy and artificial ventilation can take place. If the lungs do not respond to conventional treatments, a bronchoscopy may be ordered to exclude the possibility of lung cancer. Six weeks after recovery, another chest x-ray should be ordered to make sure the pneumonia is totally gone.

Success rating of standard medical treatment: very good. Bacterial infections respond well to antibiotic therapy. Lives can be saved by administering specific antibiotics for pneumonia infections.

HOME SELF-CARE:

◆ Increase fluid intake to thin secretions in the lungs, which encourages a productive cough.
◆ Increase air moisture with a cool mist vaporizer. Make sure that bed clothes and linen are changed often to prevent chilling.
◆ Coughing should not be suppressed with cough medicines. Coughing brings up

sputum and mucus and should be encouraged unless it becomes too irritating.
- Apply a heating pad or hot water bottle to the chest to ease pain.
- Hang the top half of your body off the bed and stay that way for 5 to 15 minutes to promote mucus drainage.

NUTRITIONAL APPROACH:

- Drink large amounts of fluid in the form of water, vegetable juices, fruit juices, soups, broths, fresh lemon juice in water and herb teas.
- Avoid caffeine, nicotine, alcohol, sugar, and rich greasy foods.
- Limit your sugar consumption.
- *Vitamin C with bioflavonoids:* Vitamin C is much more effective against pneumonia if started on the first or second day of the disease. If taken later, vitamin C can help decrease the severity of the infection.
- *Vitamin A:* Helps to boost the immune system when fighting an infection and is necessary to maintain the health of the respiratory tract. Beta carotene can help protect the lungs from free radicals.
- *Acidophilus:* Very important if undergoing antibiotic therapy, which kills friendly intestinal bacteria.
- *Vitamin E:* Helps to protect lung tissue.
- *Zinc:* Good for immune function and tissue repair. Zinc lozenges are recommended.
- *Liquid chlorophyll:* Can be taken in juice or tablet form.

HERBAL REMEDIES:

The use of botanical expectorants has a long history in the treatment of lung disorders. Lobelia, licorice, gumweed, wild cherry bark, white horehound, coltsfoot and sundew are all considered herbal expectorants which can decrease the viscosity of mucus and promote its expulsion.
- *Comfrey and fenugreek:* Helps to break up mucus in the lungs.
- *Slippery elm:* Can be mixed with juice and taken to coat the throat for the control of a dry, irritating cough.
- *Garlic:* Has antibiotic properties and helps to fight infection.
- *Golden seal:* Fights both viral and bacterial infection.
- *Elecampane:* Considered a tonic for the lungs.
- *Thyme:* Especially good for lung infections that create an abundance of mucus.
- Pleurisy root powder mixed with the herb boneset and freshly grated ginger is given to induce sweating in lung infections.
- *Hyssop:* Helps control coughing and loosens lung congestion.

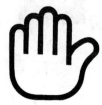

PREVENTION:

- A vaccine is now available that can offer protection against some 23 strains of pneumonia, which make up approximately 80 percent of pneumonia cases in the

United States. It is recommended that everyone over 65, with their doctor's approval, should receive this vaccine along with the influenza vaccination.

◆ Don't smoke or consume alcohol. Both of these habits can increase the risk for pneumonia as well as other respiratory illnesses.

◆ Keep your immune system healthy by eating nutritious foods that are high in raw fruits, vegetables, and fiber and low in sugar and meat.

◆ Make sure to get an adequate daily supply of vitamin C.

◆ Taking garlic every day can help to fight potential infections.

Poison Ivy

DEFINITION:

No one really knows the true definition of itching unless they have had a good case of poison ivy. Poison ivy can turn a simple romp in the forest into a date with disaster. Poison ivy refers to a skin rash which usually results when the sap or oily resin of the poison ivy plant called urushiol makes contact with the skin. This oily substance is one of the most potent natural toxins on earth. It only takes a very minute amount of the oil to provoke a violent allergic reaction on human skin.

Poison ivy can also be contracted through touching an object or animal that has made prior contact with the plant and has retained some of the urushiol on its surface. In highly sensitive people, just inhaling smoke which comes from burning the plant can cause the rash to appear. If the leaves are accidently eaten, mouth poisoning can result. The most common areas affected by poison ivy are the hands, arms and face. If the urushiol oil is left on your hands, touching other parts of your body can spread the rash. Contrary to popular belief, poison ivy cannot spread by just scratching the blisters and then touching other parts of the body. Urushiol oil must be present in order to spread the rash.

Poison ivy is found in various parts of the United States and is responsible for over 350,000 cases of skin rashes each year. It is estimated that around half of all Americans are sensitive to the plant. The sap or oil which causes poison ivy can stay active on any surface, including dead plants for up, to 5 years. Often people are not affected after only one or two exposures to urushiol, while several exposures will usually result in the development of a sensitivity to the sap. Poison ivy usually lasts approximately two weeks.

CAUSES:

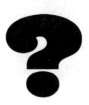

The oily sap (urushiol) contained in the bark, roots, leaves and stem of the poison ivy plant can be extremely irritating to human skin if a sensitivity to the substance exists. This substance is considered one of the most powerful toxins, requiring only a very small amount to cause a strong reaction.

SYMPTOMS:

Physical: Redness, extremely itchy rash, swelling, blistering, burning, and sometimes weeping skin. Symptoms of poison ivy can appear hours or up to a week after contact. Severe cases of poison ivy may cause a fever and acute inflammation. While scratching the blisters will not spread the rash, excessive scratching can result in infection.

MEDICAL ALERT:

For severe cases, special medical treatment may be required. If you have any of the following symptoms, go to an emergency room: fever, difficulty breathing, severe swelling, or a rash that involves the eyes, mouth or genitals.

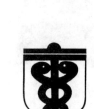

STANDARD MEDICAL TREATMENT:

After identifying the rash as poison ivy, your doctor will probably prescribe a steroid cream stronger than over-the-counter preparations. In very severe reactions, oral steroids such as prednisone may be recommended. Injections of corticosteroids may be prescribed in some cases. Antihistamines such as Benadryl or Cistaril can be used for itching.

Note: Any steroid preparation should be used with caution and should not deviate from the label or prescription. Corticosteroid creams should not be used on children unless approved by your doctor.

Side-effects: Steroid creams: These creams when used for a prolonged period of time, can cause a secondary "steroid rash," a worsening of some infectious skin conditions, permanent skin damage in thinning of the skin with blood vessels becoming more visible, and in some cases, the adrenal glands may become damaged.

Success rating of standard medical treatment: fair. Unless poison ivy is unusually severe, it can best be treated at home. Oral and topical steroids can have significant side-effects and should not be used unless absolutely necessary. Several over-the-counter poison ivy preparations are ineffective and may induce allergic reactions.

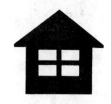

HOME SELF-CARE:

If you know or suspect that you have come in contact with poison ivy, wash the area as soon as possible. Laundry soap is recommended. Wash with it and rinse several times, letting running water pour over the area. Alcohol-based premoistened wipes can be used if nothing else is available. A washcloth that has been soaked with rubbing alcohol can effectively remove the oil.

◆ Make sure you launder everything that may have come in contact with the plant or repeated contamination may occur.

◆ For mild areas of poison ivy, apply hot compresses which can be soaked in Burow's solution (Domeboro, Burveen, Bluboro) which has been diluted (1 pint of solution to 15 pints of water).

◆ Very hot showers are also effective in removing the histamine from the rash, which is what causes the itching. During the shower, itching will become intense and then subside. Several hours of relief from itching can be obtained in this method. Try this before retiring at night.

◆ Soft ice packs are recommended for more serious rashes and can help decrease inflammation and itching. Frozen bags of vegetables work well if conventional ice bags are not available.

◆ Make compresses of baking soda and water or epsom salts and water to calm the itching of poison ivy. A cool epsom salt bath can also be helpful. If you have Milk of Magnesia on hand this can also be applied in compress form and will help to reduce itching. Witch hazel is also considered a drying agent and can help to stop oozing.

◆ Rinsing the area with a solution of lemon juice and water or vinegar and water also helps with itching.

◆ Take a bath with Aveeno or oatmeal to calm itching.

◆ Sweating can aggravate itching so keep cool and take frequent baths.

◆ A compress of ice cold milk can also help to sooth the itching and promote healing. Rinse with cool water.

◆ Calamine lotion may be helpful. Other products that help to relieve itching are Antivu lotion, Calamatum spray and Surfadil lotion. Zinc oxide ointment can also decrease itching. Avoid caladryl and zyradryl. These preparations can cause an allergic reaction in some individuals.

◆ Hydrocortisone creams such as Cortaid or Lanacort may also help control inflammation and itching; however, relief is not immediate.

◆ Keep nails short on children and use gloves or place socks over their hands at night.

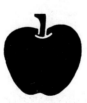

NUTRITIONAL APPROACH:

◆ Drink plenty of fluids especially in the form of fruit juices, to help cleanse the system.

◆ *Vitamin C:* Helps to fight infection and is considered a natural antihistamine which can help with itching and inflammation.

◆ *Vitamin A:* Helps to heal and generate new tissue. Considered a booster of the immune system.

◆ *Vitamin E:* Use internally and externally. Can help promote healing and minimize possible scarring.

◆ *Zinc:* Helps to repair damaged tissue.
◆ An old remedy for the itching of poison ivy is to apply a very thin slice of onion to the rash.

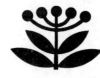

HERBAL REMEDIES:

◆ *Aloe vera gel:* Helps to heal and relieve itching and pain. If you have a fresh plant, break open the stems and apply it directly.
◆ *White oak bark:* Use this herb with lime water in a wet compress form and apply to infected areas.
◆ *Echinacea and chaparral:* Take internally in capsule form to help fight the spread of the infection.
◆ *Jewelweed:* Considered the classic herbal remedy for poison ivy. Applied externally, it soothes the rash and promotes drying of the blisters. Jewelweed is also known as the impatiens plant. Using the leaves in a compress or applying juice from the stems can be very beneficial to the rash.
◆ *Milkweed:* Juice from the milkweed is also good for itching control.
◆ *Golden seal:* Can also be used in a paste form or made into a tea and used as a compress. This helps to fight inflammation.
◆ *Gum weed:* A good herb for any kind of skin disorder. Considered an antidote in the treatment of poison ivy and poison oak.
◆ *Heartsease:* Especially good for weeping rashes. Can be used in tincture or cream form externally.
◆ *Slippery elm:* Make a paste with water and apply to infected areas.
◆ *The following herbs in combination used externally:* Comfrey, golden seal, myrrh, plaintain, chickweed and St. John's wort.

PREVENTION:

◆ Learn to recognize the poison ivy plant. It grows in a set of three leaves with the central leaf at the end of the stalk and two on either side.
◆ Anyone going into forested areas should wear protective clothing including long pants, long sleeves, shoes, socks and gloves.
◆ Use commercial poison ivy repellents such as ivy shield if going into wooded areas. If you do not have these, antiperspirant works in the same way to protect the skin. Do not use on the face area.
◆ Never burn poison ivy or any other poisonous plants. Dispose of plants in a sealed plastic bag or use an herbicide to kill them and then bury them. Do not expose your skin to the plants even when dead.

Pregnancy-Related Problems/ Morning Sickness

DEFINITION AND CAUSES:

Pregnancy can be a time of emotional elation and physical well-being. It is also true that due to the dramatic changes which are taking place in your body over the 280 days that comprise pregnancy, a number of medical problems and discomforts can occur. Changes in hormones, as well as weight, physiological factors, and nutrition-related conditions cause these problems, which can range from minor annoyances to life-threatening conditions.

The pressure from the growing fetus places stress on the abdomen and bladder and can cause gas, heartburn and frequent urination. Increased pressure from the enlarged uterus on major blood vessels can cause feelings of dizziness. The rise in estrogen which accompanies pregnancy can also result in swelling which is usually seen in the hands and feet, and the presence of progesterone can result in conditions like constipation.

It is important to keep in mind that many of these pregnancy-related problems are perfectly normal and just come with the territory. It's safe to predict that when you're holding your sweet bundle of joy, a great many of these afflictions will be quickly forgotten.

PROBLEMS ASSOCIATED WITH PREGNANCY:

Physical: Pregnancy typically causes constipation, gas, heartburn, nausea, vomiting, backache, and sleeping difficulties. In addition, anemia, groin spasms, leg cramping, varicose veins, dizziness, fatigue, bleeding gums, hemorrhoids, and mood changes can occur.

Shortness of breath, pigmentation spots, urinary tract infections, incontinence, nosebleeds, miscarriage, stretch marks, sore ribs, skin disorders, sweating, frequent urination, swelling, edema, and high blood pressure are all conditions that are associated with pregnancy.

Serious problems associated with pregnancy are toxemia, Rh incompatibility, ectopic pregnancy, spontaneous abortion, hemorrhaging, placenta previa, placenta abrupta, or a premature rupture of the membranes which may result in premature birth.

Psychological: Pregnancy can be a time of great joy and anticipation and cause a wide variety of emotional reactions ranging from resentment and fear to well being and euphoria. Most pregnant women are prone to mood swings and will find themselves crying for no apparent reason. The circumstances surrounding each pregnancy greatly help to determine individual emotional reaction. Unwanted pregnancies can create periods of significant depression and lethargy. In addition, a deficiency of certain nutrients in pregnancy can occur if the diet is not adequate. This in itself can further aggravate negative mental attitudes. Taking prenatal classes is recommended to prepare for childbirth both mentally and physically.

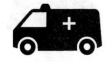

MEDICAL ALERT:

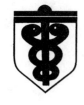

If you are pregnant and have any of the following symptoms, see your doctor immediately: bleeding, swelling of face and hands, persistent headache, blurred vision, a rise in blood pressure, sharp abdominal pains, early contractions, fever, or an absence in fetal movement.

STANDARD MEDICAL TREATMENT:

Your doctor will routinely prescribe certain antacids, prenatal vitamins, bed rest, salt-restricted diets and specific exercises to help alleviate the many discomforts that can accompany pregnancy. Regular visits to a physician are recommended. During these visits, weight and blood pressure will be monitored. At times, blood samples will be taken to check for anemia and iron supplements may be prescribed. Urine samples will be checked for the presence of sugar. Regular medical care can help to detect problems like toxemia that are potentially life threatening.

Success rating of standard medical treatment: very good. Pregnancy is a time that should be spent under the care of a qualified physician. The most controversial medical treatment associated with pregnancies is the growing number of caesarian sections. There is significant evidence that up to half of the caesarian sections performed in the United States each year are not necessary. The threat of potential lawsuits is thought to be one reason for the increased number of caesareans. The use of this option should be carefully discussed with your doctor and should not take place unless a threat exists to mother or baby. Contrary to some notions, vaginal births can occur after caesarian births.

MEDICAL TESTS USED DURING PREGNANCY:

Ultrasound: In this procedure, sound is projected off of the developing fetus through the use of high-frequency sound waves. This test is called a sonogram and produces an outline image of the baby, placenta and other structures. The image is transmitted to a video screen where a physician can assess fetal position, the maturity of the fetus, check the heart rate, sex and placental health. There is some controversy as to the safety of this procedure. It is widely accepted that the test should not be routinely done without sufficient medical cause. Recent investigations done at the University of Missouri have concluded that, if you don't have a pregnancy risk factor, you don't really need an ultrasound exam.

Amniocentesis: Through this procedure, the health of the developing baby can be evaluated. A local anesthetic is used after which a long, hollow needle is inserted into the uterus through the abdominal wall. Amniotic fluid is removed for subsequent cellular analysis. This test poses a considerable risk to both mother and baby and should be done only when an obstetrician feels it is warranted. Some possible risks are infection of the amniotic fluid, a blood exchange between mother and baby, injury to the baby, placental damage and premature labor.

Non-stress test, estriol excretion studies and oxytocin challenge test: These tests are use to evaluate the health of the unborn baby. They are used in special cases such as those involving a diabetic mother and can usually assess how well the baby will withstand the stress of labor. Discuss these tests with your obstetrician.

Chorionic villi sampling (cvs): A small sample is taken of the chorionic tissue which is found on the embryonic sac to determine whether any genetic abnormalities exist. It can be done earlier than amniocentesis. Possible risks of the procedure are fetal bleeding, uterine bleeding, infections and spontaneous abortion.

Warning: Do not take any medications, herbs, or vitamins without your doctor's approval. Avoid the following medications which can inhibit fetal development: antihistamines, cough medicines, estrogens, and mineral oil. Aspirin has been associated with excessive bleeding. Aspartame found in Nutrasweet, and Phenylalanine should also be avoided. Certain studies suggest that they may alter brain growth in the developing fetus. Certain antibiotics such as tetracycline can also cause birth defects.

MEDICAL UPDATE:

At team at the Jubilee Hospital in Belfast Ireland has concluded that snacking during labor may hasten delivery. In addition, the research suggests that babies born to mothers who ate during the early stages of labor had stronger heartbeats and better muscle tone than those who fasted. Foods eaten included scrambled eggs, toast and ice cream.

A new study done in Ireland indicates that pregnant women need even larger amounts of B-vitamins than previously thought. Pregnant women metabolize nearly 0.7 mg. of folic acid daily during the second trimester of pregnancy and 0.5 mg. during the third. The new advised dose of folic acid for pregnant women is 0.6 mg. per day.

Research at McGill University in Canada has shown that night-shift work can increase the risk for a miscarriage. Scientists speculate that by interrupting the 24 hour cycle of sleep, night work may produce hormonal imbalances. Stress related to working at night may also interfere with fetal development.

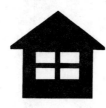

HOME SELF-CARE:

◆ Wear low shoes with good arch supports to minimize stress on the legs and back. Do not stand for long periods of time.

◆ Walking is an excellent exercise while pregnant. It can help minimize back pain, increase circulation, help to control swelling, promote better digestion, lessen constipation, lessen muscle cramping and promote a better night's sleep.

◆ If you are prone to dizziness or lightheadedness, do not get up from a sitting or lying position too quickly.

◆ A mild exercise for backache involves getting on your hands and knees and arching your lower back a few consecutive times. When you relax, do not allow your back to sag.

◆ Certain stretching exercises that can be obtained from your obstetrician can help control side cramping and muscle spasms caused by the expansion of uterine muscles.

◆ To help avoid hemorrhoids, keep your feet and legs elevated while having a bowel movement. Do not strain and do not remain on the toilet for long periods of time.

◆ Warm, not hot, sitz baths can help with hemorrhoids.

◆ If you have trouble sleeping, arrange pillows under your stomach, placing one between your legs to give added support.

◆ Leg cramps can be treated with a heating pad or hot water bottle. Leg massage is also helpful.

◆ Do not use nasal sprays or nose drops. If you have trouble with nosebleeds use a saline solution designed to relieve dry nasal membranes.

◆ Stretch marks that develop on the breasts or abdomen can be treated with vitamin E and vitamin A oil. Elastin cream is also recommended. Using these types of preparations before stretch marks appear may help to minimize them.

◆ Do not use hot tubs or saunas while pregnant. An increase in temperature can be harmful to the developing baby. It can also promote excessive sweating.

◆ Do not use over-the-counter laxatives unless specifically prescribed by your physician.

◆ Wear support hose if you have trouble with varicose veins. Special hose can be recommended by your obstetrician if the problem is severe. Put support hose on first thing in the morning before you get out of bed.

◆ Be careful when walking on ice. A fall can cause the placenta to detach which can be fatal to the fetus.

◆ Do not douche when pregnant. At least one major study has linked douching with ectopic pregnancies. In addition, some of the chemicals found in douches may endanger the health of the fetus.

Warning: Do not take any over-the-counter preparations for morning sickness without first consulting your physician.

◆ Get out of bed slowly. Take time to wake up. Often rising too quick can bring on a wave of nausea. Keep crackers by your bed and nibble a little before you get out of bed. Bagels, melba toast and saltines are good.

◆ Take a walk sometime during the day. Walking is good for cardiovascular health, muscle tone and can help to decrease stress, which also aggravates morning sickness.

◆ The value of acupressure and acupuncture should be investigated. The Chinese have identified various trigger points that directly affect the stomach.

◆ Take a warm, relaxed bath in the morning and evening.

◆ Emetrol, an over-the-counter medication, is a high-carbohydrate preparation that can help control waves of nausea but should not be taken without your doctor's approval.

◆ Do not take you prenatal vitamin supplement on an empty stomach.

◆ Take a daily nap. Morning sickness seems to increase when fatigue is present.

NUTRITIONAL APPROACH:

A note about weight gain: Today the consensus on minimum weight a pregnant woman should gain is 24 pounds. Anything below this weight may increase the risk of low birth weight babies, who are more prone to infections and other problems. If you are overweight when you become pregnant, do not use this time to lose weight. Eating a good nutritious diet is vital to the health of the developing baby. While low-fat products are encouraged, unsaturated fats are needed for proper growth.

Eat a diet high in nutrients and fiber found in whole grains, lean meats, and fresh fruits and vegetables. Adequate protein consumption is essential and should be obtained through eating lean meats, legumes and low-fat dairy products. Avoid high-sugar, high fat foods which can lead to digestive distress and excess weight gain. Adding dried prunes or bran to your diet, and drinking 6 to 8 glasses of water per day can also prevent constipation. Raw almonds are an excellent source of protein and calcium.

◆ Psyllium supplements can help with chronic constipation. Check with your doctor before using them.

◆ Decrease your salt intake. Salt can induce water retention, which can raise blood pressure. Watch your ingredient labels. Many processed foods are high in salt avoid processed cheeses, bacon, chips, etc. Do not use diuretics unless prescribed by your physician.

◆ Do not smoke or drink alcohol: Both of these activities are extremely harmful to the developing fetus and can result in low birth weight or even retardation.

◆ Don't use caffeine.

- Steam and bake your foods. Fried foods can cause heartburn and gas.
- Eating small meals throughout the day can help with nausea and vomiting. Dry snacks upon rising can help to control morning sickness. Avoid acid based foods in the morning, such as orange juice. Pass up greasy, fried or high fat foods which can cause nausea and heartburn.
- Foods high in potassium and calcium can help control leg cramps: Emphasize bananas, grapefruit, oranges, cottage cheese, yogurt, sardines, almonds, and green leafy vegetables.
- *B complex:* The B vitamins are extremely important not only to ensure the health of the developing baby and mother but to also help avoid the mood changes which can result from a lack of B vitamins. Foods rich in natural iron can also help combat fatigue. Extra B6 can help treat morning sickness.
- *Vitamin C:* Increase your intake during pregnancy through the consumption of citrus fruits, cabbage, broccoli, green peppers and berries. Do not take megadoses of this vitamin. Vitamin C helps with excessive bleeding, is vital for good collagen tissue growth and enables iron to be absorbed. It also helps promote uterine muscle strength.
- *Vitamin D:* Necessary for good bone and teeth development in that it allows for the absorption of calcium.
- *Vitamin A:* Promotes growth and helps to protect against toxins.
- *Calcium/magnesium:* Vital to the proper development of bones. A lack of these minerals can also contribute to leg cramps and insomnia.
- *Vitamin E:* Good for the health of all reproductive organs and can help to prevent miscarriage.
- *Vitamin K:* Good for excessive bleeding.
- *Iron:* Essential for the development of healthy blood cells.
- *Zinc:* Needed for the proper growth of the baby. It also helps heal stretch marks and other scars.

Note: A lack of zinc, manganese and folic acid and an imbalance of proteins have been linked to birth defects, including mental retardation.

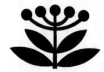

HERBAL REMEDIES:

Note: Do not take any herbs without your doctor's consent and always stay within recommended dosages.
- *Red raspberry leaf tea:* Promotes uterine muscle health. This herb is well known for its use in pregnancy. It helps to decrease bleeding after delivery and is believed to shorten the duration of labor.
- Papaya mint, ginger and alfalfa tea are all good for heartburn.
- *Shepherd's purse:* Good for proper uterine contractions. Helps to tone the uterus.
- *Nettle:* Considered a good prenatal tonic. It also helps to decrease anemia.

- *Aloe vera gel:* Good for stretch marks. Use it on the abdomen and breasts before the marks appear and as a treatment for existing marks.
- *Squaw vine:* A uterine tonic and stimulant. Best if taken the last two months of pregnancy. American Indian women use this herb all through pregnancy to facilitate a safe delivery. It also promotes lactation.
- *Blue cohosh:* This herb has been traditionally used by North American Indian women prior to childbirth to expedite delivery.
- *Alfalfa:* Contains protein and is high in vitamin K, which is good for the control of bleeding.
- Chamomile and lemon balm tea can help with insomnia. Use honey and lemon to sweeten and flavor the tea.
- *Ginger and peppermint:* Good for the nausea caused by morning sickness.
- *Sage oil:* Massaging diluted sage oil into the abdomen during the last three weeks of pregnancy can help to tone muscles for delivery.
- *Ginger:* Ginger enjoys a long tradition of use as a treatment for nausea and gastrointestinal distress. Helps to prevent vomiting and alleviate nausea.
- *Red raspberry, catnip or peppermint tea:* Good for any kind of stomach upset. Add honey and fresh lemon to herb teas.
- *Black horehound:* Helps to prevent vomiting.
- *Roman chamomile:* Reduces nausea and calms the stomach.
- *Lemon balm tea:* Suggested for its soothing effect on the stomach.
- *Alfalfa mint tea:* Helps to quiet stomach spasms.
- *The following herbs in combination may be useful:* kelp, dandelion and alfalfa.
- *To help avoid miscarriage, the following herbs in combination:* Wild yam, squaw vine, false unicorn and cramp bark.

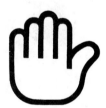

PREVENTION:

Some problems associated with pregnancy are inevitable and should be expected to some extent. The best way to avoid or minimize your risk for other problems is to routinely visit your doctor, eat a nutritious diet, take a good vitamin and mineral supplement and to keep yourself physically active and mentally healthy.

Premenstrual Syndrome (pms)

Definition:

You know that PMS has finally reached the forefront of awareness when it can be legally used as a courtroom defense for assault and battery. If it's a couple of days before your period, and you feel like hurling your china through your picture window, you probably have PMS.

Within the last 15 years, PMS has been officially recognized as a legitimate disorder than can have significant physical and mental effects on women who suffer from it. PMS can affect any woman who has menstrual cycles and usually occurs one to two weeks prior to menstruation. It has been linked to a number of disorders, and in severe cases can seriously affect its victims and their families. PMS involves emotional, physical and behavioral symptoms. It generally affects women between the ages of 24 and 40.

Over 2 million women in the United States suffer from PMS. For many women, PMS is most severe two to five days before the menstrual period begins; however, the syndrome can begin much earlier and persist until the last day of the period. Over 150 symptoms have been associated with PMS. Fortunately, today there is a wealth of information and resources on PMS.

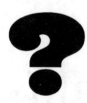

Causes:

PMS is considered to result from a hormone imbalance. High levels of estrogen can act as a stimulant to the central nervous system, producing anxiety and nervousness. Progesterone helps balance the effects of estrogen; however, in some cases, progesterone levels decrease and hormonal balance is disrupted. Other possible causes of PMS are: food allergies, low blood sugar levels, edema, yeast infections, lead poisoning, nutritional deficiencies and both physical and mental stress. There is some evidence to suggest that thyroid dysfunction can also cause PMS.

Symptoms:

Physical: Cramps, bloating, water retention, skin eruptions, headaches, backache, breast tenderness, food cravings, increased appetite, insomnia, fatigue, constipation or diarrhea, heart palpitations, joint pain and weight gain.

Psychological: PMS can cause mild to severe personality changes including depression, lethargy, irritability, agitation, sleep disturbances, nervousness, anxiety, short temper, violent outbursts, a desire to run away, a withdrawal of affection and thoughts of suicide. Virtually every community has PMS support groups. Contact your local woman's health center and participate in PMS reduction programs. Counseling may also offer some benefit through self-help groups.

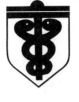

STANDARD MEDICAL TREATMENT:

There is no single treatment that can relieve all the symptoms associated with PMS. Your doctor may prescribe synthetic progesterone in an attempt to obtain hormonal balance. It is usually given during the last part of the menstrual cycle. Oral contraceptives may be prescribed to inhibit ovulation. Anti-prostaglandin drugs and diuretics are also routinely used. In addition, analgesics, tranquilizers and antidepressant drugs are used to treat PMS.

Success rating of standard medical treatment: fair. PMS is difficult to diagnose and to effectively treat. The use of hormonal therapy and diuretics has significant side-effects; however, in very severe cases of PMS these drugs may be warranted. Becoming dependent on tranquilizers, sleeping pills or antidepressants is not recommended. A nutritional and herbal approach should be carefully followed before resorting to these treatments.

HOME SELF-CARE:

◆ Exercise can be an invaluable tool against PMS. Take a brisk walk on a regular basis to release endorphins, which are brain chemicals that ease pain and create a sense of well-being. Exercise also helps to reduce breast tenderness, food cravings, water retention and depression.
◆ Try to keep a positive mental attitude through yoga, breathing exercises, or visualization therapy.
◆ Discuss PMS with your family and let them know when you are experiencing it. Keep a record of PMS on your calendar and learn to recognize it for what it is.
◆ Keep your stress levels as low as possible. Take walks, listen to soft music, get a massage, or soak in an herbal bath. Try not to schedule high-stress events during PMS times.
◆ Don't take diuretics, which can increase stress on the body by depleting it of essential minerals.

NUTRITIONAL APPROACH:

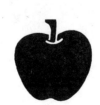

◆ Stay away from salt, caffeine, nicotine, alcohol, red meats, high-fat dairy products like butter, sugar and junk foods.
◆ Eating fatty foods can actually increase PMS symptoms and pain.
◆ Ingesting salt can aggravate bloating and water retention. Processed foods including some boxed cereals are often high in salt.

◆ If you are craving sweets like ice cream or chocolate, substitute these foods with complex carbohydrates like whole grains, pasta or bagels.

◆ Eating high-fiber foods has been found to help clear excess estrogen from the system which can cause symptoms of PMS.

◆ Not consuming caffeine can also be very beneficial for PMS victims. Caffeine is a stimulant which can contribute to anxiety and nervousness. It has also been linked to an increase in breast tenderness. Read labels on painkillers and avoid those that contain caffeine.

◆ Avoid alcohol. Alcohol can act as a diuretic and deplete the system of needed nutrients. It can significantly increase depression.

◆ Eat plenty of fresh fruits and vegetables, whole grains, cereals, legumes (beans, peas, lentils) nuts, broiled turkey, chicken and fish. Eating raw almonds as a high-protein snack is recommended.

◆ Drink plenty of water.

◆ *Calcium/magnesium:* This combination is vital in the treatment of PMS. It can decrease depression, headaches, insomnia and nervousness. It also helps to lessen menstrual cramping. Blood calcium levels can drop as much as 10 days before menstruation if estrogen levels are not adequate. A magnesium deficiency has been linked to PMS.

◆ *Zinc:* Helps the body regulate prostaglandins, which can cause menstrual cramps, and helps with stabilizing blood sugar levels.

◆ *Iron:* Helps to eliminate anemia which can result from heavy periods. Fatigue and depression can result from a low hemoglobin count, which occurs in anemia.

◆ *Chromium:* Helps to regulate and stabilize blood sugar levels, which can fluctuate more during PMS.

◆ *Selenium:* Good for menstrual cramps and breast tenderness.

◆ *Potassium:* Helps to regulate water balance in the tissues and can be lost if diuretics are taken.

◆ *Vitamin A and D:* Can help to control the acne that is sometimes associated with PMS.

◆ *Vitamin B6:* An invaluable supplement for controlling mood swings, fluid retention, breast tenderness, sugar cravings and tiredness.

◆ *Vitamin B complex:* can play a major role in preventing PMS. The B vitamins help to regulate hormone levels. A lack of the B vitamins can result in depression, fatigue, weight fluctuations and breast tenderness.

◆ *Vitamin C:* Considered an antistress vitamin which also helps to control allergies, which can sometimes intensify during PMS.

◆ *Vitamin E:* This vitamin has been referred to as a hormonal tonic and helps with depression, insomnia, breast tenderness and reproductive organ health. Olive, safflower and corn oil are good sources of vitamin E.

◆ *Acidophilus:* Acidophilus has been shown to inhibit the enzyme which converts healthy estrogen to toxic forms of the hormone.

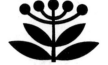

HERBAL REMEDIES:

◆ *Black cohosh*: Is believed to contain hormones precursors and minimizes menstrual cramping.
◆ *Sarsaparilla*: Believed to stimulate progesterone production.
◆ *Ginseng*: Considered a glandular tonic that helps to fight depression.
◆ *Blessed thistle*: Helps to balance hormones and can decrease the intensity of cramps.
◆ *Dong quai*: A Chinese herb used traditionally for female complaints and has been referred to as the "queen of all female herbs." This herb helps to relieve pain, bloating and vaginal dryness.
◆ *Evening primrose oil*: Helps relieve breast tenderness, mood changes, headaches, fluid retention and irritability.
◆ *Red raspberry*: Helps to strengthen the uterus and relieve painful periods.
◆ *Queen of the meadow*: A natural and effective diuretic.
◆ *Cramp bark*: Considered a uterine sedative and antispasmodic.
◆ *White willow bark*: considered a natural sedative which relieves pain.
◆ *Unicorn root*: A traditional folk remedy for female disorders, this herb has an estrogen like effect on the body.
◆ *The following herbs in combination may be useful:* Dong quai, uva ursi, valerian, licorice root, black cohosh, and cramp bark.

PREVENTION:

◆ PMS can be avoided or minimized by eating a nutritious, well-balanced diet that is high in fiber, fresh fruits and vegetables and low in fat and sugar.
◆ Regular exercise works wonders in preventing or decreasing PMS. Walking every day can help to alleviate a number of PMS symptoms.
◆ Increasing your intake of calcium/magnesium, the B vitamins, zinc and potassium prior to your period may also help to minimize PMS.
◆ Making sure that your diet is adequately supplemented with vitamins and minerals all month long also helps to control PMS.
◆ Taking herbal supplements all month long that specifically target the female reproductive system may be indicated in severe PMS.

Prostatitis

DEFINITION:

Whereas women have to face the perils of menopause, some men have to deal with prostate gland problems as they grow older. Statistics tell us that four out of every five men over the age of 50 will eventually develop an enlarged prostate, which can cause a variety of symptoms. If the prostate gland becomes inflamed, then you have what is called prostatitis.

Prostatitis can be an acute or chronic inflammation of the prostate gland and usually affects men between the ages of 30 and 50. It is most often caused by a bacterial infection that can be transmitted through sexual contact. It can afflict young men who have a tendency to get frequent urinary infections also. Elderly men with enlarged prostate glands are also susceptible to getting prostatitis.

Anyone who has experienced prostatitis has an increased chance of contracting it again. The prostate gland is the most common site of genitourinary problems in males. Prostatitis can result in a partial or total block of urine flow. Consequently, in some cases of prostatitis, the bladder can become distended, weak and susceptible to infection. Men over 40 are encouraged to have their prostate glands examined yearly.

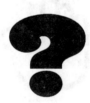

CAUSES:

Prostatitis occurs from a bacterial infection that can spread to the prostate gland from the urethra or other area of the body through the blood. It can result from sexual contact, venereal disease or from the presence of a urinary catheter. Some health care professionals believe that constipation and the consumption of alcohol is linked to prostatitis. Diets deficient in zinc are also thought to contribute to the incidence of the disease.

Taking antihistamines and decongestants for prolonged periods of time may also increase the risk of developing prostatitis from an increase in urinary retention. Exposure to pesticides and heavy metals is also linked with prostate disease. The effects of stress on prostate disorders is probably underestimated. Increased adrenalin, which is typical in unmanaged stress, causes both the neck of the bladder and the prostate gland to react, which can also make urination more difficult.

Note: High cholesterol levels are thought to promote prostate enlargement by cholesterol metabolite accumulation within the gland itself. Lowering cholesterol levels is believed to reduce the risk of prostate disorders.

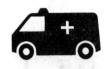

SYMPTOMS:

Physical: Prostatitis can cause pain or burning when urinating, dribbling urine, increased frequency of urination, fever, chills, penile discharge, pain in the lower abdomen, around the rectum or scrotum and in the lower back, blood or pus in the urine, and impotence. The retention of urine can increase the risk for bladder infections.

MEDICAL ALERT:

If you are experiencing any of the above symptoms, see a urologist as soon as possible to rule out the presence of prostate cancer. If you cannot urinate at all, go to the nearest emergency room. Excessive urine retention is potentially life-threatening.

STANDARD MEDICAL TREATMENT:

Your physician will examine the prostate gland manually by inserting a gloved finger into the rectum. The gland will be tender to the touch and enlarged. Lab tests will be ordered to classify the infection using urine samples and urethral secretions, which can be obtained through the manual massage of the prostate gland.

Antibiotic treatment will be initiated, and recovery is usually slow. In severe cases, antibiotics will be administered intravenously. Unfortunately, the prostate gland has a poor blood supply, making it difficult for antibiotic therapy to reach the area. Nalidixic acid is also prescribed for prostatitis. Painkillers are also routinely prescribed. If an abscess develops, surgical drainage may be required.

Surgical options: If the infection does not respond to antibiotic therapy, an operation to drain out infected fluids may be required. It is considered fairly simple and requires a short hospital stay.

Side-effects: Nalidixic acid. Visual disturbances, diarrhea, itching, nausea, vomiting, halos around lights, and rash.

Success rating of standard medical treatment: fair to good. In medical disorders involving bacterial infection, antibiotic treatment is often necessary. Unfortunately, antibiotic therapy will not cure prostatitis and in some cases, seems to increase the chances of its recurrence.

HOME SELF-CARE:

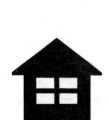

◆ Avoid sexual intercourse until the infection is gone. Intercourse may further irritate the prostate gland and prolong recovery.
◆ Mild exercise is recommended to increase circulation; however, riding a bicycle is not advised.

◆ Avoid exposure to very cold temperatures. For some reason, urination difficulties and retention are more common in cold climates.
◆ The kneeling pose in yoga is recommended for any prostate disorder.
◆ Take a neutral sitz bath which involves sitting for 15 minutes in water that is 92 to 99 degrees Fahrenheit (avoid chilling).
◆ Try not to take antibiotics for more than two weeks. Often, after antibiotic therapy, prostatitis reoccurs.
◆ Empty your bladder before going to bed and limit your intake of fluid after 6:00 pm.

NUTRITIONAL APPROACH:

◆ Increase fluid intake by drinking large quantities of distilled water daily to stimulate urine flow. Parsley juice mixed with apple juice is also recommended.
◆ Eat plenty of artichokes and asparagus, which help to cleanse the prostate gland and also act as diuretics. Watercress and parsley are also recommended for the same reason.
◆ *Zinc:* A lack of zinc has been associated with prostatitis. The prostate gland contains a concentration of zinc 10 times greater than most other organs in the body.
◆ *Essential fatty acids:* Vital to the healthy function of the prostate gland. Linseed oil, sunflower oil, evening primrose and soy oil are all good sources of essential fatty acids.
◆ *Calcium/magnesium:* Necessary for the normal functioning of the prostate gland.
◆ *Acidophilus:* Important to take if on antibiotic therapy to replace friendly bacteria which help to fight infection.
◆ *Vitamin C:* Promotes healing and also fights infection.
◆ *Vitamin B6:* Helps to promote normal cholesterol metabolism
◆ *Glycine, alanine and glutamic acid:* These amino acids taken in capsule form can help relieve nighttime urination and frequency.
◆ *Pumpkin seeds or pumpkin seed oil:* Recommended for all prostate disorders. Pumpkin seeds are rich in zinc.
◆ *Bee pollen:* Several studies suggest that using bee pollen supplements helps to significantly reduce prostate inflammation and infection. Flower pollens have been used to treat prostatitis in Europe since the early 1960s. Do not take bee pollen if you have any kind of allergies. Make sure you are not sensitive to it by taking a small amount initially.

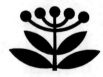

HERBAL REMEDIES:

◆ *Golden seal root:* An herbal antibiotic which fights bacterial infection.

- *Garlic capsules:* Considered a natural antibiotic, garlic fights bacterial infection.
- *Horsetail and hydrangea:* Good to help control frequent urination and help control prostate enlargement and inflammation. Can be added to hot bath water in a cheesecloth sack.
- Parsley, uva ursi, juniper berries and slippery elm are all considered diuretics and are beneficial to the genitourinary system.
- *Alfalfa:* Helps to lower serum cholesterol and reduce inflammation.
- *Buchu leaves:* are especially good for relieving prostate distress and irritation.
- *Panax ginseng:* A natural tonic for male reproductive organs by increasing testosterone levels and decreasing prostate gland size.
- *White deadnettle:* Helps to reduce benign prostate enlargement.
- *Gravel root:* An herbal diuretic that soothes urinary mucous membranes.
- Echinacea, chaparral and saw palmetto are recommended for their anti-inflammatory properties and their ability to fight bacterial infection. Saw palmetto has a specific hormonal action on the male reproductive system and can help reduce benign prostate enlargement. It is particularly beneficial for all prostate disorders.
- *The following herbs in combination may be useful:* Golden seal, parsley, marshmallow, ginger, capsicum, juniper berries, pan pien lien, uva ursi and queen of the meadow.

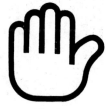

PREVENTION:

- Eat a diet high in zinc and take a zinc picolinate supplement once a day.
- Avoid becoming constipated by eating plenty of high-fiber foods and getting adequate exercise.
- Do not consume alcohol, coffee, tobacco, caffeine, red pepper or acidic foods which are considered prostatic irritants.
- Drink plenty of water. Becoming dehydrated can stress the prostate gland.
- Avoid red meats and rich foods, which may be high in uric acid. Uric acid is believed to cause prostate irritation.
- Prolonged jarring to the seat area which results from too much sitting, riding a horse, motorcycle or bike can increase the risk of prostate infection.
- If you are allergic and must use an antihistamine, discuss taking Hismanal or Seldane, which do not contain antihistamines, with your physician.
- Having frequent sexual intercourse can empty the prostate of secretions and promote better prostate health.
- Having a vasectomy has been linked to the incidence of prostate disorders, including cancer. Some studies report the risk of prostate cancer for males who have had a vasectomy is three times greater than those who have not.
- Keep cholesterol levels normal to prevent the accumulation of cholesterol metabolites in the prostate gland.

- Avoid exposure to pesticides, heavy metals or any toxic substance.
- Take an supplement of essential fatty acids every day.

Psoriasis

DEFINITION:

Psoriasis is a baffling skin disease that has no cure and has never been fully understood by medical science. It occurs when, for some reason, skin cell production gets out of control. It is a common skin disorder that is characterized by thickened patches of inflamed skin.

Psoriasis occurs in approximately 2 percent of the population of the United States and Europe. For unknown reasons, psoriasis is less common in certain populations such as Asians and Blacks. Both men and women are equally affected by psoriasis, which usually appears between the ages of 10 and 30.

The disorder results from the abnormally fast production of new skin cells. A healthy skin cell takes four weeks to complete its cycle of production, while a psoriatic cell takes less than four days. This abnormal production of cells causes skin cells to accumulate, forming thick patches sometimes referred to as plaques.

Psoriasis can affect large areas of the skin, causing a great deal of physical discomfort. Psoriasis may take different forms, therefore requiring specific treatment for each type. The disease is less common in the summer and can disappear for long periods of time. Psoriasis is considered a long-term disorder without a permanent cure. Most attacks of psoriasis can be well controlled with the appropriate treatment. The belief that psoriasis is contagious is one of the myths that surrounds this rather mysterious disease.

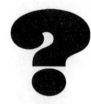

CAUSES:

The exact cause of psoriasis is unknown, although you can trace the disease in family trees, making heredity a significant factor.

Attacks of psoriasis have been linked with emotional stress, surgery, physical illness, the faulty utilization of fat, immune dysfunction, alcohol consumption, impaired liver function, incomplete protein digestion, and trauma to the skin. In addition, psoriasis attacks can be triggered by poison ivy, sunburn, and certain drugs such as lithium and beta-blockers.

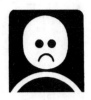

SYMPTOMS:

Physical: Psoriasis generally causes the appearance of thick patches of red, inflamed skin that has a silvery, scaly surface. It usually affects the elbows, knees, scalp, genitals and buttocks, although it can appear in any part of the body. Toes and fingernails which are affected can develop pits and ridges, and itching can be present. Joint tenderness can also accompany psoriasis.

THERE ARE THREE MAIN TYPES OF PSORIASIS:

Discoid or plaque psoriasis: Thick, scaly patches appear on the trunk and the limbs. The elbows, knees and scalp are particularly susceptible. In addition, the nails may become pitted or thickened and can separate from the nail bed.

Guttate psoriasis: This type occurs most frequently in children and consists of small patches of red, inflamed skin that can develop quickly and spread, especially following an infection.

Pustular psoriasis: Small pustules form in this type of psoriasis and can appear anywhere on the body or can stay confined to the palms or soles of the feet.

Psychological: Like acne, the worst part of this skin disorder is how it looks. Embarrassment commonly accompanies psoriasis, and those who suffer from it avoid any recreational activity in which the patches would become exposed.

Emotional stress is also a significant factor in causing attacks of psoriasis. It is common for someone suffering from psoriasis to have experienced a specific stressful event within one month prior to their outbreak. For this reason, hypnosis and biofeedback may be of some value as treatment options.

STANDARD MEDICAL TREATMENT:

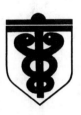

It is important to treat new patches of psoriasis promptly. In mild cases of psoriasis, ultraviolet lamp exposure (phototherapy) may be helpful. Emollient creams are also routinely prescribed by most doctors. For more severe cases, ointments which contain coal tar or anthralin may be recommended by your doctor. Corticosteroid drugs, and methotrexate, an anticancer drug, are also used. Hydroxyurea and other drugs referred to as retinoids are currently being studied. Cyclosporine drugs have had some good results, although they are not approved by the FDA for treating psoriasis. Rocaltrol is currently being tested for its potential benefits.

Freezing smaller areas of psoriasis with liquid nitrogen is also being researched. Skin patches such as Actiderm can more effectively treat affected areas. Some drugs such as Legison can have significant side-effects and should be discussed with your doctor. Oxsoralen-ultra, a liquid preparation, is also routinely used in the treatment of psoriasis.

If joint swelling is present, your doctor may want to use non-steroidal anti-inflammatory drugs. Injecting cortisone directly into an old thick patch of psoriasis can help to remove it. In severe cases, intensive ultraviolet therapy may require hospitalization.

SIDE-EFFECTS: Methotrexate (Rheumatrex): Warning; Methotrexate is highly toxic and should be prescribed only by a physician who is familiar with the drug. It can cause the death of a developing fetus, trigger a potentially fatal lung disease, severe liver and blood cell damage, and intestinal perforation. Nursing mothers should not take this drug or should switch to bottle feeding.

Other side-effects: Liver irritation, loss of kidney function, reduction of blood cell count, nausea, vomiting, diarrhea, itching, rash, hair loss, dizziness, and increased susceptibility to infection.

Success rating of standard medical treatment: fair to good. Most doctors can effectively control psoriasis with tar ointments and corticosteroid preparations. Unfortunately, stronger and stronger cortisone ointment preparations may be required over time. Retinoids and anticancer drugs have very bad side-effects and should be used only after more benign treatments have been attempted.

HOME SELF-CARE:

◆ Keeping the skin moisturized cannot be overemphasized. Apply cream onto patches of psoriasis and wrap the area in plastic overnight. Petroleum jelly can be used, or Lacticare or Eucerin creams are also recommended.

◆ Zostrix, an over-the-counter cream for the treatment of shingles, has been found to effectively treat psoriasis; however, it has not been approved for that purpose yet and should only be used with your doctor's approval. Applying the cream results in significant burning.

◆ Sensitize your skin with tar before you use ultraviolet lamps or expose the area to sunlight. Apply cortisone ointments in the morning and tar ointments at night.

◆ Spend time in the sun every day. Exposure to sunlight greatly reduces the severity of psoriasis. Dry, desert climates are especially beneficial. Protect unaffected areas with sunscreen. Do not get a sunburn. Sunburns can cause psoriasis to worsen.

◆ Maintain an optimum weight. Being overweight seems to make psoriasis worse.

◆ Applying flaxseed oil or kochia oil to affected areas can help to soften the patches. Linseed oil can be taken internally also.

◆ For cracked skin, bag balm, an ointment used to treat cow udders, is quite effective and can be purchased through a pharmacy.

◆ Cosmetic cover-up ointments can help to conceal unsightly areas and should be used only with your doctor's approval.

◆ Use oatmeal-based soaps, which do not dry the skin.

◆ For itching, make a wet compress of baking soda and water. Apple cider vinegar and water is also recommended.

◆ Keep stress levels to a minimum through hypnotherapy, breathing exercises, and yoga.

◆ Protect yourself from infection. Often a strep throat can be followed by an attack of psoriasis.

◆ Some studies indicate that acupuncture can help to control psoriasis. Discuss this with your doctor and a qualified acupuncturist.

NUTRITIONAL APPROACH:

◆ Avoid fats from meat and dairy products. Both of these foods contain arachidonic acid, a natural inflammatory substance which can turn psoriatic patches red.

◆ Avoid alcohol: Alcohol aggravates the symptoms of psoriasis and should be completely eliminated.

◆ Eliminate white sugar, white flour, processed foods and citrus fruits. Avoid tomato-based foods and caffeine.

◆ Emphasize fish (sardines, tuna, salmon), raw food, soybeans, sesame seeds and fiber. Fiber helps to reduce cholesterol levels, which have been found to be abnormally high in some psoriatic skin. Fiber helps to promote good bowel elimination. Some studies suggest that psoriasis may be caused by a toxic build-up in the colon.

◆ Use ginger or yarrow in bath water. Get into the bath and then add a couple of teaspoons of olive oil which has been added to a glass of milk to the bath water.

◆ *Fish oil or primrose oil:* Can help to inhibit arachidonic acid, which can make psoriatic lesions turn red. These oils also help to prevent skin dryness and can be taken in capsule form.

◆ *Vitamin A:* Required for healthy skin, hair and nails.

◆ *Vitamin D:* Helps to heal skin. Activated vitamin D, which is available by prescription only, has been used with some success.

◆ *Vitamin C:* Participates in the proper formation of connective tissue and collagen.

◆ *Lecithin:* Works to emulsify fats and protects cells. Helps to clean out fatty deposits like cholesterol, which has been found to be abnormally high in some psoriatic skin. Use sunflower oil, which contains lecithin.

◆ *Zinc:* Required for proper healing of the skin. A zinc deficiency has been found in psoriatic patients.

◆ *Vitamin B complex:* Helps to maintain healthy skin.

◆ *Vitamin C, folic acid, and vitamin B12:* Used in combination by Russian Medical scientists for the treatment of psoriasis.

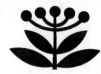

HERBAL REMEDIES:

- *Lavender:* Helps to stimulate cell growth. Mixed with olive oil, it can be applied externally.
- *Chaparral poultice:* Make a paste or patch and apply to affected areas.
- *Dandelion:* Strengthens the liver, which can be impaired in chronic skin diseases.
- *Golden seal:* Inhibits the formation of polyamines that result from improper protein digestion, and may be linked with psoriasis.
- *Yellow dock:* Helps to clear toxins from the body, and can be used in salve form externally for inflammation and itching.
- *Red clover:* Make a wet compress with red clover tea to control inflammation.
- *Figwort:* Good for chronic skin inflammations. Can be taken internally.
- *Milk thistle:* Helps to detoxify the liver, which may help to control psoriasis. It also inhibits inflammation and reduces excessive cellular proliferation.
- Chaparral and comfrey poultice made with powdered herbs and water can be applied to affected areas.
- *The following herbs in combination may be useful:* Echinacea, Oregon grape root, sarsaparilla, burdock, kelp and peach bark.

PREVENTION:

While there is no known cause for psoriasis, the following factors are believed to decrease the risk of an attack:
- Keep stress levels controlled through biofeedback, exercise, yoga etc.
- Eat a diet high in fish oils and fiber and low in animal fats and sugar.
- Don't consume alcohol.
- Make sure your diet is high in zinc and lecithin.
- Avoid becoming badly sunburned.
- Keep the immune system healthy through a nutritious diet and avoid exposure to infections.

Reye's Syndrome

DEFINITION:

The existence of Reye's syndrome has made a great majority of parents switch from giving children who have a fever aspirin to acetaminophen. Reye's syndrome is a relatively rare disorder that causes brain and liver damage and can be fatal. Several studies have indicated that up to 95 percent of children who get Reye's syndrome had been given aspirin during a viral infection. In addition, the amount of aspirin given seems to determine the severity of the disorder.

The symptoms of Reye's syndrome are similar to encephalitis, and it typically occurs after an upper respiratory infection, chicken pox or case of the flu. Reye's syndrome is almost exclusively confined to children under the age of 15. A serious attack of Reye's syndrome may result in death or serious brain damage. The death rate from the syndrome has dropped from 60 percent to 10 percent in recent years, probably due to the raised public awareness of its connection with aspirin.

CAUSES:

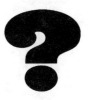

The exact cause of this disorder remains unknown. Evidence suggests that Reye's syndrome is almost always related to giving a child aspirin during a viral infection.

WARNING: Do not give children aspirin at any time. Use acetaminophen to reduce fever and discomfort. Some manufacturers of aspirin have removed their children's variety due to the emergence of Reye's syndrome.

SYMPTOMS:

Physical: The symptoms of this syndrome will appear as a child is recovering from another infection. These symptoms include prolonged uncontrollable vomiting, fever, lethargy, weakness, double vision, paralysis, hearing loss, speech impairment, delirium, disorientation, seizures, coma, abnormal heart rhythms, breathing difficulties, and jaundice.

MEDICAL ALERT:

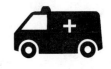

Be aware of the warning signs of Reye's syndrome and seek medical help immediately. These are: Prolonged and uncontrollable vomiting, drowsiness which occurs as the child is recovering from the flu or chicken pox, delirium or restlessness, fatigue or disorientation.

Note: A child that has the above symptoms may go into a coma within four days. Prompt treatment can prevent death and brain damage.

STANDARD MEDICAL TREATMENT:

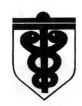

Intravenous solutions of glucose and electrolytes are given to replace minerals lost in vomiting. If the brain is involved, swelling is controlled by corticosteroid drugs and infusions of Mannitol.

In some cases, dialysis or blood transfusions may be required if liver damage has resulted. If breathing has stopped, a ventilator will be used.

Success rating of standard medical treatment: good to very good if the condition is caught in time. If the child has gone into a coma, the risk of death or brain damage is greatly increased. Recent awareness of this syndrome has significantly reduced the death rate from Reye's syndrome.

PREVENTION:

◆ Do not give anyone under the age of 21 aspirin. Use acetaminophen medications to treat fevers, aches, colds, and viral infections such as chicken pox and influenza.

◆ Avoid giving the following herbs to children: black haw, which contains salicin, also found in aspirin compounds, meadowsweet, and white willow. These herbs are related to aspirin.

◆ Keeping a child's immune system healthy through supplementation with vitamin A, vitamin C with bioflavonoids and vitamin D is recommended.

Sexual Rejuvenation/Depressed Sexual Drive

DEFINITION:

Today, sexual inadequacies are usually considered ailments that primarily affect the aging person, who may have lost his or her interest in the subject. To the contrary, diet deficiencies and bad habits frequently compromise the sexual desire and experience of people of all ages. The value of sex therapists and their psychological approach to sexual dysfunction is vital for many people who suffer from sexual problems; however, the role of nutrition and herbs has traditionally been a neglected one.

In the same way, spiritual components that should undoubtedly underpin romantic relationships have not been sufficiently addressed. The notion of pleasure and fulfillment alone in sexual relationships can often become obsessive, which minimizes the true purpose of sexual love. Sexual relationships are best when they are based on genuine, mutual love.

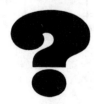

CAUSES:

A variety of physical ailments can greatly diminish one's desire and ability for sexual relationships. Some of these include migraine or tension headaches, back problems, decreased stamina from coronary artery disease, depression, mouth and gum disease, TMJ syndrome, PMS or menopausal changes, bladder infections, varicose veins, and obesity.

Symptoms:

Psychological: The emotional factors which affect sexual desire and performance are numerous and can be extremely powerful. Most therapists agree that a good sex life is at least 50 percent mental. Issues of self-esteem, dominance, commitment, are all vital to the creation and sustenance of a healthy sexual relationship, and will not be explored in depth here.

Standard Medical Treatment:

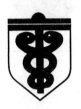

Hormone therapy is often chosen by physicians to treat impotence, frigidity and other sexual problems. While hormones may be indicated in certain cases, there are other alternatives which should be explored first. Psychiatric counseling is also routinely recommended.

Side-effects: Refer to chapter on impotence.

Home Self-Care:

◆ Keep yourself as healthy and attractive as possible. Often physiological factors such as obesity, halitosis, and intestinal disturbances can decrease appeal and dampen the desire for close physical exchange.
◆ Exercise routinely to keep yourself invigorated, control weight and build stamina.
◆ Avoid becoming constipated, which can produce bloating and fatigue. A sluggish colon can release toxins into the bloodstream which can cause a host of ailments, not to mention creating an overall feeling of malaise which is not conducive to romantic encounters.
◆ Keep your skin well-scrubbed and moisturized. Use herbal oils and give your partner a deep massage on a regular basis to relieve stress and tension, which are enemies to sexual rejuvenation.
◆ Avoid alcohol, coffee, tea and tobacco. All of these substances can interfere with normal sexual function and in some cases, can actually dull the senses. Stay away from any druglike substance you can avoid. Keep your mind clear and active.
◆ The combination of alcohol, wheat and dairy products can cause a host of intestinal ailments. Eating too much sugar can also cause wild fluctuations in blood sugar, which can contribute to feelings of depression.
◆ Skin brushing with a special brush which can be purchased at a health food store can help to remove old skin, eliminate waste products and increase circulation.
◆ Take long, leisurely herbal oil baths to relax and invigorate a tired body. Using

natural sponges can help to soften skin. Several herbal body oils have particularly nice fragrances.

◆ The Kegel exercise is excellent for women who have lost muscle tone around the vagina. During urination, try to stop and start the urine flow and repeat this several times to strengthen the pubo-coccygeus muscle. Contracting and relaxing this muscle can be done anywhere and at anytime.

NUTRITIONAL APPROACH:

◆ Eat a diet high in raw foods including fruits, vegetables, nuts, and whole grains, and use olive and safflower oil. Eat less protein in the form of lean meats and drink plenty of water. Eating grains, nuts, and seeds can improve stamina and provide protein without eating fatty meats or rich dairy products.

◆ Sunflower and pumpkin seeds: Stimulate male potency and help to heal prostate gland inflammations.

◆ For centuries, shellfish have been considered powerful aphrodisiacs these include: oysters, lobster, crab, clams, winkles, cockles, shrimp and mussels.

◆ *Vitamin A:* Lack of vitamin A may cause a lack of sex hormone production. Vitamin A is also essential for healthy mucous membranes and skin.

◆ *Vitamin B complex:* Essential for the maintenance of energy and proper sugar and hormone balance in the body. Caffeine consumption destroys vitamin B1. Lacking energy is one of the main causes of decrease in sexual desire. The B vitamins also promote circulation and actively participate in the production of neurotransmitters which control feelings of pleasure and well-being.

◆ *Choline:* Plays an important role in sexual arousal by contributing to neurotransmitter production in the brain.

◆ *Vitamin E:* Involved in fatty acid production, which is essential to the formation of hormones. Vitamin E also treats symptoms typically associated with the menstrual cycle or menopause. Vitamin E is also considered a male energizer which helps to build male sex glands and achieve hormonal balance.

◆ *Vitamin F:* Needed by the prostate gland, adrenal glands and the thyroid gland for healthy function.

◆ *Calcium/magnesium:* Helps to correct hormone production and can calm jittery nerves and reduce stress and tension.

◆ *Silicon:* Some nutritionists believe that a healthy sex life is not possible without silicon.

◆ *Zinc:* Stimulates the prostate gland and spermatozoa. Studies have indicated that a zinc deficiency may cause male sterility and may also contribute to a reduction in sex drive.

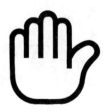

HERBAL REMEDIES:

◆ *Fenugreek tea:* Contains diosgenin, which is used in the synthesis of sex hormones. Roasted fenugreek seeds have been used for generations as an aphrodisiac. Fenugreek also keeps the urinary tract free from mucus and can decrease the risk of bladder infections which can result from sexual intercourse.

◆ *Siberian ginseng:* Stimulates energy and stamina. This herb also contains testosterone and is a good treatment for impotence. Studies have confirmed that ginseng significantly contributes to sexual potency.

◆ *Damiana:* Helps to balance female hormones and can help improve male performance and sperm count.

◆ *Vervain:* reported as being magical by ancient Romans, Egyptians and Chinese, this herb has been thought of as an aphrodisiac for centuries.

◆ *Saffron:* A traditional Assyrian aphrodisiac which was also used by the Greeks and Phoenicians. It is also a uterine stimulant.

◆ *Sarsaparilla:* Contains progesterone and testosterone precursors for balancing hormones and also stimulates circulation.

◆ *Gotu kola:* Increases stamina and helps to revitalize nerves. It also contributes to stabilizing hormone levels in the body.

◆ *Fennel:* Used by Roman warriors for strength, it was famous for its ability to provoke sexual vigor.

◆ *Mint:* Peppermint is considered a valuable treatment for impotence and decreased libido by the Arabs.

◆ *Saw palmetto:* Considered a hormonal tonic. It is believed to increase breast size and contributes to reproductive organ health.

◆ *Chickweed:* Helps to keep plaque from forming in arteries, which can impair male sexual performance and contribute to impotence.

◆ *Dong quai:* Helps alleviate a number of female problems and is good for treating menopausal symptoms. This herb may also enlarge breasts.

PREVENTION:

◆ Preventing the loss of sexual desire requires a variety of both emotional and physical factors. Proper nutrition, regular exercise and maintaining a healthy lifestyle that includes a positive mental attitude can keep one sexually young indefinitely.

◆ Get off of any drugs that you don't absolutely need to take. Several medications depress your sex drive, and doctors don't always discuss this side-effect with you. Some of them are tranquilizers, birth control pills, antidepressants, high blood pressure drugs, ulcer drugs, appetite suppressants, migraine medications, and steroids.

Sinusitis

DEFINITION:

Sinus problems plague thousands of Americans, who spend a literal fortune on over-the-counter sinus medications. Sinusitis is not just a case of congested sinuses but involves some infection as well, adding insult to injury. Sinusitis technically refers to an inflammation of the mucous membranes of the sinuses. It commonly affects the frontal and maxillary sinuses, and usually occurs as a complication of a cold or other viral infection of the nose or throat. It is commonly caused by an infection of bacterial origin.

When the sinuses become obstructed from a cold, allergy, or dental problem, mucus flow is impaired and bacterial invasion can take place. A blocked sinus cavity is the perfect breeding habitat for bacteria. Sinusitis is a common disorder; however, some people are lucky enough to never get it.

CAUSES:

Sinus infections occur when a sinus outlet is obstructed by a swelling of the nasal lining. Air and mucus build up and cause an increase in pressure and a perfect environment for bacterial invasion.

Bacterial sinusitis is typically caused by an upper respiratory tract infection such as the common cold or influenza. Allergies can also predispose one to sinus infections. Other factors which can result in sinusitis are underlying dental infections; sudden changes in pressure, which can occur in flying, swimming and diving; smoking; fumes; foreign bodies in the nose; damage to the nasal bones; asthma; nasal deformities such as a deviated septum; and the presence of pneumococci, streptococci and staphylococci. Sensitivity to birth control pills or to aspirin can also cause the sinuses to close and increase the risk of infection.

Note: The notion that a sluggish colon can indirectly cause sinusitis has been proposed. Chronic constipation or the incomplete emptying of the bowel are thought to result in a buildup of toxins in the system. These toxins may cause mucus to be retained and infection to occur. While mainstream medicine probably refutes this connection, avoiding constipation through proper diet is a factor that should not be overlooked.

SYMPTOMS:

Physical: In an acute sinus infection, nasal congestion and discharge will usually come from one nostril only. Other possible symptoms include a sensation of heaviness around the eyes and behind the nose, a nasal speaking tone, tearing, fever, chills, frontal headaches, pain in the cheekbones, tenderness and swelling over the sinus area, a non-productive cough, a musty odor, bad breath, or a bad taste in the mouth.

In chronic sinusitis, a post-nasal drip may be present; however, pain is usually absent. In the cases of chronic sinusitis, permanent mucosal damage can occur.

The notion of a "sinus headache" is considered more myth than truth. Persistent headaches due to chronic sinus problems or allergies are considered rare. A real sinus headache will feel worse if you bend over.

MEDICAL ALERT:

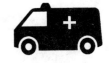

A sinus infection requires prompt medical attention. See your doctor if you have pain which radiates from your sinuses to the eye area or beneath the forehead. You may also have a fever or develop bad breath or have a bad taste in your mouth. If left untreated, a sinus infection can lead to serious complications.

STANDARD MEDICAL TREATMENT:

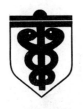

Sinusitis is difficult to distinguish from a cold. Your doctor will examine your nose, ears, throat and teeth. In some cases, an x-ray may be ordered. Antibiotic therapy will be initiated if a bacterial infection is present.

Some doctors point out that removing the nasal obstruction through decongestants or surgery will sometimes clear up the infection.

Over-the-counter nasal decongestants in both pill and spray form will be recommended, along with the application of heat and steam. In rare instances, puncturing the sinuses may be necessary to relieve pain and pressure. Irrigating the infected sinus passages is also routinely done.

Surgical options: For chronic sinusitis, a surgical procedure in which the infected tissue is removed to facilitate permanent nasal drainage may be indicated. If a deviated septum is causing the problem, it can be surgically corrected.

HOME SELF-CARE:

◆ If you smoke, stop. Chronic sinusitis is often related to smoking.
◆ Get plenty of rest. Stay in bed if necessary to get the kind of rest required to fight infection.
◆ Applying moist hot packs to the nasal area can facilitate drainage.
◆ Alternating soft ice packs and hot packs can also bring relief.
◆ Avoid using decongestant nasal sprays such as Afrin over a long period of time. Over-the-counter nasal sprays are among the most addictive drugs around. They can also damage the nasal lining and impair the normal function of nasal cilia and membranes. Nasal sprays can cause a rebound effect in which nasal

congestion returns with increased swelling and pressure than was originally present. Using these sprays sparingly in the early stage of a sinus infection can help to promote drainage.

- Sudafed, Sine-Aid, Sinarest, and Drixoral are recommended by some physicians but should not be taken if driving, operating machinery or if heart or kidney disease is present.
- Nasal saline sprays designed to moisten the nose can be purchased or made at home by mixing 1/4 teaspoon salt with 1/4 teaspoon baking soda in a glass of warm water. The saline will not clear up congestion.
- Do not blow your nose too forcefully. Gently blow your nose after you have used steam inhalation or a decongestant. Blowing one nostril at a time is recommended and can prevent a buildup of pressure in the ears. Gently sniffling helps to drain the sinuses and should be encouraged.
- Raise the head of the bed or sleep with extra pillows. Lying flat can increase pressure in the nasal passages and cause more discomfort.
- Use a cool mist vaporizer to add humidity to the air.
- Certain yoga exercises can help to drain fluids and decrease congestion. Neck and eye exercises, corpse pose and shoulder stand are recommended.
- Exercise can help to clear sinus passages by releasing adrenaline. Avoid swimming.

NUTRITIONAL APPROACH:

- A short fruit juice fast (two days) is initially recommended. Use plenty of orange, grapefruit, lemon, pineapple or grape juice. After two days, add plenty of raw vegetables and broths. Drink plenty of fluids.
- Sipping hot herb teas or broths can help to facilitate mucus flow.
- Eating hot peppers can also initiate mucus flow. Horseradish is a traditional treatment for sinus congestion. Jalepeno peppers and cajun spice have the same effect.
- Eliminate dairy products and wheat, which can cause nasal congestion and mucus production.
- Avoid alcoholic beverages. Fermented alcohol can actually clog up nasal passages.
- *Vitamin C with bioflavonoids:* Take a supplement every two hours to fight infection.
- *Vitamin A:* Essential for proper immune system function when fighting an infection.
- *Vitamin B complex:* Helps to fight infection.
- *Zinc lozenges:* Take for one week only, as prolonged use of these may lead to immunosuppression.
- *Zinc supplements:* Especially beneficial for nasal membranes.

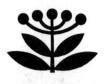

◆ *Coenzyme Q10:* A powerful immune system stimulant.

HERBAL REMEDIES:

◆ *Golden seal:* An effective botanical remedy for acute bacterial sinusitis due to its antibiotic-like action.
◆ *Garlic:* A natural antibiotic that fights both viral and bacterial infection.
◆ Swabbing the sinus passages with oil of bitter orange can help relieve swelling and promote drainage.
◆ *Comfrey:* Helps to promote mucous flow in the upper respiratory system.
◆ Make a tea of bayberry bark or golden seal, bring it to a simmer, and inhale the vapors.
◆ Sage and eucalyptus can be added to steam inhalations. Both of these herbs soothe inflammation and are antibacterial.
◆ *Burdock:* Has antibacterial properties.
◆ *Slippery elm:* Good for tissue repair and healing.
◆ *White oak bark:* Helps to shrink mucosal membranes.
◆ Use a menthol or eucalyptus pack over the sinus membranes.
◆ Rubbing Chinese essential oils on the nose are can help relieve congestion (do not use near the eyes).
◆ *Mullein:* Soothes inflamed of mucous membranes and can help reduce nasal congestion.
◆ *Aloe vera:* Helps to heal damaged tissue.
◆ *Fenugreek:* Works to liquify mucous and promote drainage.
◆ *The following herbs in combination may be useful:* Echinacea, golden seal, yarrow and capsicum.
◆ Other herbs that are beneficial include: Horehound, mullein, eucalyptus, coltsfoot leaves and wild cherry bark.

PREVENTION:

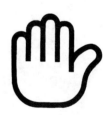

◆ If you have a cold or the flu and your sinuses swell, use decongestants so that your sinuses do not remain obstructed for long periods of time.
◆ Try to control allergies so that nasal mucosa are not constantly irritated and blocked. Irrigating the nose on a regular basis with saline solutions can help remove allergens that cause irritation.
◆ Use good dental hygiene and take care of tooth problems promptly to avoid developing sinusitis as a complication of dental disease.
◆ Keep your colon functioning well by eating plenty of foods that are high in fiber, raw fruits and vegetables and avoiding fatty junk foods, rich dairy products, white sugar and white flour. The notion that poor intestinal function can cause the production of mucus and lead to subsequent infection should not be dismissed.

Snoring and Sleep Apnea

DEFINITION:

If you sleep with someone who snores badly, you may want to hit them rather than "hit the sack." People who snore rarely appreciate with what their companions have to put up with every night. There are over 100 million Americans who snore. Snoring usually occurs during non-REM sleep and is caused by the rattling of the air passageways as air is inhaled and exhaled.

Sleep apnea is a potentially dangerous condition that affects 50,000 or more Americans. It refers to a condition in which the sleeper stops breathing temporarily and snores very loudly to compensate for air. Breathing can cease for up to 10 seconds or longer. As a result of this erratic breathing, oxygen deprivation can occur.

Sleep apnea typically affects overweight, middle-aged men and in severe cases, can be life-threatening. Prolonged sleep apnea can lead to excessive fatigue, high blood pressure, stroke, and personality changes. Victims of sleep apnea usually do not feel rested in the morning and may experience difficulty staying awake or concentrating. Sleep apnea has been linked to some cases of infant death syndrome.

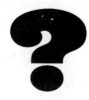

CAUSES:

Possible causes of snoring include congested sinuses; swollen sinuses, adenoids, or tonsils; a deviated septum; chronic allergies; a nasal obstruction; being overweight; and sleeping on your back, which causes tissue in the upper airway and the tongue to vibrate upon breathing. Nighttime drinking can also aggravate snoring. Sleeping pills and tranquilizers can also produce snoring and should be avoided if possible.

Certain antihistamines can also cause one to snore. Smoking can also contribute to snoring by causing respiratory tract tissue to thicken and produce more mucus. Smoking is particularly damaging for someone with sleep apnea, because it further decreases the body's oxygen supply.

Other factors which can cause sleep apnea include: physical abnormalities of the chest, back or neck; brain disorders; obesity; hypothyroidism; acromegaly; consuming alcohol; and taking sleep inducers. People who typically snore very loudly can also be prone to sleep apnea. Some cases may be the result of a malfunction of the medulla in the brain, which causes disrupted breathing patterns.

Note: A lack of sleep can cause snoring and aggravate the cycle of sleep apnea. Try to go to bed early and rise early so that the quality of sleep improves.

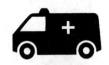

MEDICAL ALERT:

Sleep apnea is a condition that warrants a visit to your physician. If you feel fatigued and know that you are a heavy snorer who stops breathing from time to time in between snores, see your physician.

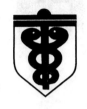

STANDARD MEDICAL TREATMENT:

For sleep-related disorders, your doctor will probably refer you to a sleep disorder clinic. Your physician will first examine you to see if you have a nasal obstruction, swollen adenoids, a deviated septum or enlarged tonsils which can cause snoring. Any physical obstructions or anatomical deformities will be addressed. A device that forces air under pressure into the nose and the back of the throat and keeps the airway from collapsing may be suggested for victims of sleep apnea. In addition, a steady supply of oxygen which is inhaled while sleeping is also sometimes prescribed.

An antidepressant drug called protriptyline (Vivactil) benefits some victims of sleep apnea. If a malfunction of the medulla exists, medroxyprogesterone (Provera) may be prescribed to stimulate breathing.

Surgical options: Removing tissue, adenoids, or nasal obstructions or creating a special opening in the windpipe may be necessary in severe cases of sleep apnea. In extreme cases which are due to brain disorders, a pacemaker may have to be implanted in the diaphragm to stimulate breathing.

Side-effects: Protriptyline(Vivactil): Blood pressure changes, abnormal heart rates, hallucinations, disorientation, anxiety, restlessness, numbness, tingling in the limbs, dry mouth, convulsions, and lack of coordination are only a few of the documented side-effects of this family of drugs.

Warning: Pregnant women or nursing mothers should not take this medication unless specifically instructed to do so by their physicians.

Success rating of standard medical treatment: fair. Usually, losing weight will benefit the victim of sleep apnea more than any other medical treatment. Surgical corrections are sometimes effective and supportive measures such as oxygen administration while sleeping may help to avoid future complications.

MEDICAL UPDATE:

New surgical procedures have recently been used to treat sleep apnea and should be investigated. New laser treatments are currently under study at several U.S. medical centers. Surgery to alleviate snoring is usually expensive and requires general anesthesia. A new laser approach trims excess tissue from the tonsils, soft palate and the uvula and can be done on an outpatient basis using a local anesthetic. Patients will need two to five 30-minute treatments and can return to work the same day. Researchers are hoping to have this laser surgery available this year.

HOME SELF-CARE:

◆ Attach a rolled-up sock to the back of your pajamas so that when you lie on your back when sleeping, it creates enough discomfort that you roll over.

◆ Keep humidity levels in the bedroom high enough so that mucous membranes do not dry out.

◆ Go to bed at the same time each night and get an adequate amount of sleep.

◆ Sleep with a pillow that is designed to support your neck, which can be purchased at a medical supply house.

◆ Use a firm mattress. Soft and saggy mattresses can contribute to airway obstruction and poor sleeping posture.

◆ Sleeping with an oxygen mask is sometimes recommended in severe cases of sleep apnea to avoid deprivation when breathing stops.

◆ Self-hypnosis and biofeedback may prove valuable in treating both snoring and sleep apnea. The power of suggestion has proven valuable in controlling snoring and should be investigated.

NUTRITIONAL APPROACH:

◆ Avoid eating foods that can cause allergies such as wheat, dairy products and seafood. These food may cause nasal congestion, which can result in snoring.

◆ *Calcium lactate or chelate and magnesium:* Helps to relax the nerves and muscles and promotes sleep.

◆ A lack of the B vitamins, especially pantothenic acid and inositol can cause fitful, unrestful sleep.

◆ Eat foods that are naturally high in tryptophan to promote restful sleep including turkey, bananas, dates, yogurt and whole grains.

◆ Do not consume caffeine, alcohol, white sugar, or chocolate and do not use nicotine.

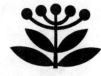

HERBAL REMEDIES:

◆ *Catnip:* Helps to induce sleep.

◆ *Hops:* Calms the nerves and is considered a natural hypnotic.

◆ *Skullcap:* A traditional herbal remedy for insomnia and other sleep-related disorders.

◆ *Valerian root:* Valerian root helps to relieve tension, anxiety and stress and promotes sleep without the side-effects associated with commercial or over-the-counter sleeping pills.

◆ *A combination of the following herbs may be useful:* Skullcap, catnip, passion flower and chamomile.

PREVENTION:

◆ Don't consume alcohol, which can play a major role in snoring.
◆ Switch from antihistamines that cause drowsiness to ones that contain terfrnadine (Seldane) to treat hay fever.
◆ Lose weight. Being obese is a major contributing factory to both snoring and sleep apnea.
◆ Don't sleep on your back. Retrain yourself to sleep on your side or stomach.
◆ Do not smoke. Smoking can cause respiratory irritation and contribute to snoring.
◆ Exercise regularly. Exercise helps to make the entire cardiovascular system more efficient and promotes a more restful sleep.
◆ Keep your nasal passages from becoming congested.
◆ Don't eat right before going to bed.

American Sleep Disorders Association
604 Second Street SW
Rochester, MN 55902

Sore Throat

DEFINITION AND SYMPTOMS:

Most of us rarely notice how often we swallow until we have the misfortune of getting a sore throat. Having a sore throat can also make you feel sick all over.

In technical terms, a sore throat refers to a raw or painful sensation which usually occurs in the back of the throat and causes discomfort when one swallows. It is an extremely common condition and can result from a number of factors. Throat pain that is accompanied by swollen lymph glands is usually a sign of either a viral or bacterial infection. Coughing does not usually accompany strep throat, and white spots can appear on the tonsils in both strep and viral infections. The intensity of the pain of a sore throat does not always indicate its seriousness. A simple sore throat usually lasts for 3 to 5 days.

CAUSES:

A sore throat can be caused by pharyngitis, tonsillitis, colds, influenza, laryngitis, infectious mononucleosis and other viral illnesses such as measles, mumps and chicken pox. Some sore throats result from a bacterial infection caused by the streptococcal bacteria. If this particular type of sore throat is left untreated, it may result in rheumatic fever, which can cause subsequent heart valve damage (refer to chapter on rheumatic fever). Strep throat usually affects children.

Sore throats experienced by adults will rarely have a bacterial cause. Other possible causes of sore throats include mouth breathing, allergies, smoking, dust, fumes, chemical agents, very hot foods, abrasions, or a tooth or gum infection. Coughing for extended periods of time or clearing the throat too often can also cause throat irritation. In some instances, an earache will cause pain upon swallowing if the eustachian tube is irritated. These types of sore throats occur on one side only.

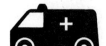

MEDICAL ALERT:

Any sore throat that is accompanied by difficulty in breathing, excessive drooling, a temperature of 101 degrees F. or greater, joint pain, a lump in the neck, prolonged hoarseness, blood in the saliva, pus in the back of the throat, or a rash should be seen by a doctor immediately. An untreated strep throat can result in a throat abscess, an inflammation of the kidneys and rheumatic fever.

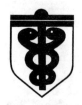

STANDARD MEDICAL TREATMENT:

Your doctor will almost always take a throat culture, and examine the nose, ears and throat. A throat culture can only detect the presence of the beta-strep bacteria, which is treated with penicillin. Routinely, antibiotics (some form of penicillin) will be prescribed regardless of the type of sore throat present. In the case of repeated sore throats in children, a tonsillectomy will sometimes be suggested.

Success rating of standard medical treatment: poor to good. Most doctors are quick to treat every sore throat with antibiotics, whether the infection is bacterially or virally caused. Antibiotics are useless against viral infection. Using antibiotics for sore throats caused by the strep bacteria is very effective and highly recommended to prevent more serious infections.

Removing the tonsils to decrease the frequency of sore throats in children is often ineffective. Unfortunately, the tonsillectomy is an operation that is often unnecessary.

Note: If a throat culture is performed, ask your doctor whether the infection is viral or bacterial. If it is viral, you may want to skip antibiotic treatment. Taking antibiotics can weaken the immune system, trigger an allergic reaction, and kill friendly intestinal bacteria. If there is a history of rheumatic fever in your family, or if you have scarlet fever or an outbreak of rheumatic fever has occurred, then immediate antibiotic treatment of a sore throat is warranted and prudent.

MEDICAL UPDATE:

◆ Home throat culture kits may soon be available that enable anyone to check for the presence of a strep infection without going to their doctor's office.

HOME SELF-CARE:

Warning: Do not give children aspirin to avoid the possibility of contracting Reye's syndrome.
◆ Gargles are an excellent way to treat most sore throats. For bacterial infections, gargle with a mixture of half water and half hydrogen peroxide.
◆ Other gargles that are good for sore throats include liquid chlorophyll and sea salt, salt and warm water and liquid vitamin C, and lemon and honey.
◆ Sucking on cold popsicles or fruit bars can help soothe the pain of a sore throat. Lozenges that contain phenol can help to numb the pain of a sore throat (phenol-containing sprays are not as effective or long lasting as the lozenges). Recommended over-the-counter lozenges are Ricola, Mentholyptus, and natural black licorice drops.
◆ Apply a soft ice bag covered in flannel to the throat.
◆ Foot massage, acupressure, chiropractic treatments and reflexology have all been used for sore throats and have received mixed reviews. Try some of these approaches. These systems unquestionably improve circulation, which can boost the body's defense mechanisms against invading pathogens.
◆ Take a stiff bristle hairbrush and tap your lymph glands and throat area several times a day. External stimulation with the pointy bristles helps to bring more blood to the area, which can facilitate healing.
◆ Keep your environment humidified to prevent sore throats that occur from too much dryness in the air. Inhaling cool mist from a cool mist vaporizer can also help to soothe irritated throats.
◆ The lion position in yoga is considered a good treatment for recurring sore throats.

NUTRITIONAL APPROACH:

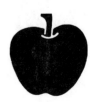

◆ Eat cloves of raw garlic to fight both viral and bacterial infection. Capsulized garlic is also recommended.
◆ Increase your intake of fluids through citrus fruit juices (orange, lemon, limes, grapefruits), carrot juice, herbal teas and vegetable broths. Forcing fluids helps to cleanse the lymph system and eliminate toxins.

- Avoid caffeine, which acts like a diuretic and can deplete your body of much-needed fluids.
- Decrease solid foods and concentrate on liquid forms of food for the first two days of a sore throat.
- *Vitamin C with bioflavonoids:* Helps to heal damaged tissue and detoxify the body during any kind of infection. Use powdered vitamin C in fruit juice several times a day.
- *Vitamin A emulsion:* Can enter the system quickly, and helps in the healing of inflamed tissue and in strengthening the immune system.
- *Zinc lozenges:* Helps to kill bacteria and promote tissue healing. Can also help with pain. Use zinc gluconate or a lozenge that contains zinc. Do not take zinc for longer than a few days, or it may deplete your body of other minerals.
- *Chlorophyll drinks:* Helps to potentiate the immune system to fight infection.
- *Acidophilus:* Vital if taking any kind of antibiotic. Acidophilus will help to replace friendly bacteria which is killed during antibiotic therapy.

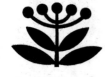

HERBAL REMEDIES:

Note: Any of the herbs listed can be used as gargles if made into a strong tea.
- *Echinacea:* A natural antibiotic that fights both viral and bacterial infection and boosts the immune system.
- *Golden seal:* A strong herbal antibiotic that has none of the side-effects of commercial antibiotics.
- *Marshmallow:* Helps to heal irritated mucous membranes.
- *Slippery elm:* Good for irritated throat tissue. Taken as a tea, slippery elm can help coat and soothe inflamed throats.
- Make a gargle out of chamomile and slippery elm tea.
- Combining horehound tea, honey, a pinch of cayenne pepper and a teaspoon of honey is also recommended as a tried-and-true sore throat remedy.
- A hot chamomile compress placed on the throat can help with pain.
- Strong clove tea flavored with honey can be sipped several times a day for sore throat.
- *Agrimony:* Acts as an astringent and healing agent for irritated mucous membranes.
- *Hyssop:* Works to help heal throats and fights infections which may be present.
- *Lady's mantle:* Works to reduce inflammation and is also good for laryngitis.
- *Loosestrife:* A natural astringent that helps soothe inflammation and is particularly good if a fever accompanied the sore throat.
- *Echinacea:* An antibacterial herb that is good for sore throats caused by tonsillitis.

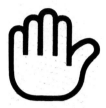

PREVENTION:

◆ Don't sleep with your mouth open. If you need to shrink swollen nasal membranes, consult your doctor and evaluate your options.

◆ Eat a diet high in fresh fruits and vegetables and take a vitamin C supplement every day to ward off infection.

◆ Change your toothbrush often to prevent bacteria which could cause recurring throat infections.

◆ Don't smoke: Smoking constantly irritates mucosal lining of both the throat and the lungs. If you don't smoke, stay away from smoke-filled environments.

◆ Keep your home well humidified, especially during the winter months, and don't overheat the house while sleeping.

Sprains and Strains

DEFINITION:

Both sprains and strains usually occur when you least expect it. A harmless looking dip in the lawn can cause you to abruptly twist your ankle and go flying. The irony of both sprains and strains is that frequently, they can cause more pain and discomfort than a fracture. To effectively treat these kinds of muscle injuries, you must learn the difference between a sprain and a strain.

A strain occurs when a muscle is stressed beyond its capability due to putting excess weight on the muscle or overusing it. Strains are also referred to as pulled muscles. Strains typically occur in the hamstring, quadricep muscles of the thigh, groin muscles and shoulder muscles. A sprain, on the other hand, results when a ligament which connects bone to muscle is stretched to the point of tearing. In this case, the soft tissue which surrounds the joint may become inflamed.

Strains and sprains are treated much the same way, except that in strains, heat can be initially applied to promote healing. In the case of a severe sprain, treatment should be the same as for a fracture or a broken bone. Any joint can become sprained and the severity of that sprain depends on the extent of the ligament tear. Knees, ankles and fingers are especially susceptible to injury. Most people will refer to any painful joint injury as a sprain, although that may be technically incorrect. The majority of strains and sprains heal within two weeks.

CAUSES:

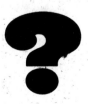

Sprains occur from unexpected movements or twisting motions typical of falls or athletic injuries. Muscles commonly become overstretched during vigorous exercise. Sprains also commonly occur when dancing, playing tennis, soccer, hiking, or during downhill skiing. If the demands placed on a muscle are excessive, a ligament tear results.

Strains are milder than sprains and usually result in a muscle that contracts and becomes stiff and painful. Strained or pulled muscles commonly result when lifting a heavy weight, playing golf or stretching to catch a baseball.

SYMPTOMS:

Strains: A strained muscle will feel sore and stiff but will not swell or become black and blue like a sprained one. Strains usually impair mobility.

Sprains: Pain and tenderness in the joint area is typical of a sprain, although the joint will usually still function to some extent. Other symptoms include swelling, which usually occurs quickly due to bleeding into the tissue surrounding the joint. Bruising is also common, and in severe cases, a deformed appearance to the joint may occur.

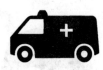

MEDICAL ALERT:

If pain and swelling persist for over two days, see your physician immediately to eliminate the possibility of a fractured or broken bone. Frequently people assume they have a sprain when, in fact, a break in the bone has occurred.

FIRST AID:

First aid for strains: Use heat initially on the strained area with a heating pad or hot water bottle for 15 minutes several times a day.

For sprains:
◆ Do not use the injured part.
◆ Elevate the affected area using pillows or a sling.
◆ Apply the cold pack for several hours, and the pain and swelling will reduce.
◆ After 24 hours, heat may be applied.
◆ Support the joint involved with an elastic bandage and do not put any weight on the area for at least two days.

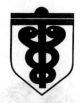

STANDARD MEDICAL TREATMENT:

In cases of severe sprains, an x-ray will be ordered by your doctor to rule out a fracture, and the joint may be casted. Watching for swelling is important if casting has occurred, because it can decrease circulation. Analgesics may be prescribed for pain and in extreme cases, nonsteroidal anti-inflammatory drugs may be recommended. Occasionally, surgery may be required to repair badly torn ligaments.

In these cases, future physical therapy will be recommended to restrengthen the joint and restore mobility.

Success rating of standard medical treatment: good. Most strains and sprains can be treated at home; however, in severe cases, casting may be required. The debate between the use of cold vs. hot therapy is still ongoing, with varying opinions on the value of both.

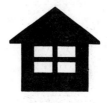

HOME SELF-CARE:

◆ If you suspect a sprain, which is identified by swelling and bruising, rest the joint by elevating it to drain fluids and apply ice packs to reduce swelling.
◆ With a strain, which does not swell or bruise, apply a hot water bottle or heating pad to the area for 15 minutes several times per day. Heat increases the circulation to the area and promotes the production of collagen, which is crucial to proper healing.
◆ Do not place any weight on the injured area.
◆ Let pain be your guide to activities. If it hurts, don't do it.
◆ An elastic bandage can be used to wrap a sprain and provide support; however, make sure that it is not so tight as to impair circulation. The Ace bandage should be firm but not tight. There should not be any purple or bluish color to the area. Do not stretch the bandage as you wind it on. The stretchiness is for mobility purposes. Wrap the bandage as you would a roll of gauze.
◆ Tumeric and hot water can be combined to form a paste that can be applied to the sprained or bruised area with a gauze dressing to reduce swelling. Clay poultices can accomplish the same thing.
◆ Apple cider vinegar compresses are also good to help reduce swelling and pain.

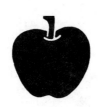

NUTRITIONAL APPROACH:

◆ *Bromelain:* Drink plenty of pineapple juice immediately after the injury. Pineapple has an enzyme called bromelain which helps with bruising and can promote healing.
◆ *Vitamin B complex:* Important for any tissue repair.
◆ *Calcium/magnesium:* Essential for the proper healing of bone and connective tissue.
◆ *Potassium and silicon:* Helps to promote calcium absorption and contributes to connective tissue repair and strength.
◆ *Vitamin C:* Functions in connective tissue repair and works as a natural anti-inflammatory. It also helps to strengthen and repair broken capillaries, which can speed the healing of bruises.
◆ *Zinc:* Promotes tissue repair.

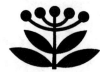

Herbal remedies:

◆ Mullein poultice or paste applied to the sprain can help control swelling.

◆ *Thyme:* Stimulates blood flow to injured tissues. Use an oil to add to a warm compress after swelling has gone down.

◆ *Arnica:* Comes from the high mountains of western North America and is a traditional remedy used for bruising and sprains. Use it externally in cream or tincture form to decrease bruising and discoloration. Arnica can be purchased in some drugstores and in herb shops. Do not take internally.

◆ A paste made from five egg whites, cayenne pepper, and thyme leaves can be applied on a gauze bandage to the sprain to promote circulation.

◆ *Comfrey:* Comfrey has been traditionally used for centuries as a bone knitter and wound healer. Soak the ankle or affected area in comfrey tea and take internally for its healing properties. Comfrey encourages cell growth in the connective tissues and the bones.

◆ *Horsetail:* Beneficial for bone and connective tissue health. Promotes healing in both.

◆ *The following herbs in combination may be useful:* Comfrey, mullein, pan pien lien, white oak bark, marshmallow root and queen of the meadow.

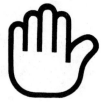

Prevention:

◆ Strengthening weak muscles through proper exercise can help avoid strains and sprains. Stretching before exercising and staying flexible are important preventive measures. Staying fit is probably the best deterrent to sprains and strains.

◆ Use good, supportive shoes that fit well during athletic activities.

◆ Walk or jog in well-lit areas to avoid falling in divots and hidden ruts.

◆ Don't overdo when exercising and avoid violent twisting motions.

◆ Use elastic supports around areas susceptible to injury such as ankles or knees.

Stress

DEFINITION:

Unfortunately, becoming "stressed out" is a normal part of our hurry-up-and-wait kind of lives. Most of us are busier than we should be and, in addition, have to deal with money pressures, traffic jams, irritable bosses, whiny children, and car trouble. While our pioneer ancestors may have had to endure more physical stress, we have to carry the everyday mental burden of being aware of crime, wars, pestilence and calamities all over the world (not to mention following everyday politics).

While in and of itself stress in not necessarily bad, individual reaction to stress can produce undesirable and detrimental results, such as prolonged states of anxiety, or even a host of medical disorders. Some doctors believe that the majority of their patients have stress-related complaints.

Unquestionably, stress-related medical and emotional problems have dramatically increased over the last few decades and testify to the fast-paced, demanding lives that most of us lead. The fact that Valium and Tagamet are among the most widely prescribed drugs in the world indicates that stress-related disorders truly exist in epidemic proportions.

CAUSES:

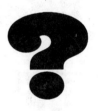

Stress can be the by-product of several things which can become a routine part of some life-styles. These include death of a loved one, financial problems, alcoholism, job-related pressures, deadlines, problematic family relationships including marital discord, difficult in-laws, and teenagers. Stress and anxiety can result from crowded environments, high traffic areas, loneliness, medical concerns, divorce and single parenting, PMS, and the overscheduling of one's life.

Long-term stress is typical of caregivers of the elderly and physically or mentally handicapped. When the body fails to effectively manage stress, various physical and mental symptoms can result. During periods of prolonged stress, the body can react by increasing adrenalin, which elevates heart rate, shuts down digestion and results in elevated blood pressure and faster breathing. In addition, fats, cholesterol and sugars can be released from body stores. Internalizing stress can keep the mind agitated and throw the nervous system off. A number of biological changes can be initiated by stressors.

SYMPTOMS:

Physical: Stress related ailments include ulcers, colitis, high blood pressure, heartburn, headaches, backaches, neck aches, diarrhea, loss of appetite, dizziness, asthma, skin rashes, hives, heart palpations, impotence, hair loss, TMJ syndrome, and lowered immunity.

More serious diseases which are thought to be associated with prolonged stress or anxiety are angina, autoimmune diseases, cancer, Crohn's disease, diverticulosis, heart disease, impotence, menstrual irregularities, migraine headaches, rheumatoid arthritis and pancreatic disease.

Psychological: Under periods of prolonged stress, one can become anxious, fearful, angry or depressed. Stress can induce the following symptoms irritability, short temper, insomnia, over-or undereating, panic attacks, forgetfulness, crying or a decline in productivity.

Counseling one-on-one or in support groups can be of great value if coping with stress becomes too difficult. Psychotherapy alone doesn't make life easier. It can, however, provide coping skills and relaxation techniques in combination with providing a controlled setting in which to unload emotional baggage.

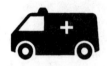

Medical alert:

Seek medical help if you are experiencing the following symptoms:
- blackouts or dizzy spells
- trembling
- hives
- chronic pain
- racing pulse or palpitations
- overwhelming anxiety or panic

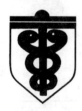

Standard medical treatment:

Drug therapy is commonly used by doctors to treat stress-related disorders. The most common are the benzodiazepines, which include Valium, Librium, Xanax and Ativan. Because insomnia typically accompanies anxiety, sleeping pills are also routinely prescribed. Triazolam (Halcion) is a benzodiazepine most commonly used as a sedative. Your doctor may also advise counseling through psychotherapy.

Side-effects: Benzodiazepines (Valium, Librium, Xanax, Ativan): This family of highly addictive depressants interferes with normal mental function. If benzodiazepines are taken over a long period of time and stopped, significant withdrawal symptoms may occur. Side-effects of benzodiazepines include drowsiness, confusion, depression, lethargy, headache, slurred speech, stupor, and tremors.

Warning: Do not take this drug for the first three months of pregnancy. These drugs can increase the risk of birth defects and create a dependency in the developing baby. Do not breast feed if taking a drug from this family of drugs.

Triazolam (Halcion): Side-effects Drowsiness, headache, dizziness, nervousness, light-headedness, poor muscle coordination, nausea, vomiting, and confusion.

Warning: This drug should not be used by pregnant or nursing women or anyone under the age of 18.

Note: Recently halcion has been implicated as a factor in precipitating suicide. New investigations have refuted this correlation and the FDA considers Halcion a safe drug according to its criteria.

Success rating of standard medical treatment: fair. Medical science usually approaches the management of stress with drug therapy. While in severe cases, tranquilizers, antidepressants and sleeping pills may be necessary, frequently, these therapies are counterproductive and have significant negative side-effects. Managing stress through good diet, exercise, relaxation techniques and counseling is preferable to becoming dependent on drugs.

HOME SELF-CARE:

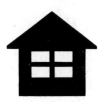

- Exercise regularly. The importance of exercise in relieving stress cannot be over emphasized. Exercise releases endorphins in the brain, which create a sense of well-being as well as provide a release for pent-up tension.
- The conscious regulation of breathing can be an invaluable technique for achieving relaxation. Exhale completely through your mouth slowly. Inhale through your nose to the mental count of four. Hold your breath for a mental count of seven. Exhale slowly and completely through your mouth to a mental count of eight. Repeat the cycle three more times. This exercise can act as a natural tranquilizer.
- Learn yoga techniques to control breathing, relax muscles and meditate. Transcendental meditation can be of great benefit in relieving tension.
- Get a regular professional massage. Massage therapy is wonderful for easing tension and soothing the nerves. A good massage is relatively inexpensive and a skilled therapist can work wonders.
- Leave your job at work and make a commitment to leave work promptly.
- Don't be afraid to say no. Stay in charge of your life and your calendar. It is better to underschedule than to overdo it.
- Get a dog or cat to care for. Petting a dog can ease tension and lower blood pressure.
- Avoid taking any over-the-counter or prescription drug you don't need. Several drugs can cause agitation and anxiety. Over-the-counter antihistamines can cause extreme restlessness and depression.
- Get away from urban areas into the country or the mountains and let nature work its magic on your nerves.
- Take long, warm baths or get a spa.
- Listen to soothing classical music when driving through traffic.
- Avoid listening to the news, the radio or reading the newspaper if these

activities produce stress or anxiety.

◆ Don't react to irritating comments from others. Avoid political or religious topics that make you feel volatile.

◆ Unplug the telephone during dinner or in the evening and invest in some soothing music.

◆ Make sure you set a strict bedtime for children so you can count on some quiet evening time for yourself.

◆ Join a bowling league or involve yourself in some other hobby or group activity.

◆ Try hypnotherapy, yoga, biofeedback or music therapy to relax and meditate. Deep breathing exercises are very good for relieving tension.

◆ Pray and regularly attend a worship service. The power of prayer and the role of spirituality have been sadly undervalued by health care providers in our society. People who have a solid spiritual foundation are generally much more able to cope with stressors that all of us experience at one time or another.

◆ Make your bedroom a restful, quiet place where you can relax and unwind.

◆ Get professional counseling if you need extra coping skills.

◆ Don't wear tight or uncomfortable clothing or shoes.

◆ Keep your environment cool rather than too warm.

◆ If you need to, change jobs, relationships, or move to a new location. Career-oriented people who had decided to climb the corporate ladder in large urban areas sometimes abandon their original plan, move to a small urban community and settle for a much lower salary. They compensate for their money loss with more peace of mind.

◆ Learn to see the humor in life and laugh heartily and often. Laughing releases endorphins in the brain which make us feel better and happier. When you find yourself in a stressful situation, such as a traffic jam or waiting in an eternal line at the division of motor vehicles, find the humor in it. Keep humorous cassettes in the car and pop them in when you feel tension mounting.

Nutritional approach:

◆ Avoid alcohol, caffeine and nicotine. These in and of themselves can create stress on the body and the emotions. Coffee, tea, chocolate, and caffeine drinks can alter mental states and increase internal stress. Caffeine and nicotine can actually raise adrenalin levels in the body and make us feel nervous and on edge.

◆ Avoid eating white sugar products, heavily spiced foods, colas, fried foods, MSG, and high-fat junk foods. These foods can heighten the stress response.

◆ Eat plenty of complex carbohydrates to keep blood sugar levels stable and supply energy.

◆ Eat a nutritious breakfast and don't eat a heavy meal before going to sleep.

- The adrenal glands are directly responsible for our reaction to stressors. Proper diet helps to keep these glands functioning properly.
- *Vitamin B complex:* The 17 vitamins which belong to this category are considered stress vitamins and are essential for maintaining good mental health and the proper function of the nervous system.
- *Pantothenic acid:* Important for healthy adrenal gland function, which is vital to coping with stressors. It is also considered a natural antidepressant which can reduce anxiety and help to promote sleep.
- *Vitamin E:* Helps to protect the glands, especially during periods of stress.
- *Vitamin C:* Helps to stimulate adrenal function, which may become impaired during prolonged periods of stress.
- *Zinc and calcium/magnesium:* Both help to calm and control feelings of nervousness.
- *Potassium:* Helps to relieve insomnia and boosts glandular function.
- *L-tyrosine:* An amino acid which helps to reduce stress and promote sleep.
- *GABA:* An amino acid plus inositol that acts as a tranquilizer.
- *Lecithin:* Helps to protect nerve fibers.

HERBAL REMEDIES:

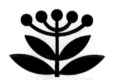

- *Chamomile and peppermint tea:* Relaxes and calms the nerves.
- Lavender, basil and rosemary oil massage can relax tense muscles.
- *Passion flower:* A natural tranquilizer which is not sedating and can be taken in tincture form.
- *Valerian root:* Relaxes the nervous system and helps to reduce nervous tension.
- *Mistletoe:* Tones the nerves and is considered a natural tranquilizer.
- *Wood betony:* An herbal nervine which can be taken in tea form.
- *Lobelia:* A powerful herbal nerve relaxant.
- *Scullcap:* A restorative and relaxant for the central nervous system.
- *Hops:* A natural sleep inducer and nervous system relaxant.
- *Suma:* Helps the body cope with environmental and psychological stress.
- *Neroli oil:* An antidepressant and sedative that can help combat panic attacks or palpitations resulting from anxiety.
- *Gotu kola:* Counteracts depression.
- *Vervain:* A relaxing herbal nervine.
- *The following herbs in combination may be useful:* Lobelia, scullcap, hops and ginseng. These are considered tonics for the adrenal glands, which improve the body's ability to function under stressful conditions.

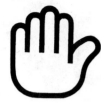

PREVENTION:

Preventing stress-related disorders involves becoming self-aware and incorporating good habits into everyday routines. Many of the self-help suggestions and nutritional guidelines work as preventive measures as well.

◆ A nutritious diet, regular exercise and the ability to recognize "red flags" which indicate that stress levels are too high can contribute to preventing anxiety.

◆ Learning to relax is vital. Today there are a number of ways to control stress and lessen its detrimental effects. Some of these are biofeedback, yoga, music therapy, self hypnosis, breathing exercises, music therapy and stretching exercises. Taking time every day to relax is essential to the maintenance of good mental and physical health.

◆ Find some spiritual direction, and establish a routine in which you pray or meditate regularly.

Stroke

DEFINITION

While most people believe that a stroke usually strikes without warning, in most cases there are specific identifiable stroke risk factors. Today we know that a high cholesterol count can significantly raise your risk for strokes. Once again, Western life-styles and high-fat diets have significantly contributed to the incidence of strokes.

Strokes are caused by a reduction in blood flow to a particular area of the brain which results in oxygen starvation of brain cells and tissue death. Strokes cause a significant amount of disability and death in the United States, although they are half as common as they were 25 years ago due to better high blood pressure control.

Strokes commonly strike older people between the ages of 60 and 80. Many of the risk factors for a heart attack apply to strokes as well. Strokes are more common in people who have diabetes and a high cholesterol count. As in the case of heart attacks, the damage from a stroke can vary with each individual. In mild strokes, full recovery is common. Moderate strokes will usually leave some permanent effect ranging from a minor speech impediment to total paralysis. Specific damage is determined by the location and extent of the stroke. Each year in the United States 170,000 people die from strokes. Approximately 50 percent of stroke cases experience a full or partial recovery within a few months.

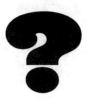

CAUSES:

Blood flow to the brain can be obstructed by clogged or narrowed arteries, by the rupture of a blood vessel or by the lodging of a clot or piece of plaque within an artery. Blood clots cause half of all strokes. Arteriosclerosis, high blood pressure, a cerebral embolism, and cerebral hemorrhage can all result in a stroke.

Coronary artery disease (atherosclerosis) is the most common cause of stroke. Factors that increase the risk of having a stroke are diabetes, obesity, irregular heart beats, damaged heart valves, a recent heart attack, smoking, high blood cholesterol and possibly birth control pills.

Note: A person with even a moderate elevation in blood pressure runs six times the risk of experiencing a stroke than someone with normal blood pressure.

SYMPTOMS:

Physical: Frequently, a stroke is preceded by a number of warning signs brought on by temporary spells of impaired brain function caused by brief reductions in blood flow. These may include temporary weakness, fainting, loss of memory, paralysis, loss of vision, difficulty speaking, numbness, clumsiness, blurred vision, dizziness, loss of hearing and disorientation.

These warning signs are called TIA's (transient ischemic attacks) and last a short time because the blockage is temporary. Contrary to popular belief, headaches are uncommon with strokes. A full-blown stroke may cause a loss of consciousness, paralysis on one side of the body, the inability to speak, double vision, memory impairment, confusion, and numbness. Unlike the warning symptoms of a stroke, these will persist for at least 24 hours or longer.

Psychological: One of the worst complications of a stroke is the depression that can follow. In most cases this depression passes and is considered very treatable.

Being aware that this is a normal reaction in a stroke patient helps both the stroke victim and his family deal with the stroke in a more productive manner. Emotional support at this time is vital to recovery. Stroke patients require a great deal of patience while they relearn old skills. Feelings of anger and frustration are normal following a stroke. A positive attitude can greatly enhance recovery.

MEDICAL ALERT:

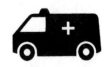

If you notice any of the above warning signs of a stroke, contact your doctor or a hospital immediately. Anticlotting agents may be prescribed to prevent the onset of a stroke. Any unexplained fainting, dizziness, paralysis or visual or hearing disturbances need immediate medical attention.

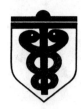

STANDARD MEDICAL TREATMENT:

Brain scans such as CT scanning can now pinpoint the exact location of a stroke and rule out the possibility of a brain tumor, abscess or subdural hematoma. A carotid arteriogram, which is a special x-ray of the arteries, may be required to assess whether surgery to prevent further strokes is possible.

Other tests that your doctor may order are chest x-rays, an ECG, and MRI. To make sure stroke victims are well-nourished, your physician may want to use intravenous feedings and nasogastric tubes. In addition, preventing infection, and bedsores and keeping the limbs mobile, will also be high on the medical priority list. To prevent the accumulation of fluid within the brain, corticosteroid drugs may be used.

Drugs can control high blood pressure and keep the blood thin. In rare occasions, surgical repair of a damaged artery or manually removing a clot may be possible. Physical therapy is important in stroke patients who have lost the use of a limb. Vocal therapy can help to retrain vocalize skills and pronunciation. Your doctor will recommend various specialists who are skilled in these areas.

Success rating of standard medical treatment: fair. Stroke patients often require hospitalization and they should get immediate medical attention. Unfortunately, medical science cannot cure strokes. Adopting a healthy life-style can go a long way toward preventing strokes. For impaired mobility following a stroke, proper physical therapy is essential to keep muscles from withering.

MEDICAL UPDATE:

◆ Sensitive ultrasound screening can detect lesions in the arteries, which are considered silent predictors of stroke. This procedure locates potentially dangerous changes in the carotid artery which could result in a stroke. An Angioview 600 ultrasound machine is used for this purpose and has only become available within the last two years. Ideally, in the future, people at high risk for a stroke could have this kind of examination on a periodic basis.

◆ Recent studies have confirmed that cigarette smoke inhibits two components that clear excess cholesterol from artery walls and that it also damaged HDL's or "good" cholesterol.

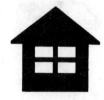

HOME SELF-CARE

The positive and supportive attitude of caregivers for the stroke patient is the one most important factors in promoting recovery. Patience is vital. The relearning of speech and movement take time.

◆ Take advantage of community rehabilitation organizations. Contact your hospital or health centers for sources.

◆ Social workers and physical therapists can make home visits. Make sure they are accredited and check Medicare coverage policies.

◆ You may need to have ramps and handrails installed in strategic places during the recovery process. If you are in a wheelchair, often just changing the hinges on a door can allow for a complete swingback of the door, allowing the wheelchair to move freely.

◆ Keep your environment barrier-free.

◆ Put grab bars near the toilet and tub areas.

◆ Get rid of throw rugs, large floor pillows, boxes, stools and furniture that gets in the way.

◆ Supervised swimming is an excellent exercise for recovering stroke victims and can also provide valuable physical therapy.

◆ Board games can help sharpen mental skills.

◆ Working at the computer can gradually develop hand-eye coordination.

◆ Keep yourself attractive by dressing nicely and keeping hair clean.

Suggestions for the caregiver:

◆ Encourage the stroke survivor to do things independently, but keep your expectations realistic.

◆ Keep family life structured, with regular meals, sleep schedules, and activities.

◆ Watch for signs of depression and be a constant source of encouragement. Talk to a stroke survivor often, even if his or her response is limited.

◆ Learn some basic sign language skills to improve communication.

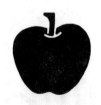

NUTRITIONAL APPROACH:

◆ Eat a diet high in fiber including whole grains such as oat, wheat, barley, millet, buckwheat, cornmeal and brown rice. Eat plenty of raw fruits and vegetables. Add generous amounts of onion and garlic to your diet.

◆ Do not consume alcohol, nicotine or caffeine.

◆ Avoid all animal fats, butter, ice cream, white sugar, white flour, greasy fried foods, high-fat cheeses, and red meats. Eat fish, white meats such as skinless turkey or chicken breast, and drink plenty of fluids.

◆ *Vitamin A and E:* Considered antioxidants, these vitamins can help oxygenate cells and promote tissue repair.

◆ *Vitamin C with bioflavonoids:* Helps to protect the capillaries and cleans and strengthens the veins and arteries.

◆ A chelation combination of vitamins and minerals can help to control plaque deposits in the arteries. Such a combination includes vitamin A, B complex, vitamin C, vitamin E, magnesium, manganese, chromium, potassium, selenium, choline, methionine, zinc, cysteine, iodine, iron and bioflavonoids.

- *Potassium:* Helps to control blood pressure raising factors such as salt. One study suggests that by eating fruits high in potassium, your risk of stroke can be significantly reduced.
- *Chlorophyll:* Helps to rebuild muscle and purify the blood.
- *Lecithin:* Is good for the proper utilization of fats and inhibits the accumulation of fatty deposits in the arteries.
- *CoQ10:* Helps to oxygenate tissues and cells and is good for the cardiovascular system.
- *Germanium:* A tonic for the circulatory system.
- *Salmon oil:* Has essential fatty acids which can help to prevent heart disease.

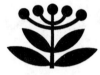

HERBAL REMEDIES:

- *Capsicum:* Helps to clean veins and strengthen artery walls.
- *Burdock:* Improves overall circulation.
- *Ginkgo:* Helps to enhance mental function and clarity.
- *Gotu kola:* An herb which feeds brain cells.
- *Hawthorne:* Works to regulate high blood pressure and prevent hardening of the arteries.
- *Alfalfa:* Can help control blood cholesterol levels.
- *Yarrow:* Relaxes peripheral blood vessels and improves blood flow.
- *Linden:* Helps to prevent arteriosclerosis and promotes the healing of blood vessels.
- *Chickweed:* Helps to dissolve plaque buildup in blood vessels.
- *The following herbs in combination may be useful:* Hawthorne berries, pan pien lien and capsicum.

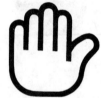

PREVENTION:

- Keep your blood pressure within the normal range. Have it checked frequently. High blood pressure promotes the formation of plaque in the arteries and increases the risk that a weak artery will burst, which can cause a stroke. High blood pressure medication may be necessary.
- Keep blood cholesterol low by eating a high-fiber, low-fat diet. Have your cholesterol levels checked often. Diet is the single most important factor for the prevention of atherosclerosis, which is a leading cause of stroke. Avoid eggs, animal meats, ice cream and butter.
- Keep your salt intake low. In some people, a salt sensitivity can cause blood pressure elevation.
- Don't smoke or drink alcohol. Smoking causing spasms in the artery walls and contributes to a cholesterol buildup in the arteries. Not smoking can decrease

your risk of stroke. Cigarette smoking is directly associated with a hardening of the arteries, which can lead to strokes.

◆ Control stress levels in your life through daily relaxation techniques such as yoga, biofeedback, and self-hypnosis.

◆ Keep your weight within optimum levels by eating right and exercising daily. Aerobic exercise is recommended.

◆ Low doses of aspirin taken daily may help to prevent a stroke if you are at high risk. If you are at high risk for a stroke, other anticoagulant drugs may be prescribed indefinitely. Discuss these options with your doctor. Do not routinely take aspirin without your doctor's approval.

◆ Bypass operations, which reroute blood flow impeded by an obstructed artery, can prevent strokes.

◆ Surgery in which blood vessels are repositioned to supply the brain with adequate oxygen can decrease one's risk for stroke. Another operation done under a local anesthetic is able to open up a roughened section of the carotid artery and clean out any deposits.

◆ Women who smoke should not use birth control pills, which can increase the risk of a stroke due to the formation of blood clots.

FOR MORE INFORMATION CONTACT:

Evergreen Stroke Association
9423 Southeast Thirty-Sixth Street
Mercer Island, WA 98040

Courage Stroke Network
Courage Center
3915 Golden Valley Road
Golden Valley, MN 55422

CAREGIVER SUPPORT:

Children of Aging Parents
2761 Trenton Road
Levittown, PA 19056

Barrier Free Environments
PO Box 30634
Water Garden Highway 70 West
Raleigh, NC 2762280.

TMJ (TMD) (temporomandibular joint syndrome or disorder)

DEFINITION:

TMJ syndrome, (now known as TMD) has become a household term over the last 10 years, and it seemed for a while that almost everyone thought they had it. If your jaw clicks, you can't open your mouth very wide and it hurts to eat corn on the cob, you may be a victim of TMJ syndrome.

TMJ treatments, which range from the sublime to the ridiculous, abound, and finding the right dentist or oral surgeon to treat true TMJ is vital. The sudden awareness of this jaw problem over the last few years is thought by some professionals to be another sign that we live in an age when stress-related disorders are on the increase.

TMJ syndrome refers to pain and a variety of other symptoms found in the facial area which are thought to result from a malfunction of the temporomandibular joint of the jaw, and the muscles that operate the joint. Approximately 10 million Americans suffer from TMJ. True TMJ syndrome can cause a great deal of pain and discomfort, and can be treated by the right specialist.

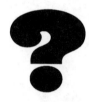

CAUSES:

The most common cause of TMJ syndrome is a spasm of the muscles that control chewing. Factors that can bring about these spasms are teeth grinding or a misaligned bite, which continually places stress on these muscle groups; injuries to the jaw, head or neck; impacted wisdom teeth; emotional stress; nail biting; or chewing the inside of the cheek. In some cases, osteoarthritis and damage to the disc or pad that cushions the joint can also cause TMJ symptoms.

SYMPTOMS:

Physical symptoms are usually more severe in the mornings and can include: frequent headaches, tender jaw muscles, facial pain, pain around the ear, ringing in the ears, toothaches, eye pain, neck pain, clicking or popping jaw joint, difficulty opening the mouth, jaws that get locked or feel as if they have become unhinged, pain upon yawning or chewing, and a fluttering sound in the ears.

Psychological: TMJ is often seen as a stress-related disorder. Stress management, in combination with supportive therapy, can help to control nervous habits which compound TMJ. Clenching or grinding the teeth when under stress can cause significant injury to the jaw joint. Awareness of these habits is crucial to treating and preventing future TMJ problems (refer to chapter on stress).

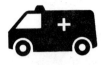

MEDICAL ALERT:

If you cannot eat properly, brush your teeth or are suffering severe headaches, see your physician or dentist.

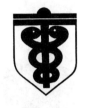

STANDARD MEDICAL TREATMENT:

A combination of moist heat and muscle relaxants may be tried initially by your dentist. If symptoms persist, a bite splint may be prescribed, which fits over the teeth to prevent clenching or grinding. An arthroscope, in which dye is injected into the joint and then viewed with a fluoroscopy, may be required to fully examine the joint. Your doctor will order this test, which is usually done by a radiologist in the x-ray department of a hospital.

If the bite needs correction, an orthodontic appliance may be indicated and in severe cases, jaw surgery may be required to properly align the teeth and jaws. Non-steroidal anti-inflammatory drugs such as Naprosyn, ibuprofen and aspirin are routinely prescribed for TMJ pain. In some cases, a cortisone injection will be administered directly into the temporomandibular joint to relieve inflammation and pain.

Success rating of standard medical treatment: fair to good. TMJ syndrome has become a widespread condition that is often mistreated by dentists, chiropractors and physicians. These treatments can be costly and not particularly effective. The use of splints or surgery should be considered only as last resorts. Jaw joint surgery has had limited success when the meniscus or disc needs replacement. Breaking the jaw to realign the bite is a major operation and involves a significant amount of trauma, pain and discomfort. Relaxation techniques, and proper diet should be employed first and other treatment options assessed.

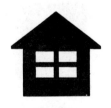

HOME SELF-CARE:

◆ If you are clenching your teeth due to emotional stress, make time for relaxation. Wear a splint if you need to break the habit of grinding or clenching the teeth and keep a record of the times when you engage in the behavior.
◆ Cut food into small, easy-to-chew pieces and eat slowly.
◆ When yawning, be careful not to open the mouth too wide.
◆ Apply soft ice packs to the jaw area that hurts. Moist heat is also recommended, although cold seems to be more beneficial.
◆ Don't bite into an apple, corn on the cob or eat chewy candies like caramels, which can throw your jaw joint into a lock. Avoid hard-to-chew foods such as

bagels, and don't chew gum.

- Don't sleep on your stomach, which puts pressure on one side of your face and can push your jaw joint out of alignment. Using a cervical pillow can encourage sleeping on your back and promote the relaxation of jaw muscles.
- Don't lie on your back and prop your head up at a sharp angle to watch TV.
- Don't try to hold the phone between your head and chin
- Don't wear a heavy shoulder bag that can throw your body alignment off.
- Try biofeedback and controlled breathing exercises to promote relaxation and reduce tension.
- Acupuncture can provide pain relief.

NUTRITIONAL APPROACH:

- Eat nutritious foods that do not stress the jaw joint such as steamed vegetables, soft fruits, fruit and vegetable juices, whole grain cereals and breads, fish, skinless turkey and chicken, yogurt, low-fat cottage cheese, and soups.
- Avoid foods that stress the body such as candy, colas, potato chips, pies and rich pastries, fried and fatty foods and red meats.
- *Calcium/magnesium:* Use citrate or gluconate variety as a muscle relaxant.
- *Vitamin B complex with extra pantothenic acid (vitamin B5):* Helps to control nervousness and stress.
- *L-tyrosine:* An amino acid that helps to promote sleep and fight depression and anxiety.
- *Vitamin C:* Vital to maintaining the health of connective tissue and enabling the body to cope with stress.

HERBAL REMEDIES:

- *Hops:* Helps to promote sleep and minimize tooth grinding.
- *Valerian root:* Considered a natural tranquilizer.
- *Scullcap:* Relieves emotional tension and nervousness.
- *Passion flower:* Relaxes the body and alleviates tension.
- *Gentian:* Works to relieve joint inflammations.
- *Devils' claw:* A powerful botanical anti-inflammatory.
- *Thyme:* An antispasmodic which can help to control muscle cramping.

PREVENTION:

Avoid habits that can damage the jaw joint or initiate muscle spasms. Here are some recommended don'ts:

- Don't chew gum for long periods of time.

- Don't clench or grind your teeth or move your jaw from side to side.
- Don't sleep on your stomach or side.
- Learn to relax and manage tension every day.
- Don't hold your head up by propping your chin in your hands for long periods of time.
- Eat well-balanced meals that fortify the body to manage stress more effectively.
- Don't use alcohol, tobacco or caffeine. These substances can increase stress and deplete the body of essential nutrients.
- Protect your jaw joints from injury by not opening your mouth too wide when yawning or biting down on hard candies.
- Use a cervical pillow, which can train you to sleep on your back.
- If you do heavy weightlifting, don't clench your teeth while lifting.
- Learn to manage stress by taking time to relax each day. Monitor nervous habits that surface when under tension and replace them with deep breathing and other relaxing practices.

Toxic Shock Syndrome

DEFINITION:

Toxic shock syndrome is a newly defined and relatively rare disease which usually affects menstruating women in their late teens or early twenties. It has been linked to the use of highly absorbent synthetic fiber tampons, which trigger infection by the staph bacteria. Toxic shock syndrome can occur in children, older women and men, although cases are rare.

The disease strikes suddenly and in 1985, 114 women died from it. Interestingly, once you've had toxic shock syndrome you have a higher risk of getting it again. Toxic shock itself is not new. It can strike whenever staph organisms form in large enough numbers and recovery from this type of infection can be long and difficult.

After certain types of tampons were taken off the market, toxic shock no longer received the kind of publicity we saw during the 80's. Today, several hundred cases are reported each year, although now, menstrual toxic shock comprises only a quarter of cases. The mortality rate from toxic shock is approximately 3 percent.

CAUSES:

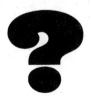

The staphylococcus bacteria is believed to enter the body through a break in the skin and is sometimes present in the nose and mouth areas. Some women carry this bacteria within the vagina. The exact link of tampon use to the disease is unclear. One theory explaining the relationship of tampons to the infection is that they trap bacteria and provide a breeding ground in which they multiply rapidly.

Leaving a tampon in for long periods of time affords the bacteria an opportunity to reproduce quickly. Another theory is that synthetic, absorbent fibers of some tampons can cause tiny lacerations in the vagina which allow for the transmission of the bacteria and the toxin it produces into the bloodstream.

Toxic shock syndrome has also been associated with vaginal barrier contraceptives (diaphragms or contraceptive sponges), and there have been some reports of sexual partners both contracting the disease. Toxic shock can occur as a result of a staph infection of the skin, wounds, as a complication of surgery, influenza, pneumonia and from infections related to childbirth. Some cases of toxic shock syndrome have been linked to nasal packing to control nosebleeds.

SYMPTOMS:

Physical: Toxic shock syndrome is characterized by nausea, diarrhea, dizziness, possible headache, sore throat, aching muscles and a sudden high fever. Initial symptoms are subsequently followed by a red, peeling rashthat resembles a sunburn, typically found on the palms and soles of the feet. At this stage, possible shock, kidney failure, unconsciousness, paralysis and even death can occur.

A dramatic drop in blood pressure is another symptom typical of toxic shock syndrome. In mild cases, only one or two symptoms may be present.

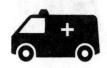

MEDICAL ALERT:

Any woman who is wearing a tampon and begins to experience any of these symptoms should immediately remove the tampon and seek medical attention as soon as possible.

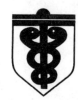

STANDARD MEDICAL TREATMENT:

Diagnosis is made by culturing a blood sample and secretions which are obtained from the vagina. Antibiotic therapy is initiated, which usually involves a semisynthetic penicillin or a cephalosporin drug. Intravenous fluids are given to replaced lost fluids, fever is controlled and blood pressure is raised. It is important to realize that antibiotic treatment has no effect on the illness itself, which is a result of toxins which have already been released into the body.

Success rating of standard medical treatment: good. This rating would be higher but due the nature of this bacterial infection, once the toxins are produced, killing the bacteria does not affect the physical damage already done. Antibiotic therapy seems to reduce recurrences of toxic shock syndrome, which used to affect 30 percent of patients. Today, the risk of a recurrence is approximately 5 percent.

Note: Nutritional and herbal suggestions are offered as supportive treatments. Toxic shock syndrome needs immediate medical treatment and requires the facilities of a hospital.

NUTRITIONAL APPROACH:

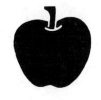

◆ Eat a diet high in fish, broccoli, cabbage, cauliflower, chicken, apples, apricots, bananas, green beans, berries, melons, fresh peas, brown rice, buckwheat and pineapple to strengthen the immune system.
◆ Take vitamin A supplements, which can increase one's resistance to disease and protect against infection.
◆ *Vitamin C with bioflavonoids:* Very important for tissue repair and the ability to fight viral and bacterial organisms.
◆ *Vitamin B complex:* Helps increase resistance to disease.
◆ *Zinc:* A booster for the immune system.
◆ *Magnesium:* This mineral produces properdin, a blood protein that can help fight invading bacteria and viruses.
◆ *Acidophilus:* Important if on antibiotic therapy for the replacement of friendly bacteria.
◆ *Chlorophyll:* Helps to clear the blood of toxins.

HERBAL REMEDIES:

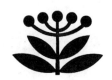

◆ *Burdock:* Helps to remove toxins from the bloodstream.
◆ *Golden seal:* Considered an herbal cleanser and healer. It also has natural antibiotic properties.
◆ *Garlic:* Take capsules to fortify the immune system.
◆ *Chaparral:* Helps to detoxify cells that have been infected or exposed to toxins from bacteria and viruses.
◆ *Echinacea:* A lymphatic and blood cleanser.
◆ *Pau d'arco:* Helps to rid the body of poisons and protects liver function.
◆ *The following herbs in combination may be useful:* Red clover, peach bark, sheep sorrel, prickly ash bark, barberry, buckthorn, licorice and rosemary leaf.

PREVENTION:

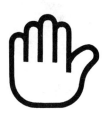

◆ Tampons should be changed often, and alternating tampons and pads is recommended.
◆ Do not use tampons overnight.

- Anyone who has had toxic shock syndrome should not use tampons, vaginal sponges or diaphragms.
- Don't use tampons for minor vaginal discharges.
- Don't leave a contraceptive sponge in the vagina for more than 24 hours.
- Don't pack your nasal passages for long periods of time to control nosebleeds.
- Keep your immune system healthy through a nutritious diet and by avoiding alcohol, caffeine, tobacco, and unnecessary drugs. If your body has to undergo surgery or experiences illness, a strong immune system can help to fight subsequent staph infections, which occur as secondary complications to these conditions.

Ulcers (peptic, duodenal or gastric)

DEFINITION:

At one time, having an ulcer was considered a liability of success in the dog-eat-dog business world. Today, we know that ulcers can develop from factors other than stress, and the way that we view and treat ulcers has drastically changed.

Technically, an ulcer is an open sore that forms on the skin or any mucous membrane such as the lining of the stomach. It may be shallow or deep, and is characterized by pain and inflammation. Most ulcers are found within the upper digestive tract and are comprised of peptic, duodenal and gastric ulcers. Ulcers usually form in the duodenum first, which is the initial section of the small intestine. They may also occur in the stomach lining itself.

An estimated 5 million Americans suffer from ulcers. With drug therapy, peptic ulcers usually heal within eight weeks. The chances of an ulcer recurring without continuing treatment is between 60 and 70 percent. Gastrointestinal ulcers can occur at any age.

CAUSES:

Stomach ulcers occur when the mucous lining that normally protects the stomach from the damaging effects of stomach acid breaks down. While the effect of stress on the stomach is debated by some doctors, tension unquestionably causes an increase in the production of stomach acid and a decreased blood flow to the stomach.

The belief that too much acid in the stomach causes ulcers has been questioned. The mystery behind stomach ulcers lies in why the mucous membrane breaks down and permits acid damage in the first place. Certain prescription drugs such as nonsteroidal anti-inflammatories can increase the risk of developing ulcers by damaging mucous membranes.

Mucous lining damage may also result from cigarette smoke, a genetic predisposition (people with type O blood have a higher rate of duodenal ulcers), and the possibility of bacterial infection. The notion that stress and anxiety can weaken the immune system, allowing for the development of ulcer-causing bacteria, has received more attention and credibility lately.

Irregular, hurried meals have also been associated with ulcer formation. Some studies have also linked food allergies with the development of peptic ulcers.

SYMPTOMS:

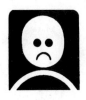

Physical: Only around 50 percent of all people who suffer from stomach ulcers have tell-tale symptoms. Symptoms of a duodenal or peptic ulcer include heartburn, nausea, a gnawing sensation below the breastbone that is relieved by eating food but then recurs two to three hours after a meal, intense pain, passing dark stools or throwing up dark vomitus. If an ulcer bleeds for a prolonged period of time, anemia can result.

Psychological: Although the stress connection to gastric ulcers has been doubted by some medical doctors, the link is unquestionably valid. High-stress jobs, relationships, and certain personality traits do increase the risk for developing ulcers. This association may not be the result of an increase of stomach acid, but rather from lowered immunity, which can cause the stomach lining to be more vulnerable to ulceration. Learning to relax and cope with everyday stressors is vital to decreasing one's risk of developing ulcers (see chapter on stress).

MEDICAL ALERT:

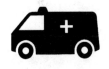

If you spit up blood which looks like coffee grounds or have dark tarlike stools, contact your doctor immediately. These symptoms may indicate gastro-intestinal bleeding and should be immediately addressed. Bleeding ulcers can be life-threatening. A perforated ulcer constitutes a medical emergency and occurs when an ulcer perforates through the abdominal wall, spilling its contents into the abdominal cavity.

STANDARD MEDICAL TREATMENT:

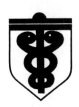

Diagnosis of an ulcer is confirmed by an x-ray and by viewing the lesion directly through a gastroscopy, in which a tube is threaded through the mouth into the intestinal tract. Your doctor will probably order a barium swallow to examine the stomach lining under an x-ray.

Lab tests to analyze stomach acid content and a bowel movement analysis may be done to check for internal bleeding. Sucralfates (Carafate) is recommended by some physicians as the best drug choice in treating ulcers. It produces a thick paste that protects the ulcerated tissue. Because it coats the stomach so efficiently, sucralfate succeeds in healing 80 percent of ulcers within the first six weeks of treatment.

Other drugs routinely prescribed are H2 blockers i.e. cimetidine (Tagamet, Zantac, Axid, Pepcid), which all suppress the production of stomach acid. Antispasmodics may also be used. Prostaglandin drugs are now used to treat ulcers caused by taking anti-inflammatory drugs like ibuprofen for prolonged periods of time.

For peptic ulcers, histamine-2 receptor antagonist drugs are used (cimetidine, famotidine, rantidine). These block the effects of histamine, which causes inflammation. Lowering histamine levels in the stomach reduces the formation of stomach acid, which promotes ulcer healing.

Antacid drugs are also commonly prescribed. Once the ulcer is healed, maintenance drugs may be prescribed. A fairly new drug called Misoprostol is currently being used in several other countries for the treatment of peptic ulcers.

Surgical options: Partial gastrectomy: If the ulcer does not heal after 8 weeks of treatment, an operation to remove the portion of the stomach which contains the ulcer may be advised.

Side-effects: Sucralfates (Carafate): Constipation, diarrhea, nausea, upset stomach, dizziness, indigestion, dry mouth, rash, itching, back pain and sleeplessness. The incidence of reported side-effects with this drug is low.

Warning: Do not use this drug if pregnant or nursing unless specifically instructed to do so by your doctor. The use of this drug for children is not recommended, as studies have been limited to adults only.

Side-effects: H2 blockers: Cimetidine: mild diarrhea, muscle pains, cramps, dizziness, skin rash, nausea, headache, confusion, drowsiness, and vomiting.

Note: Cigarette smoking reverses the effect of cimetidine on stomach acid.

Warning: While cimetidine has not been linked with birth defects, it should be avoided by pregnant or nursing women unless deemed essential by a physician.

Success rating of standard medical treatment: good. New drugs can help to heal ulcers and significantly reduce their discomfort, however, ulcers have a high tendency to recur. In most cases, even without treatment, ulcers will heal themselves within six weeks. Unfortunately, medical science does not effectively get to the root of why the stomach tissue remains susceptible to ulcers. Most doctors fail to teach their ulcer patients life-style modifications that will minimize their chances of further ulcer development.

MEDICAL UPDATE:

Recently, evidence has pointed to the presence of bacterial infection as a possible cause of peptic ulcers. As a result, antibiotic treatment has produced encouraging results. Discuss this option with your physician.

Antibiotics combined with traditional ulcer medication appears to be the best way to treat an ulcer, according to studies done in Vienna, Austria. Gastroenterologists at the Hanusch Hospital found that ulcers recurred in 8 percent of 50 patients that were treated with such a combination as opposed to a recurrence rate of 86 percent in patients who were not. Zantac or glaxo plus two antibiotics such as amoxicillin and metronidazole, was the effective combination used. As a result of this study, it has been recommended that every ulcer patient should be checked for the presence of H. pylori infection, which can be treated with antibiotics. H. pylori bacteria was first detected 10 years ago in cases of gastritis, and has been linked to not only stomach ulcers, but to stomach cancer as well.

HOME SELF-CARE:

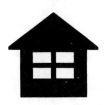

- The majority of ulcers heal on their own with bed rest and proper diet.
- Pepto-Bismol contains bismuth, which can kill bacteria that invade the stomach and are thought to cause ulcers. If the theory that bacteria causes stomach lining vulnerability to ulcers is valid, this approach may be worth trying.
- Taking over-the-counter antacids can provide some relief and help to promote healing; however, long-term use of these preparations may cause diarrhea or constipation. Some studies suggest that calcium carbonate antacids (Tums, Alka-Z) may actually produce more gastric acid secretion if taken routinely. The prolonged use of sodium bicarbonate antacids (Rolaids, Alka-Seltzer, Bromo-Seltzer) may cause chemical imbalances. The antacids most frequently recommended for ulcers are aluminum-magnesium compounds (Maalox, Mylanta, Digel). These may cause a depletion of calcium and phosphorus and contain aluminum, which may be toxic.
- While some doctors are skeptical that stress can cause ulcers, there is enough credible evidence that the connection is a valid one. People who live in high-stress cities have a greater incidence of ulcers. Keep stress levels controlled through biofeedback, visualization therapy, yoga, controlled breathing, and exercise.
- Slow down your pace of living, including the speed in which you eat and drink. Don't eat under stress.
- Stop smoking. Smokers are twice as likely to get ulcers as non-smokers. Smoking also inhibits ulcer healing and increases your chances of having recurring ulcers.
- Avoid taking aspirin and ibuprofen. These medications, along with other nonsteroidal anti-inflammatory drugs, should not be taken by anyone suffering

from an ulcer. They can cause further deterioration of the stomach lining. Acetaminophen is recommended.

NUTRITIONAL APPROACH:

- Avoid the following foods: Dairy products (drinking milk or cream was recommended in the past to control acid, but can actually aggravate the production of stomach acid), fatty foods, soda pop, caffeine, alcohol.
- For years, bland diets have been prescribed for ulcers, although there is some question as to whether this is a valid approach. White sugar and flour may also increase the production of stomach acid and are discouraged.
- Eat frequent, small meals. Up to six meals a day are recommended. The presence of food can help to neutralize stomach acid; therefore, don't go for long periods of time without eating.
- High-fiber diets are recommended for their therapeutic use. Fiber promotes mucin secretion and delays gastric emptying.
- Coffee including decaf must be strictly avoided.
- Avoid taking large doses of vitamin C, which can create more stomach acid.
- Taking iron supplements is not recommended if you have an ulcer. Iron is a gastric irritant.
- Potatoes and almond milk are recommended for their acid-neutralizing properties.
- Barley helps to rebuild the lining of the stomach.
- Foods that are recommended include low-fat yogurt, avocados, bananas, squash, yams, steamed broccoli, and carrots.
- Blue grapes are routinely used in Europe to treat ulcers.
- *Okra powder:* Acts as a demulcent to stop inflammation.
- Persimmons also facilitate healing of the stomach lining.
- *Whey powder:* Contains compounds that help to heal ulcerated tissue.
- *Vitamin U:* A recently discovered vitamin that is high in chlorophyll and helps promote healing of duodenal and peptic ulcers.
- *Vitamin E:* Relieves pain and reduces stomach acid.
- *Vitamin A:* Helps to heal ulcerated tissue and protect the stomach lining from irritation.
- The combination of vitamin A and vitamin E has been shown to inhibit the formation of stress ulcers in rat experiments.
- *Cabbage juice:* Promotes healing of the mucous membranes. Freshly juiced cabbage is best.
- *Vitamin K:* Helps to control bleeding.
- *Calcium/magnesium:* Helps to soothe the nerves and control stress.
- *Zinc:* Helps to promote healing of ulcers. Studies have indicated that ulcer patients who take zinc sulfate heal faster than those who do not. Take zinc

supplements with food.
◆ *Potassium:* Helps to balance excess acid.
◆ *L-glutamine:* An amino acid that is excellent for healing peptic ulcers.
◆ *Pectin:* Helps to heal duodenal ulcers.

HERBAL REMEDIES:

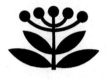

◆ *Aloe vera:* Promotes healing of damaged tissue. Stay within recommended dosages to avoid irritation. Take aloe vera juice after meals.
◆ *Garlic oil:* A natural antibiotic.
◆ *Licorice:* a natural anti-inflammatory that produces viscous mucus, which protects the stomach wall and reduces acid production. Use the DGL form of licorice.
◆ *Meadowsweet:* Reduces stomach acid production and heals the stomach lining.
◆ *Papaya:* Contains enzymes which promote good digestion and heal the stomach lining.
◆ *Slippery elm:* Soothes irritated mucous membranes.
◆ *Fennel:* An anti-inflammatory that promotes digestion.
◆ *Peppermint tea:* Drink frequently to soothe the lining of the digestive tract.
◆ *Flaxseed tea:* Coats the digestive tract and protects the ulcers from irritation.
◆ *Lemon balm:* Has a sedating effect which helps to calm a nervous stomach.
◆ *Golden seal:* A natural antibiotic that fights bacterial infection and promotes healing in the digestive system.
◆ *White oak bark:* Helps to heal ulcers in the gastrointestinal tract.
◆ *Capsicum:* Can help to anesthetize and heal ulcers.
◆ *Pau d'arco:* A powerful antibiotic which can fight the presence of bacterial infection in ulcers.
◆ *Hops:* A nervine that can tranquilize the nerves.
◆ *The following combination of herbs may be useful:* golden seal, capsicum and myrrh.
◆ *The following herbs in combination:* Marshmallow, echinacea, golden seal, cabbage, slippery elm, echinacea, and American cranesbill.

PREVENTION:

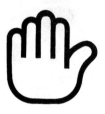

◆ Stress in all its forms is unquestionably a contributing factor to ulcers. Reduce stress through daily relaxation using methods such as music therapy, stretching, yoga, and biofeedback exercise. Change jobs or locations if stress is severe.
◆ Don't smoke: Smoking greatly increases your risk for developing ulcers as well as a whole other host of serious diseases. Smoking constricts the blood vessels that supply nourishment to the stomach lining.
◆ Eat regular meals and don't overeat.
◆ Avoid alcohol, which can result in stomach lining irritation.

◆ Avoid taking corticosteroids, ibuprofen, aspirin, Indomethacin, Prioxicam, and Naproxen for long periods of time.
◆ Keep your immune system healthy by eating nutritiously and supplementing your diet with garlic capsules, which fight both bacterial and viral infection.
◆ Taking daily supplements of zinc has a protective effect against the formation of ulcers.

Vaginitis

DEFINITION:

Any woman who has experienced a vaginal infection knows the true meaning of aggravation. Unfortunately, the vaginal canal, under certain circumstances, provides an excellent environment for bacteria and other microbes to thrive in. The itching and discomfort that can result from a yeast infection, which is a form of vaginitis, can try your patience to the limit. Fortunately, there are several steps you can take to help relieve these miserable symptoms.

Vaginitis, or vaginal infections in general, are commonly experienced by women and account for approximately 7 percent of all visits to gynecologists. Vaginitis refers to any inflammation of the vagina which can result from a variety of causes. Vaginal infections are most commonly caused by the fungus Candida albicans (yeast infections) and most vaginal infections result from a change in the normal vaginal environment.

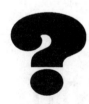

CAUSES:

Vaginal infections result from a variety of microbial invaders. A common fungus which normally inhabits the vagina can cause yeast infections. The use of antibiotics can increase the risk of this type of vaginal infection by killing good bacteria which keep it controlled.

High blood sugar found in diabetics can greatly increase the risk of vaginal yeast infections. Sugar from the urine can help to feed the infection. Increased risk for yeast infections has also been linked to using birth control pills, although low-dose pills seem less prone to do so.

Pregnancy can increase the risk of vaginitis. Other factors linked to vaginal infections include high stress levels; prolonged use of corticosteroids; regular douching, which can upset the normal chemical and microbial balance of the vagina; tampon use; wearing nylon tights; hormonal changes associated with menstruation; lack of estrogen; chemical irritants; allergens; and the presence of foreign bodies. Injuries caused by physical agents, trauma or sexual activity can also cause vaginitis.

SYMPTOMS:

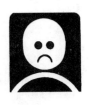

Physical: Vaginitis can cause burning, irritation and itching in the vaginal area. It can also result in a vaginal discharge which may or may not itch, burn or have a foul odor. In yeast infections, a discharge may or may not present. In other kinds of vaginal infections, the discharge can be an abnormal color. Painful urination or intercourse may also be present.

In some instances, vaginitis may be a symptom of a more serious condition such as a chronic inflammation of the cervix or a sexually transmitted disease. Pelvic inflammatory disease can sometimes cause symptoms thought to be vaginitis and requires immediate medical treatment. Chlamydia, gonorrhea and syphilis may produce similar symptoms and need prompt medical attention.

Note: After menopause, the lining of the vagina can become dry and thin, making it more susceptible to inflammation.

Psychological: Women with recurring vaginal infections may be responding to emotional stress. Anyone who has routine vaginal infections and is in good overall health may want to assess her life-style and try implementing daily relaxation techniques such as regulated deep breathing.

MEDICAL ALERT:

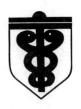

See your doctor immediately if you have pelvic pain, a fever or swollen glands in the groin area. Any sores in the vaginal area should also be examined by a physician.

STANDARD MEDICAL TREATMENT:

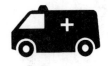

A laboratory analysis of vaginal discharge can easily diagnose the presence of a vaginal infection. If you have a yeast infection, your doctor will most likely prescribe nystantin (Mycostantin, Nilstant) and imidazole creams or suppositories. Varieties of this treatment include miconazole (Monistat), terconazole (Terazol), clotrimazole (Gyne-Lotrimin, Mycelex), and econazole. All of these are thought to be equally effective in treating a yeast infection.

Mycelex-G is also routinely used to treat vaginal infections. In cases of post-menopausal vaginitis, estrogen supplements may be recommended. Ketoconazole (Nizoral) has also been prescribed in pill or cream form for the treatment of fungal infections of the vagina.

Note: Using vaginal creams or douching prior to the lab test can make microscopic analysis difficult.

Side-effects: Nystatin (Mycostatin, Nilstant): Side-effects are rare and usually mild with this preparation. The only side-effect reported is intravaginal irritation.

Success rating of standard medical treatment: good. In some cases, doctors will recommend antibiotics to clear up vaginitis which can actually trigger or worsen some vaginal infections. In addition, while prescribed or over-the-counter preparations are usually effective at clearing up vaginitis, inexpensive douches and home self-care techniques are often effective and will save you a great deal of money.

MEDICAL UPDATE:

Vaginal itching that appears just before your period may be a condition called cytolytic vaginosis, which is caused by bacteria that grow in the presence of elevated levels of estrogen. This type of vaginal disorder is not considered a true infection and can be remedied with a baking soda douche rather than a strong drug. Mix 2 tablespoons of baking soda in a quart of warm water and douche two times a day.

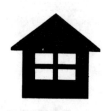

HOME SELF-CARE:

◆ Douching with acidophilus solutions diluted with warm water can have remarkable results in fighting yeast infections. Adding garlic oil to the douche has also been recommended, but only in small amounts or burning can occur. Using acidophilus or yogurt is only recommended for yeast infections. If a bacterial infection is present, this treatment may actually make the infection worse.
Note: Do not use douches if pregnant.
◆ Wear white, cotton underwear to promote the circulation of air. Avoid plastic, polyester and leather fabrics, which can trap in heat and moisture, providing a perfect environment for bacterial proliferation.
◆ Underwear can be sterilized by soaking it in bleach for 24 hours.
◆ If the itching is intense, over-the-counter preparations like Benadryl or Cortaid can help. Don't use these before going to the doctor for an examination.
◆ Tampons can be saturated with boric acid or acidophilus and placed in the vagina for treatment. Other substances which can be used in douches or on tampons include Betadine (diluted 1:1000), licorice, diluted white vinegar, or a 2% solution of zinc sulphate diluted in 1 pint of warm water.
Note: Placing yogurt in the vagina is discouraged if there is a chance of bacterial infection. In this case, the presence of yogurt can cause the infection to proliferate. Only use yogurt if you are sure the vaginitis is caused by a yeast infection.
◆ Avoid sexual activity during treatment to avoid reinfection and reduce

irritation.
◆ Warm sitz baths, using herb teas, apple cider vinegar or epsom salts can help relieve itching and burning.
◆ Don't use dusting powders. Powder trapped in the vaginal area can promote infection.
◆ During a vaginal infection don't use commercial douches, contraceptive foams or jellies, or feminine deodorant sprays. These substances can further disrupt the natural chemical balance of the vagina.
◆ Cleanse the vaginal area thoroughly with a cotton swab soaked in calendula to remove the bacterially saturated discharge.

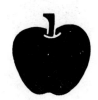

NUTRITIONAL APPROACH:

Often the internal environment of the vagina can reflect the condition and health of the entire body. The right kind of diet is important in enabling the body to keep infection under control.
◆ Food allergies have been strongly associated with yeast infections.
◆ Avoid a high-sugar diet along with alcohol, chocolate, fermented foods, cheeses, and other diary products, mushrooms, citrus fruits and gluten foods. Eat oat bran instead. Do not eat any yeast, and keep carbohydrates low until the infection is controlled.
◆ Avoid vitamin supplements that are yeast-based.
◆ The use of artificial sweeteners can increase the likelihood of yeast infections.
◆ Eat plenty of live culture, low-fat yogurt.
◆ *Acidophilus liquid or capsules:* Replenishes the friendly bacteria in the vagina needed fight infection. The lactobacillus variety has been found to be the most effective.
◆ *Vitamin A and beta carotene:* Necessary to maintain the health of the vaginal mucosa and boost the immune system.
◆ *Vitamin B complex:* Can be deficient in women with recurring vaginitis. Lack of estrogen can increase the need for vitamin B6.
◆ *Vitamin C:* Important for immune system health in fighting any infection.
◆ Vitamin C and bioflavonoids: Help to stop the spread of infection and have been useful in reducing the frequency and severity of herpes infections.
◆ *Vitamin D with calcium and magnesium:* Helps to relieve stress, which has been associated with vaginal infections.
◆ *Vitamin E:* Can be used externally for itching. A lack of vitamin E in the diet can compromise immunity.
◆ Avoid taking iron supplements while the infection is active. Iron can feed certain bacteria.
◆ *Zinc picolinate:* In some studies, zinc has been shown toxic to vaginal yeast infections. A lack of zinc can also weaken the immune system, which can

predispose one to infection. Topical zinc can also be used for itching.

- *Chlorophyll:* This substance is bacteriostatic and can soothe inflamed tissue.
- *Lysine:* Can reduce the reoccurrence of vaginal infections. Oral supplementation has been shown to decrease the frequency and severity of certain infections.

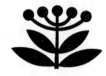

HERBAL REMEDIES:

- *Aloe vera gel:* Helps to soothe and heal irritated tissue.
- *Golden seal and Oregon grape:* Both of these herbs contain the alkaloid berberine, which is antibacterial. Can be used internally and as a therapeutic douche.
- *Garlic capsules:* Have antifungal properties that have been shown to be effective against some antibiotic-resistant organisms.
- Fennel, ginseng, alfalfa, red clover, anise, dong quai and licorice are considered to have a mild estrogenic effect, which can help maintain hormonal balance, thereby reducing the risk of vaginal infections.
- *Tea tree oil:* This oil, diluted, can be used in douche form to fight infection and sooth irritated tissue Four to five drops can be placed on a tampon and inserted.
- *Pot marigold:* An antifungal, astringent herb that promotes healing. Can be used as a douche or in cream form.
- *Damask rose:* A cooling anti-inflammatory that can help relieve vaginal itching. Use in lotion form.
- *White oak bark:* Works as an astringent, which fights vaginal infection.
- *Pau d'arco tea:* Has antifungal properties and helps to fight infections of any kind.

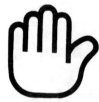

PREVENTION:

- Keeping the immune system healthy through diet, exercise and vitamin and mineral supplementation can help to prevent vaginal infections. Don't smoke, drink alcohol or use caffeine.
- Eat a diet that is low in sugar and high in fiber and fresh vegetables and fruits. Avoid artificial sweeteners, which have been linked to a higher incidence of yeast infections.
- Take acidophilus culture after meals.
- Don't wear nylon underpants. Use white, cotton underwear, which discourages the growth of infection.
- Avoid wearing tight-fitting clothing that inhibits air circulation, especially overnight.
- Wear pantyhose that have cotton crotches.
- Double rinse underwear to prevent chemical irritation from detergents.
- During periods, wear pads at night rather than tampons.
- Using a natural lubricant during intercourse to prevent irritation. Mineral oil, egg whites, petroleum jelly and plain yogurt are recommended. Baby oil contains

perfume which may prove irritating.

◆ Don't use spermicides as a contraceptive option. These can increase your risk of vaginal infections.

◆ Use unscented, uncolored toilet paper to avoid any chemical irritation.

◆ Don't use chemical douches, which disrupt the normal alkaline/acid balance of the vagina and can increase the risk of bacterial invasion.

◆ Avoid the prolonged use of antibiotics if possible.

◆ Avoid deodorant or heavily perfumed soaps.

Varicose Veins

DEFINITION:

Varicose veins plague a great number of people. They are considered unsightly and often discourage the wearing of short skirts or bathing suits. Medically speaking, varicose veins refers to veins which have become swollen due to a weakness in the vessel walls or valves, which allows for a backflow of blood to occur. As a result, blood pools in superficial veins, causing them to become stretched and puffy. The legs are more susceptible than any other area to varicose veins. Spider veins, which are usually found on the thighs, are a much milder form of varicose veins.

More than 40 million Americans suffer from varicose veins, with women outnumbering men four to one. Most varicose veins do not require medical attention but can cause considerable discomfort and embarrassment. They are considered troublesome, but rarely disabling.

In severe cases, varicose veins can cause skin ulcers which are slow to heal and need immediate medical treatment.

CAUSES:

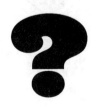

Certain conditions can create a lack of proper circulation, causing veins to respond by dilating and twisting. These include pregnancy, sitting for prolonged periods of time with legs crossed, obesity, the constricting of blood vessels with garters or tight clothing, and standing for long periods of time.

Age increases the risk of this condition, as the skin becomes less elastic, which lessens vein support. Chronic constipation, which causes straining during bowel movements, can cause anal varicose veins (hemorrhoids) and has also been linked to the formation of varicose veins in the legs. Varicose veins run in families.

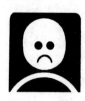

SYMPTOMS:

Physical: Varicose veins are bluish, bulgy and are often accompanied by dull, nagging pains. The most usual site for these veins is at the back of the calf or on the inside of the leg anywhere between the ankle and the groin area. Varicose veins may also form around the anus, causing hemorrhoids.

Varicose veins may cause swelling, leg sores, leg cramping, and a feeling of heaviness. They may become tender to the touch, and the skin above a varicose vein may itch. Feelings of heaviness or pressure from these veins can increase for some women just prior to and after menstruation.

Some people notice a brown discoloration of the skin near the ankles in severe cases of varicose veins. Eczema of the skin near the veins is also possible. Spider veins, which are very common, especially in the thigh area, are considered harmless. Skin ulcers can form around serious varicose veins and need medical attention.

Cutting or bruising the skin around varicose veins can cause a great deal of blood flow and will also require medical treatment. In severe cases, inflammation of the vein walls can result, which may lead to the formation of blood clots or thrombophlebitis.

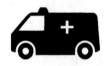

MEDICAL ALERT:

See your doctor immediately if you have varicose veins that are unusually painful or exhibit red lumping that does not decrease when you elevate your legs. This might indicate the presence of a blood clot. If varicose veins are cut or rupture around the ankle area, blood loss can be substantial. Apply finger pressure to the area and elevate it. Get medical attention immediately.

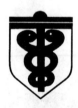

STANDARD MEDICAL TREATMENT:

Most doctors will use elastic tourniquets on your legs to determine which of the veins are damaged. Because varicose veins leak, they will stand out when blood flow is constricted. A venography can further check the performance of leg veins and is done by injecting dye in a varicose vein and watching its progress with an x-ray. Thermography records the temperature of various parts of the leg in order to produce a heat map to pinpoint the exact location of weak valves.

Your doctor may want to inject varicose veins with sclerosing agents (sclerotherapy) and wrap them firmly for a few days to help control inflammation. This procedure will eventually cause other veins to take the place of the ones treated. This is usually done on an outpatient basis and involves two to three visits. If the varicose veins are located in the thigh area, this procedure is usually unsuccessful. Stripping the veins first may be recommended in this instance.

Surgical options: In severe cases of varicose veins, surgical removal may be advised. Bulging, discolored veins may cause pain and skin ulcers. In these instances, the veins are removed by stripping them through a small incision. This operation which is performed under a general anesthetic, usually requires a week's stay in the hospital and a gradual increase in activity.

Success rating of standard medical treatment: poor to fair. Varicose veins are difficult to treat. Surgery is sometimes successful; however, it can be uncomfortable and disappointing. Prevention is the best approach to varicose veins and involves an awareness of genetic susceptibility and life-style adaptations. The role of diet has been downplayed in the case of this disorder, and may prove more significant than previously thought.

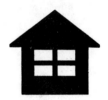

HOME SELF-CARE:

- Exercise regularly to improve circulation. Walking every day for 15 minutes is excellent.
- Avoid sitting or standing for long periods of time.
- Elevate your legs several times a day to promote better blood flow.
- Raise the foot of your bed several inches above the head to facilitate blood flow. Do not do this if you have breathing difficulties or a history of heart trouble.
- Avoid putting unnecessary stress or weight on the legs by crossing them or lifting heavy objects.
- Wear support hose, which are individually fitted and can be ordered through medical supply houses. Put on the hose first thing in the morning.
- Daily sitz baths can help with discomfort.
- If you cut a varicose vein, elevate your leg immediately and apply pressure. Get medical attention if the bleeding does not stop.
- Practicing the yoga shoulder stand is recommended to improve circulation. Yoga breathing exercises can also help relieve varicose vein pain.
- Taking aspirin every day can help with discomfort and increase blood mobility. Discuss this option with your doctor.
- Witch hazel compresses can improve circulation and help control discomfort.

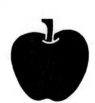

NUTRITIONAL APPROACH:

- Varicose veins are seldom seen in areas of the world where high-fiber diets are the rule. Some health care providers believe that the Western diet, which is high in refined carbohydrates and fat and low in fiber contributes to the development of varicose veins.
- Emphasize a diet high in fiber and rich in legumes, fresh fruits and vegetables, and grains.

- Avoid fatty foods and refined carbohydrates. Eat plenty of fish, fiber and raw fruits and vegetables. Don't eat margarine, animal fats, red meat, ice cream, pastries or other rich foods.
- Decrease your salt intake: Salt can cause swelling in people who are salt-sensitive.
- *Vitamin C plus bioflavonoids:* Promotes blood circulation and vein wall strength. Vitamin C also helps to prevent bruising and the formation of blood clots. Take supplements and eat dark berries.
- Consume plenty of onion and garlic.
- *Lecithin:* A fat emulsifier that aids in circulation.
- *Vitamin D, calcium and magnesium:* Help to relieve leg cramps.
- *Vitamin E:* Improves circulation and can help control feelings of heaviness in the legs.
- *Vitamin K:* Helps control bleeding and clot formation.
- *Zinc:* Aid in cell healing and is especially good if varicose ulcers have developed.
- *Bromelain:* Helps to increase fibrinolytic activity of the blood, which can reduce risk of clot formation. Bromelain may also help to prevent the hard and lumpy skin that is found around varicose veins.
- *Lysine:* Considered a circulatory tonic.
- Psyllium, oat bran, and guar gum can promote regularity and prevent bowel movement straining.

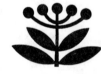

HERBAL REMEDIES:

- White oak bark compresses can be applied to varicose veins to stimulate blood flow.
- *St. John's wort* oil can be rubbed into varicose veins.
- *Redmond clay packs:* Help to heal and stimulate blood flow.
- *Capsicum, garlic, onion and ginger:* Promote blood flow by stimulating circulation, and increase fibrinolytic activity in the blood, which discourages the formation of blood clots.
- *Kelp:* Strengthens and cleans veins.
- *Butcher's broom:* Strengthens blood vessels and helps to keep them clean. It is considered a natural vasoconstrictor and can be used both internally and externally.
- *Bilberry:* Strengthens capillaries and small veins and improves circulation. It also helps reduce the risk of blood clots.
- *Horse chestnut:* Strengthens blood vessels and reduces blood vessel irritation and permeability.
- *King's clover:* Considered an herbal tonic for the veins which also has anti-inflammatory and anticoagulant properties.
- *Comfrey, vitamin E, and wood sage:* Good for the treatment of varicose ulcers. Aids tissue regeneration slow-healing wounds.

- Calendula ointment is good if itching is a problem.
- *The following herbs in combination may be useful:* hawthorne, capsicum and garlic.

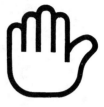

PREVENTION:

- Don't smoke: Smoking can contribute to circulatory disorders and the development of blood clots.
- Keep your weight down. Obesity significantly contributes to the development of varicose veins by putting extra pressure on soft-walled veins, which require an increased blood flow.
- Exercise regularly to promote blood flow.
- Try to rest your legs by elevating them often if you must stand or sit for long periods of time.
- Make sure your diet is high in vitamin C, which contributes to blood vessel strength.
- Don't wear tight shoes, garters, knee-highs or girdles.
- Wear support hose or compression stockings if you are at risk for varicose veins.
- Avoid constipation, which can cause straining and put pressure on the lower circulatory system.

Warts (verrucae)

DEFINITION:

Warts have always conjured up notions of toads, witches' brews, wicked spells and magic potions. Having warts can make you feel more like a frog than a human, no matter how common they are. In fact, 75 percent of the general population will have warts at one time or another and over $120 million is spent each year on wart remedies.

Warts are contagious growths which are found on the skin or mucous membranes. There are over 30 types of the papillomavirus which cause warts to develop. Warts are located on the upper-most layer of the skin and their appearance is determined by their positioning on the body. Warts can be spread by picking, biting, touching, shaving, trimming, or in the case of genital warts, through sexual contact.

The peak incidence of warts is from the ages of 10 to 19, with 70 percent of all warts occurring between the ages of 10 and 39. For unknown reasons, girls are more susceptible to warts than boys. What may look like a wart after the age of 50 is probably a raised age spot.

The incubation period for warts can be anywhere from one month to eighteen months. Warts appear to be less common in tropical areas of the world. To the dismay of most of us, warts are quite resistant to treatment and often reoccur.

The following are types of warts that exist:

Common warts: These are firm, round, or irregular sharply defined growths that can grow up to a quarter inch in diameter. They usually have a rough surface and appear in areas that are prone to injury such as the hands, knees, face and scalp. These types of warts are commonly seen in children.

Flat warts: These are flat, flesh-colored growths that occur on the wrists, the backs of the hands and sometimes the face. They may also itch.

Digitate warts: These warts are dark in color and have fingerlike projections.

Filiform warts: These warts are long and slender and usually grow on the eyelids, armpits or the neck and commonly infect overweight, middle-aged people.

Plantar warts: Found on the soles of the feet, these warts become flattened due to the weight of the body. They can cause considerable discomfort.

Note: If a wart enters a cut or an opening around the cuticle it is referred to as a periungual wart, and can be particularly difficult to treat. Use an antibiotic cream on the area and cover it to discourage further injury or inflammation.

Genital warts: See chapter on herpes.

CAUSES:

The papillomavirus causes the formation of warts. There are over 35 varieties of this virus. Children who suffer from allergies and dermatitis seem more prone to have warts. Going barefoot or wearing improper footwear have been linked with the development of plantar warts. In addition, having damp feet may also predispose one to plantar warts.

Interestingly, people who routinely handle meat have a higher incidence of warts, implying that meat may carry the wart-causing virus. Some drugs such as tetracycline, have been linked to developing warts, although there is no scientific basis for this connection.

Warts are spread by direct contact with combs, razors, swimming pools, or locker room floors. People who suffer from diseases which compromise their immune systems such as AIDS, or leukemia may become more susceptible to warts. Emotional stress has also been connected to increased vulnerability to developing warts.

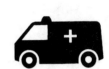

SYMPTOMS:

Psychological: In spite of scientific skepticism, warts seem to have an unquestionable psychological connection. The power of suggestion, visualization therapy and hypnosis have cured warts in a number of people. The use of placebos in treating warts is remarkably successful and indicates that warts are particularly susceptible to mental influence.

Psychoneuroimmunology is based on the premise that mental phenomena can affect immune function, and is particularly applicable to the treatment of warts.

MEDICAL ALERT:

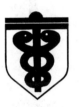

Anyone who has warts in the genital area or develops what appears to be a wart after the age of 45 should see a physician as soon as possible. Genital warts require medical attention, and wartlike growths after 54 may indicate a more serious skin condition. Warts on the face should not be treated at home.

STANDARD MEDICAL TREATMENT:

Approximately half of all warts with the exception of plantar and genital warts, will disappear in 6 to 12 months without any specific treatment. The application of liquid nitrogen (cryosurgery), in which the warts are frozen and subsequently fall off, is commonly employed by most doctors. As the frozen wart thaws, a blister forms which lifts the wart off the skin. Most physicians choose liquid nitrogen as the most effective and least expensive treatment for warts. Cantharidin liquids or plasters can also be used to create a blister on the wart.

Fulguration, in which heat is used to destroy warts, can also be effective. This approach is more frightening for children than using liquid nitrogen. Genital warts are usually removed by surgery or by the application of podophyllin, which acts like liquid nitrogen.

Injecting alpha interferon directly into warts has had some success; however, the treatment may be impractical and too expensive when a large number of warts are present. Injecting or applying bleomycin to warts has also produced some good results but is still considered inferior to the methods listed above. A product called the trans-ver-sal patch is an adhesive patch which releases a continuous dose of medication and is available with a prescription. It is considered more effective than over-the-counter patches.

Surgical options: Surgical removal of warts is done with a scalpel, a laser or an electric needle.

Success rating of standard medical procedure: good. Warts can be easily removed; however, they have a tendency to recur. No form of medical treatment is 100 percent effective. If liquid nitrogen or other toxic chemicals are not skillfully applied, healthy tissue can be damaged and scarring is possible. The advantage of medical treatment over some home remedies is the time factor. Doctors can treat warts quickly; however, those treatments are not without pain or discomfort.

HOME SELF CARE:

Note: These home remedies are not for genital warts (refer to chapter on herpes for information on genital warts).

◆ Compound-W or Vergo are non-prescription wart medications that can be applied at home. They are salicylic acid compounds and work by softening and dissolving the wart. These preparations have mixed results. If a wart is unusually large, these preparations are sometimes ineffective. Mediplast is a medicated pad which sticks directly on the wart. Careful sizing of this product is necessary to prevent injury to surrounding skin. Coat surrounding healthy tissue with petroleum jelly for added protection.

◆ Applying a crushed garlic clove to the wart and bandaging it for at least 24 hours has been successful for some people. A blister will usually form and the wart will fall off within 5 to 7 days.

◆ Apply castor oil or any sweet oil (wheat germ oil) to the warts several times a day, and use an emery board to sluff off dead skin. This same treatment can soften corns and callouses.

◆ Applying the juice of white cabbage to the warts is an old traditional treatment.

◆ Crushing an aspirin and applying it the wart, which is subsequently covered with a piece of cellophane tape, may be effective but should not be attempted by anyone with an aspirin sensitivity or allergy.

◆ Exposure to heat can sometimes cure warts, either through sunlight or by soaking the wart in very hot water for 30 minutes several times per week.

◆ Taking fresh banana skin daily to warts is a method of treatment used in Israel. This softens the wart and it can eventually be scraped off.

◆ Putting adhesive tape (waterproof) directly on warts for a week, exposing the wart to air for 12 hours and then reapplying the tape for another week may cause them to disappear within four to six weeks. In some cases and for unknown reasons, treating one wart in this manner has inhibited the growth of other warts present which were not treated.

◆ Soak a cotton ball in fresh pineapple juice or bromelain powder and tape over the wart to eventually dissolve it.

◆ A salt paste applied to the wart with a cotton ball taped to the wart can also help to dissolve the growth.

◆ Put a drop of iodine on the wart every night. This treatment is often quite successful.

◆ There is a strong belief in some circles that taking time to visualize away your

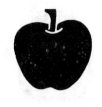

warts by imagining them shrinking and disappearing has produced remarkable results and should be attempted. Visualize for 2 to 5 minutes a day.

NUTRITIONAL APPROACH:

◆ Warts are controlled and attacked by the body's immune system. Some people are naturally resistant to warts. Keeping the immune system healthy through a diet high in vitamins and minerals and low in fat and empty calories is recommended.
◆ Get off of junk food and eat plenty of raw fruits, vegetables, and whole grains. Avoid red meat and use only low-fat dairy products. Use safflower or olive oil and get sufficient rest.
◆ Increase your intake of sulfur-containing foods such as eggs, citrus fruits, asparagus, garlic and onions. Sulfur-containing amino acids contribute to the development of antibodies that fight the polyoma virus group. Desiccated liver tablets are high in this amino acid and can be taken daily.
◆ *Vitamin C:* Has potent antiviral properties. Can be taken internally or applied as a paste to the wart.
◆ *Vitamin A:* Required for the proper formation of epithelial and mucous membranes. Applying vitamin A oil directly to warts has proven successful in some people.
◆ *Vitamin E:* Can be applied externally to warts. Helps to normalize skin tissue and prevent scarring. Impressive results have been obtained through this method and it is definitely worth trying.
◆ *Zinc:* Boosts the immune system to fight against the virus responsible for the outbreak of warts.
◆ *L-cysteine:* An amino acid which is required for normal and healthy skin processes.

HERBAL REMEDIES:

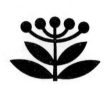

◆ *Comfrey:* Make a paste out of comfrey powder and water and apply to the wart every night.
◆ *Aloe vera gel:* Apply to the wart at least twice a day. File the wart down before applying to facilitate absorption.
◆ *Thyme, wintergreen, sassafras or thuja oil:* Can be applied nightly on the wart and subsequently scraped with a pumice stone in the morning.
◆ *Dandelion, milkweed or wheatgrass juice:* Can be applied to the wart every day with subsequent rubbings with an emery board or pumice stone. Dandelion extract has a corrosive effect and can destroy wart-infected tissue.
◆ *Arbor vitae:* A volatile herbal oil which has an antiviral effect.
◆ *Black walnut and golden seal:* Both have strong antiviral properties and can be taken as capsules and applied externally in paste form.

◆ *Tea tree oil:* Apply externally to warts. Tea tree oil has antifungal and antiviral properties.

PREVENTION:

◆ Wear cotton socks, don't go barefoot and keep feet dry and in well-fitted shoes to prevent plantar warts. Never go barefoot in public places like swimming pool areas, locker rooms, or health clubs. This also helps to avoid contracting athlete's foot.
◆ Keep your shoes dry by airing them out and changing them frequently. Use leather or canvas shoes that breathe. Vinyl shoes can trap moisture and cause sweating.
◆ Use Lysol in bathrooms. Everyday bleach can kill viruses and bacteria.
◆ Take a daily dose of vitamin C to maintain a healthy immune system.
◆ Keep your immune system healthy by not smoking or drinking alcohol and by eating a nutritious, high-fiber, low-fat diet.

Wrinkles

DEFINITION:

What woman hasn't heard someone say that wrinkles make men look wise and distinguished, and make women just look old. As today's baby boomers approach middle age, cosmetic sales are soaring. The most prevalent attitude toward aging today is, "age gracefully by fighting it every step of the way." Most bathroom cabinets are chuck full of jars, potions, elixirs and chemical peels designed to fool Mother Nature. Alas, wrinkles usually always prevail.

Unfortunately, wrinkles are a natural part of the aging process despite our obsession with somehow obliterating them. They develop due to the gradual wearing away of the outermost layer of skin called the epidermis, which is comprised of dead tissue. This skin is replaced by more dead tissue that comes from the lining base. Wrinkles are permanent features of aging skin because they originate from the dermis, which is deeper than the epidermis.

After the age of 25, the cells in the dermis begin to die off and become smaller. Skin begins to lose some of its elasticity and resiliency. Any shrinkage of tissue in the dermis causes a wrinkle in the epidermis. The dermis becomes stiffer as we age. The more the dermis is stretched, the greater the risk for developing wrinkles. Because the face and its muscles are so active, it can be the site of significant wrinkling.

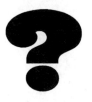

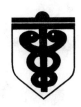

CAUSES:

Contrary to popular belief, wrinkles are not caused by dehydration or dry skin. Frowning and squinting; however, do cause wrinkling by constantly stretching the dermis. Other factors associated with an increased risk for wrinkling are smoking, radiation damage from sun exposure, scrubbing the skin with caustic or harsh substances, sleeping on your side or stomach, a lack of vitamins and minerals, and drinking alcohol.

STANDARD MEDICAL TREATMENT:

Retin-A, an acne preparation, has become extremely popular over the last few years as a treatment for wrinkles. There is significant controversy over the validity of using retin-a for this purpose. Retin-A comes with an array of side-effects which may discourage its use for this purpose (see the chapter on acne). Most doctors agree that while the benefit of Retin-A for age-related wrinkles is doubtful, Retin-A does smooth away finer wrinkles that can develop from exposure to the sun.

Chemical face peels (chemosurgery): Carbolic acid or alpha-hydroxy acids that are up to 70 percent concentrated are used for acid face peels, which remove the outermost layer of skin. Some burning of the skin results and smoother skin develops as healing occurs. The procedure involves a significant amount of discomfort and causes scabbing to form. The scab will fall off after about 10 days, exposing a new layer of unblemished skin. A red or dark color to the skin can persist but usually returns to normal after several weeks. Sun exposure is prohibited for 6 months.

Dermabrasion: A special tool is used to sand the surface of anesthetized skin located in wrinkled areas. This procedure leaves raw, pink areas that will need approximately two weeks to heal. The procedure is simple and usually takes around 30 minutes.

Surgical options: Face-lifts. Face-lifts can now be done on an outpatient basis although some situations still require a short hospital stay. The operation can be done under local or general anesthesia. It usually takes somewhere between 2 to 4 hours. Incisions are made under the hairline and around the ears, and any fatty tissue present is removed. The neck skin is subsequently tightened. Often a chemical peel or eyelid surgery accompanies this procedure. The face will remain bandaged for several days following the surgery. After two and a half weeks, swelling goes down and the incisions are significantly healed enough to resume normal activities.

Complications: Face-lifts rarely have complications, although they can occur. Possible complications include infection, scarring, facial nerve injury, loss of facial tissue, hair loss around the incisions, and hematomas.

Warning: Make sure you choose a recommended, fully licensed plastic surgeon to perform the above procedures.

Success rating of standard medical procedures: Surgery: good. Face-lifts, eyelifts, and chemical peels can have dramatic results; however, they come with a significant amount of discomfort and some risk. These operations have become extremely popular over the last decade, and when done by a skillful surgeon can be quite satisfying. Chemical peels and dermabrasion are not considered as successful as face-lifts although in some cases, the improvement is substantial. The use of Retin-A and alpha-hydroxy acids in cosmetic forms is limited. While fine lines created by sun exposure may be affected, significant wrinkles which are the natural result of aging are not.

MEDICAL UPDATE:

Cosmetic preparations containing alpha-hydroxy acids such as glycolic acid, lactic acid or malic acid are currently in great demand for their ability to supposedly melt wrinkles away. These acids are naturally occurring substances found in sour milk, citrus fruits and sugar cane. Concentrations of 3 to 5 percent are now available without a prescription and have fewer side-effects than Retin-A.

The acids work by sloughing off dead cells and exposing new skin. They are also thought to thicken underlying layers of skin and increase hyaluronic acid, which keeps cells together. Both of these help to smooth out fine lines that are usually the result of sun exposure. Companies like Avon, Estee Lauder, have jumped on the bandwagon and offer these creams at a premium price. Like Retin-A, alpha-hydroxy creams can help with tiny creases but will not reverse the natural process of aging. They are not magic elixirs, but do have credibility in their ability to eliminate fine lines.

Note: Having a face-lift or other cosmetic procedure can greatly increase one's self-esteem and confidence. If extensive wrinkles and sagging skin are making you want to withdraw socially, check out local plastic surgeons and talk to patients who have had procedures done. Just remember that having your face changed can be emotionally traumatic and may require a period of adjustment, a factor which should be discussed with your plastic surgeon.

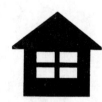

HOME SELF-CARE:

◆ Avoid sun exposure. Cells from young skin that have been exposed to too much sun look the same as cells that are old and have naturally wrinkled. Unprotected sun exposure can unquestionably cause premature aging. The midday sun is the most damaging. Avoid direct exposure between the hours of 10:00 a.m. and 3:00 p.m. Use strong sunscreens with a high SPF if you must be in the sun. Apply these 30 minutes before exposure and reapply after swimming. Highly reflective surfaces such as water, sand, and concrete can cause considerable sun damage by intensifying its effect on skin cells.

◆ Tanning booths can contribute to skin damage just as much as sunshine.

◆ Use a good moisturizer daily. While moisturizing your skin will not stop wrinkles from forming, it can significantly improve the texture of the skin, making it appear smoother.

◆ Whipping up egg whites into a meringue-like texture, applying it to your face for 30 minutes, and then rinsing can help to temporarily tighten the skin. The effect only lasts for an hour or two.

◆ Use mild soaps and cleansers that will not dry out or remove oils that help to keep the skin supple and well-nourished. Soaps such as Neutrogena are gentle enough not to disrupt the normal balance of the skin.

◆ Train yourself to sleep on your back. Sleeping on your side or stomach can create a number of unnatural creases on the face. Bunching up your pillow and nestling your face in it can scrunch up facial tissue and create lines.

◆ Don't smoke: Smokers have significantly more wrinkles than non-smokers and age faster. Smoking decreases the body's oxygen supply, which can contribute to reduced blood circulation to the face, which causes more epidermal damage. The very act of smoking causes the face to contract in various ways, which may also contribute to the formation of creases and lines.

◆ Don't drink alcohol: Drinking can cause facial swelling, which stretches the skin, thereby causing wrinkling. Alcohol can also rob your body of essential nutrients which promote healthy cell function in the skin.

◆ Wear hats and sunglasses to prevent squinting, frowning and sun damage.

◆ Use a humidifier in your home if you live in an arid climate. While moisture will not prevent or cure wrinkles, it can minimize their noticeability.

◆ Treat yourself to facial massages, which increase circulation and stimulation.

◆ Keep yourself at an optimal weight. Becoming overweight and then losing fat can create sagging, wrinkled skin.

◆ Exercise regularly. Exercise can increase circulation to skin cells and improve overall oxygenation. People who exercise routinely have better overall elasticity and density to their skin. Exercise also gives skin a healthy glow.

◆ Manage stress through relaxation techniques. People under tension frown a lot and develop unattractive ridges and furrows. Laugh lines are unquestionably preferable.

◆ The shoulder stand and mudra practices in yoga are recommended for wrinkle control.

◆ Often highly priced wrinkle creams are not what they're touted to be. Before you spend a fortune, do a little homework and compare ingredients and percentages of chemical substances in a number of brands. Often the price tag reflects on the brand name rather than its contents.

NUTRITIONAL APPROACH:

◆ A diet high in saturated fats has been linked to the development of dry skin. Eat a low-fat high-fiber diet. Use polyunsaturated and monounsaturated oils. Add essential fatty acids to your diet through OMEGA 3 oils. Good oils include safflower, sunflower, corn, sesame, pumpkin seed, olive, canola, flaxseed, almond and hazelnut. Avoid shortening, animal fats, hydrogenated oil and coconut oil.

◆ Eat a diet high in raw fruits and vegetables, lean meats, low-fat dairy products, whole grains and drink plenty of pure water.

◆ *B complex vitamins:* Essential for healthy skin. Cracks and lines that form around the lips can be a sign of a B-vitamin deficiency. The B vitamins found in chicken, eggs and whole wheat can help to promote healthy, young-looking skin.

◆ *Vitamin A and beta-carotene:* Antioxidants which can minimize cell damage. Very dry skin can be one of the first indications of a vitamin A deficiency. In some cases, applying cod liver oil, which is very rich in vitamin A, to very dry areas of skin can bring more relief than commercial lotions. Eat plenty of carrots, sweet potatoes, and tomatoes to supply vitamin A. Supplements are also recommended in safe dosages. Eating plenty of green leafy vegetables, carrots and fresh fruits helpa to promote and maintain healthy skin.

◆ *Vitamin C:* Helps to repair connective tissue, which comprises the dermis layer of the skin.

◆ *Vitamin E:* Helps to decrease scarring and aids in skin repair. It is also good for relieving dry, rough skin. Vitamin E can be directly applied to the skin. Often commercial preparations which contain vitamin E do not have rich enough concentrations of the vitamin to achieve good results. Open a capsule of the vitamin or use wheat germ oil directly.

◆ Honey facials can help to make the skin soft and supple. Smooth pure, raw honey on the face and let it stay for 15 minutes. Then rinse off with cool water and a washcloth.

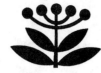

HERBAL REMEDIES:

◆ Dried peppermint leaf tea (1 pint) strained and added to a pint of apple cider vinegar makes for a wonderful facial rinse that is recommended for dry skin.

◆ Diluted myrrh extract is considered a good herbal skin conditioner.

◆ *Jojoba oil:* used for generations by the American Indians to condition skin and improve its quality. It has a similar structure to natural sebum found in the skin.

◆ *Redmond clay:* A traditional herbal treatment for toning the skin.

◆ *Aloe vera:* Helps to heal cell damage to the skin and can be used in gel or lotion form.

◆ *Irish moss, marshmallow and comfrey* are emollient herbs which help to soothe and lubricate dry skin. They can be used in strained tea form as rinses, wet compresses or used in a facial mist machine.

- *Marigold, lady's mantle and witch hazel* are considered natural astringents which can tone and refresh the skin. They can be used in tea form as a rinse or sprayed on with a fine mist atomizer.
- *Elder flowers, violet, yarrow and chamomile* make good herbal cleansers.
- *Lavender and thyme* are antiseptic herbs that stimulate the skin.
- Herbal creams and ointments that contain marigold, comfrey, marshmallow, peppermint oil and olive oil are also recommended for good skin repair.
  Note: Keep herbal liquids in the fridge in closed containers to promote freshness.

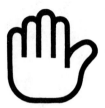

PREVENTION:

All of the suggestions listed in the home self-care and nutritional section of this chapter work as preventative measures as well. A healthy life-style and diet can go a long way to keep skin looking young and vibrant. In addition, a positive mental attitude can decrease your chances of developing frown furrows. Laugh lines and crow's feet are the kind of wrinkles that are perfectly acceptable.

Bibliography

WORKS CITED:

THE AMERICAN RED CROSS FIRST AID AND SAFETY HANDBOOK, and Kathleen A. Handal, M.D., Boston: Little Brown and Company, 1992.

Austin Phyllis, Agatha Thrash M.D., and Calvin Thrash, M.D., M.P.H. NATURAL HEALTHCARE FOR YOUR CHILD. Sunfield, Missouri: Family Health Publications, 1990.

Balch, James F., M.D. and Phyllis A. Balch C.N.C.. PRESCRIPTION FOR NUTRITIONAL HEALING. Garden City Park, New York: Avery Publishing Group, 1990.

Bricklin, Mark. THE PRACTICAL ENCYCLOPEDIA OF NATURAL HEALING. Emmaus, Pennsylvania: Rodale Press, 1976.

Castleman, Michael. THE HEALING HERBS. Alice Feinstein, ed. Emmaus, Pennsylvania: Rodale Press, 1991.

Chilnick, Lawrence, ed., THE PILL BOOK, 5TH ED. New York: Mantam Books, 1992.

Choppra, Deepak, M.D. PERFECT HEALTH. New York: Harmony Books, 1991.

Clayman, Charles B. M.D., and Jeffrey R.M. Kunz M.D., Harriet S.Meyer M.D., Eds. THE AMERICAN MEDICAL ASSOCIATION HOME MEDICAL ADVISOR. New York: Random House Publishing, 1988.

THE COLUMBIA UNIVERSITY COLLEGE OF PHYSICIANS AND SURGEONS COMPLETE HOME MEDICAL GUIDE. New York: Crown Publishers Inc. 1989.

Culpepper, Nicholas. CULPEPPER'S COMPLETE HERBAL. London: Bloomsbury Books, 1992.

Donahue, Peggy Jo and the Editors of Prevention Magazine. HOW TO PREVENT A STROKE. Emmaus, Pennsylvania: Rodale Press, 1989.

Galland, Leo, M.D. with Diane Dincin Buchman, PH.D., SUPERIMMUNITY FOR KIDS. New York: Dell Publishing, 1988.

Gittleman, Ann Louise, M.S. with J. Lynne Dodson, SUPER NUTRITION FOR WOMEN. New York: Bantam Books, 1991.

Gomez, Joan, M.B.B.S.,M.R.C.Psych.,D.B.M.. FAMILY GUIDE TO COMMON AILMENTS. London: The Hamlyn Publishing Group, 1981.

Janiger, Oscar, M.D. and Philip Goldberg. A DIFFERENT KIND OF HEALING. New York: G.P. Putnam's Sons, 1993.

Jensen, Bernard. LOVE, SEX, AND NUTRITION. Garden City Park, New York: Avery Publishing Group Inc., 1988.

Kirchheimer, Sid and the Eds. of Prevention Magazine Health Books. THE DOCTOR'S BOOK OF HOME REMEDIES II. Emmaus, Pennsylvania: Rodale Press, 1993.

Kloss, Jethro. BACK TO EDEN. Loma Linda, California: Back to Eden Publishing Company, 1992.

Kunz, Jeffrey R.M.,M.D. THE AMERICAN MEDICAL ASSOCIATION FAMILY MEDICAL GUIDE. New York: Random House, 1982.

Lieberman, Shari, M.A., R.D. and Nancy Bruning. DESIGN YOUR OWN VITAMIN AND MINERAL PROGRAM. New York: Avery Publishing Group Inc., 1990.

Maybey, Richard. THE NEW AGE HERBALIST, with Michael McIntyre,Pamela Michael, Gail Duff and John Steven, New York: MacMillan Publishing Company, 1988.

MERCK MANUAL. Merck and Co. Inc.

Meyer, Joseph E.. THE HERBALIST. Glenwood. Illinois: Meyerbooks, 1986.

Murray, Michael T. N.D., Joseph E. Pizzorno, N.D. AN ENCYCLOPEDIA OF NATURAL MEDICINE. Rocklin, California: Prima Publishing, 1991.

Ody, Penelope. THE COMPLETE MEDICINAL HERBAL. New York: Dorling Kindersley, Inc., 1993.

Oppenheim, Michael, M.D., A DOCTOR'S GUIDE TO THE BEST MEDICAL CARE. Emmaus, Pennsylvanis: Rodale Press, 1992.

Ritchason, Jack. THE VITAMIN AND HEALTH ENCYCLOPEDIA. Provo, Utah:Woodland Books, 1986.

Santillo, Humbart. N.D. NATURAL HEALING WITH HERBS. Prescott,Arizona: Hohm Press, 1993.

Scala, James, M.D., EATING RIGHT FOR A BAD GUT. New York: Penguin Publishing Group, 1992.

Scala, James, M.D. HIGH BLOOD PRESSURE RELIEF. New York: Penguin Publishing Group, 1990.

Stockwell, Christine. NATURE'S PHARMACY, A HISTORY OF PLANTS AND HEALING. Australia: Century Hutchison, 1988.

Tenney, Deanne. AN INTRODUCTION TO NATURAL HEALTH. Provo, Utah: Woodland Books, 1992.

Tenney, Louise, M.H..HEALTH HANDBOOK. Provo, Utah: Woodland Books,1987.

Tenney, Louise, M.H. NUTRITIONAL GUIDE WITH FOOD COMBINING. Provo, Utah: Woodland Books, 1991.

Tenney, Louise, M.H.. MODERN DAY PLAGUES. Provo Utah: Woodland Books, 1987.

Tenney, Louise, M.H.. TODAY'S HERBAL HEALTH. 3rd ed. rev. Provo, Utah: Woodland Books, 1992.

Tierra, Michael, C.A., N.D., O.M.D. PLANETARY HERBOLOGY. New Mexico: Lotus Press, 1988.

Tkac, Debora, ed..THE DOCTOR'S BOOK OF HOME REMEDIES. Emmaus, Pennsylvania: Rodale Press, 1990.

THE WELLNESS ENCYCLOPEDIA, from the Editors of the University of California at Berkeley, Boston: Houghton Mifflin Company, 1991.

Vickery, Donald, M.D. and James F. Fries, M.D. TAKE CARE OF YOURSELF, 4TH Ed. Reading, Massachusetts: Addison-Wesley Publishing Company, Inc., 1990.

Weil, Andrew, M.D. NATURAL HEALTH, NATURAL MEDICINE. Boston: Houghton Mifflin Company, 1990.

Zifferblatt, Steven M., Ph.D., Patricia Zifferblatt and Norm Chandler Fox. THE BETTER LIFE INSTITUTE FAMILY HEALTH PLAN. Nashville, Tennessee: Thomas Nelson Inc., 1983.

Index

Quercetin, 19, 77, 253
Radiation, 80
Rash, 92, 144, 239
Raspberry, 114, 151, 249
Red clover, 5, 83, 95, 237, 257, 314, 362
Red raspberry, 118, 138, 300, 305
Redmond clay, 366, 376
Reflexology, 248, 329
Respiratory infection, 175
Retin-A, 3, 373, 374
Retinoids, 311, 312
Reye's syndrome, 92, 116, 142, 314-316
Rheumatic fever, 328, 329
Rheumatoid arthritis, 30, 31
Ribavirin, 176
Riboflavin, 12
Ricola, 329
Ringworm, 42
Ritalin, 203
Rocaltrol, 311
Rodents, 176
Rose hips, 118
Rosemary, 88, 121, 143, 182, 339; oil, 120
Rubella, 239
Rutin, 169, 191
Safflower, 371; oil, 318
Saffron, 174, 182, 195, 261, 319
Sage, 323
Salicin, 316
Salicylic acid, 370
Saline solutions, 323
Salmon oil, 110, 344
Salmonella, 135
Salt, 344; paste, 370
Sarcomas, 78
Sarsaparilla, 8, 216, 221, 245, 305, 319
Sassafras, 5, 278, 371
Saw palmetto, 309, 319
Scarlet fever, 329
Schizandra berries, 195
Sclerotherapy, 364
Scullcap, 49, 220, 339, 348
Seizures, 152, 153, 315
Seldane, 309
Selenium, 13, 22, 24, 40, 44, 73, 82, 84, 95, 98, 103, 174, 181, 200, 244, 261, 287, 304
Self-hypnosis, 326
Semisynthetic penicillin, 350
Senility, 21
Senna, 114
Septum, 320; deviated, 321, 324, 325
Serotonin, 15
Sex drive, 318; depression of, 319
Sex hormones, 319
Sexual desire, diminished, 316
Sexual disorder, 213

Sexual intercourse, 57, 307, 309
Sexual potency, 319
Sexual Rejuvenation, 316-319
Sexually transmitted disease, 359
Shellfish, 318
Shepherd's purse, 151, 300
Shock, 15, 71
Siberian ginseng, 14, 151, 177, 269, 319
Silica, 282
Silicon, 21, 48, 55, 265, 282, 318, 333
Silymarin, 13
Sinarest, 322
Sine-Aid, 322
Sinus headache, 321
Sinuses, 324
Sinusitis, 320-323; chronic, 321
Sitting, 309
Sitz bath, 308, 361, 365
Skin cell production, 310
Skin, brushing, 317; cancer, 7; disorder, 2, 42, 144; rash, 291; ulcers, 364
Skullcap, 29, 41, 126, 156, 261, 265, 269, 326
Sleep apnea, 324-327
Sleep, lack of, 324; inducers, 324; unrestful, 326
Sleeping, pills, 324, 326, 336; posture, 326
Slippery elm, 41, 45, 49, 63, 103, 110, 115, 118, 138, 290, 294, 309, 323, 330, 357
Smoking, 320, 321, 324, 327, 331, 344, 357, 367, 373, 375
Snoring, 324-327
Soap, mild 375; oatmeal based, 312
Sore throat, 100, 327-331
Soy oil, 308
Speech impairment, 315
Sperm count, 319
Spermatozoa, 318
Spider bites, 222
Spider veins, 363, 364
Spina bifida, 53
Spirulina, 212
Sprains, 331-334
Squaw vine, 249, 301
Squinting, 373
St. John's Wort, 14, 74, 126, 147, 366
Staph bacteria, 349; infection, 350
Staphylococcus, 61, 135, 320
Steroid, 1, 90; cream, 292
Stillingia, 5
Stinging nettle, 20
Stoneroot, 191
Strains, 331-334
Strawberry, 5
Strep throat, 313, 327, 328
Streptococcal bacteria, 328

Streptococci, 320
Stress, 46, 306, 311, 314, 335-340, 352
Stretch marks, 298
Stretching, 334
Stroke, 340-346
Sucralfates (Carafate), 354
Sudafed, 322
Suicide, 122
Sulfur, 282
Sulfur-containing foods, 371
Sulphur, 24
Suma, 24, 83, 126, 201, 339
Sun, exposure, 373, 374; spots, 6
Sunburn, 310, 312
Sunflower, oil, 308; seeds, 318
Sunlight, 312
Sunscreen, 312
Support hose, 365, 367
Suppositories, 359
Sweet sumach, 56
Swimmer's ear, 140, 141
Swimming, 343
Swollen lymph glands, 327
Syphilis, 359
Tampons, 349, 350, 351, 360
Tanning booths, 375
Tar ointments, 312
Tea tree oil, 5, 45, 74, 121, 174, 362, 372
Teeth, grinding, 346
Temperature, 328
Temporomandibular joint, 346
Terfenadine, 16
Terfrnadine (Seldane), 327
Testosterone, 214, 309, 319
Tetracycline, 58, 86, 289, 368
Theophyline, 38
Theophylline bronchodilators, 38
Thermography, 364
Thiamine, 12, 132
Throat,abscess, 328; culture, 328; culture, home kits for, 329; pain, 327
Thrombolytic drugs, 179
Thrombophlebitis, 364
Thuja oil, 371
Thyme, 45, 77, 88, 121, 290, 334, 348, 371, 377
Thyroid, 206
Tick bite, 235
Timoptic, 168
Tinactine, 43
Tmj (tmd), 250, 346-349
Tonsillectomy, 328
Tonsillitis, 328
Tonsils, 324, 325, 327
Tooth decay, 50
Toothbrush, 331
Tormentil, 191
Tourniquets, 364
Toxic build-up, 313